# Biochemical and Imaging Diagnostics in Endocrinology

*Editors*

RICHARD J. AUCHUS
BARRY D. PRESSMAN
ADINA F. TURCU
ALAN D. WAXMAN

T0362299

# ENDOCRINOLOGY AND METABOLISM CLINICS OF NORTH AMERICA

www.endo.theclinics.com

*Consulting Editors*
ANAT BEN-SHLOMO
MARIA FLESERIU

September 2017 • Volume 46 • Number 3

**ELSEVIER**

1600 John F. Kennedy Boulevard • Suite 1800 • Philadelphia, Pennsylvania, 19103-2899

http://www.theclinics.com

ENDOCRINOLOGY AND METABOLISM CLINICS OF NORTH AMERICA Volume 46, Number 3
September 2017 ISSN 0889-8529, ISBN 13: 978-0-323-54550-1

Editor: Stacy Eastman
Developmental Editor: Meredith Madeira

*Endocrinology and Metabolism Clinics of North America* (ISSN 0889-8529) is published quarterly by Elsevier Inc., 360 Park Avenue South, New York, NY 10010-1710. Months of issue are March, June, September, and December. Periodicals postage paid at New York, NY and additional mailing offices. Subscription prices are USD 337.00 per year for US individuals, USD 674.00 per year for US institutions, USD 100.00 per year for US students and residents, USD 423.00 per year for Canadian individuals, USD 834.00 per year for Canadian institutions, USD 490.00 per year for international individuals, USD 834.00 per year for international institutions, and USD 245.00 per year for international and Canadian and foreign students/residents. To receive student/resident rate, orders must be accompanied by name of affiliated institution, date of term, and the signature of program/residency coordinator on institution letterhead. Orders will be billed at individual rate until proof of status is received. Foreign air speed delivery is included in all *Clinics* subscription prices. All prices are subject to change without notice. **POSTMASTER:** Send address changes to *Endocrinology and Metabolism Clinics of North America*, Elsevier Health Sciences Division, Subscription Customer Service, 3251 Riverport Lane, Maryland Heights, MO 63043. **Customer Service: Telephone: 1-800-654-2452** (U.S. and Canada); **1-314-447-8871** (outside U.S. and Canada). **Fax: 1-314-447-8029. E-mail: journalscustomerservice-usa@elsevier.com (for print support); journalsonlinesupport-usa@elsevier.com (for online support).**

*Reprints.* For copies of 100 or more, of articles in this publication, please contact the Commercial Rights Department, Elsevier Inc., 360 Park Avenue South, New York, NY 10010-1710; phone: +1-212-633-3874; fax: +1-212-633-3820; E-mail: reprints@elsevier.com.

*Endocrinology and Metabolism Clinics of North America* is covered in *MEDLINE/PubMed (Index Medicus)*, *EMBASE/Excerpta Medica*, *Current Contents/Clinical Medicine*, *Current Contents/Life Sciences*, *Science Citation Index*, *ISI/BIOMED*, *BIOSIS*, and *Chemical Abstracts*.

# Contributors

## CONSULTING EDITORS

**ANAT BEN-SHLOMO, MD**
Pituitary Center, Division of Endocrinology, Diabetes, and Metabolism, Cedars-Sinai Medical Center, Los Angeles, California

**MARIA FLESERIU, MD, FACE**
Northwest Pituitary Center, Departments of Medicine and Neurological Surgery, Oregon Health & Science University, Portland, Oregon

## EDITORS

**RICHARD J. AUCHUS, MD, PhD, FACE**
Professor, Division of Metabolism, Endocrinology, and Diabetes, Departments of Internal Medicine and Pharmacology, University of Michigan, Ann Arbor, Michigan

**BARRY D. PRESSMAN, MD, FACR**
Professor and Chair, Department of Imaging, S. Mark Taper Foundation Imaging Center, Cedars-Sinai Medical Center, Los Angeles, California

**ADINA F. TURCU, MD**
Assistant Professor, Division of Metabolism, Endocrinology, and Diabetes, Department of Internal Medicine, University of Michigan, Ann Arbor, Michigan

**ALAN D. WAXMAN, MD**
Director, Nuclear Medicine, S. Mark Taper Imaging, Cedars-Sinai Medical Center, Clinical Professor of Radiology, University of Southern California, School of Medicine, Los Angeles, California

## AUTHORS

**VIDYA ALURI, MD, MS**
Division of Endocrinology, University of Iowa, Iowa City, Iowa

**ANCA AVRAM, MD**
Associate Professor, Department of Radiology, University of Michigan, Ann Arbor, Michigan

**SARDIUS CHEN, MD**
Radiology Resident, Department of Imaging, Cedars-Sinai Imaging, Cedars-Sinai Medical Center, Los Angeles, California

**CHEE KIAN CHEW, MD**
Research Fellow, Division of Endocrinology, Diabetes, Metabolism, and Nutrition, Mayo Clinic, Rochester, Minnesota

**BART L. CLARKE, MD**
Professor of Medicine, Division of Endocrinology, Diabetes, Metabolism, and Nutrition, Mayo Clinic, Rochester, Minnesota

**JOSEPH S. DILLON, MB, BCh**
Division of Endocrinology, University of Iowa, Iowa City, Iowa

**N. REED DUNNICK, MD**
Fred Jenner Hodges Professor and Chair, Department of Radiology, University of Michigan, Ann Arbor, Michigan

**JOEL EHRENKRANZ, MD**
Associate Professor, Division of Endocrinology, Department of Medicine, University of Colorado School of Medicine, Aurora, Colorado; i-calQ LLC, Salt Lake City, Utah

**NAZANENE H. ESFANDIARI, MD, FACE**
Clinical Associate Professor, Division of Metabolism, Endocrinology, and Diabetes, Department of Internal Medicine, University of Michigan, Ann Arbor, Michigan

**HEMAMALINI KETHA, PhD**
Clinical Instructor, Department of Pathology, University of Michigan Health System, Ann Arbor, Michigan

**SIVA S. KETHA, MBBS, MPH**
Fellow, Department of Cardiovascular Diseases, Mayo Clinic, Jacksonville, Florida

**ERICA B. MAHANY, MD**
Assistant Professor, Division of Reproductive Endocrinology and Infertility, Department of Obstetrics and Gynecology, University of Michigan, Ann Arbor, Michigan

**MARK MASCIOCCHI, MD**
Assistant Professor, Department of Radiology, UMass Memorial Medical Center, University of Massachusetts Medical School, Worcester, Massachusetts

**MICHELLE MELANY, MD**
Chief of Women's Imaging, Department of Imaging, Cedars-Sinai Imaging, Vice Chair of Imaging, Greater Los Angeles VA Medical Center, Clinical Professor of Radiology, David Geffen School of Medicine at UCLA, Los Angeles, California

**MISHAL MENDIRATTA-LALA, MD**
Assistant Professor, Department of Radiology, University of Michigan, Ann Arbor, Michigan

**MARIA PAPALEONTIOU, MD**
Assistant Professor, Division of Metabolism, Endocrinology, and Diabetes, Department of Internal Medicine, University of Michigan, Ann Arbor, Michigan

**BARRY D. PRESSMAN, MD, FACR**
Professor and Chair, Department of Imaging, S. Mark Taper Foundation Imaging Center, Cedars-Sinai Medical Center, Los Angeles, California

**JOHN F. RANDOLPH Jr, MD**
Professor, Department of Epidemiology, School of Public Health, Professor, Division of Reproductive Endocrinology and Infertility, Department of Obstetrics and Gynecology, University of Michigan, Ann Arbor, Michigan

**RAVINDER J. SINGH, PhD**
Professor and Consultant, Department of Pathology and Laboratory Medicine, Mayo Clinic, Rochester, Minnesota

**ADINA F. TURCU, MD**
Assistant Professor, Division of Metabolism, Endocrinology, and Diabetes, Department of Internal Medicine, University of Michigan, Ann Arbor, Michigan

**DOUGLAS VAN NOSTRAND, MD, FACP, FACNM**
Director, Nuclear Medicine Research, Professor of Medicine, Division of Nuclear Medicine, MedStar Health Research Institute, MedStar Washington Hospital Center, Georgetown University School of Medicine, Washington, DC

**ASHLEY WACHSMAN, MD**
Attending Radiologist, Department of Imaging, Cedars-Sinai Medical Center, Los Angeles, California

**RUN YU, MD, PhD**
Associate Professor, Division of Endocrinology, Diabetes, and Metabolism, David Geffen School of Medicine at UCLA, Los Angeles, California

# Contents

**Role of Mass Spectrometry in Clinical Endocrinology**

Siva S. Ketha, Ravinder J. Singh, and Hemamalini Ketha

The advent of mass spectrometry into the clinical laboratory has led to an improvement in clinical management of several endocrine diseases. Liquid chromatography tandem mass spectrometry found some of its first clinical applications in the diagnosis of inborn errors of metabolism, in quantitative steroid analysis, and in drug analysis laboratories. Mass spectrometry assays offer analytical sensitivity and specificity that is superior to immunoassays for many analytes. This article highlights several areas of clinical endocrinology that have witnessed the use of liquid chromatography tandem mass spectrometry to improve clinical outcomes.

**Point-of-Care Endocrine Diagnostics**

Joel Ehrenkranz

Endocrinology relies on hormone and metabolite measurement for public health screening, diagnostics, and disease management. Advances in microfluidics, immunoassay technology, electronics, and software are moving in vitro endocrine diagnostics from the laboratory to the point of care. Point-of-care endocrine diagnostics provide results clinically equivalent to those produced by expensive laboratory instrumentation for a fraction of the cost and with a substantially more rapid turnaround time. Similar to the transformation of mainframe computers into laptops, tablets, and smartphones, clinical laboratories are evolving into point-of-care technologies.

**Biochemical Testing in Thyroid Disorders**

Nazanene H. Esfandiari and Maria Papaleontiou

This article summarizes the main principles for the appropriate use of laboratory testing in the diagnosis and management of thyroid disorders, as well as controversies that have arisen in association with some of these biochemical tests. To place a test in perspective, its sensitivity and accuracy should be taken into account. Ordering the correct laboratory tests facilitates the early diagnosis of a thyroid disorder and allows for timely and appropriate treatment. This article focuses on a comprehensive update regarding thyroid-stimulating hormone, thyroxine/triiodothyronine, thyroid autoantibodies, thyroglobulin, and calcitonin. Clinical uses of these biochemical tests are outlined.

Laboratory biochemical testing is critical to the clinical understanding of bone disorders. Patients with skeletal diseases have underlying themes in their pathophysiology that would be impossible to detect without biochemical assessment of serum and urine minerals, vitamin D, parathyroid hormone, parathyroid hormone–related peptide, and bone turnover markers. Bone disorders are caused by abnormalities in signaling pathways that affect bone formation and resorption. Therapies for common bone diseases were developed in direct response to underlying biochemical abnormalities.

Neuroendocrine cells are widely distributed throughout the body. They can produce, store, and secrete peptides and biogenic amines. Neuroendocrine tumors (NETs) are rare, but most are found in the intestine, pancreas, and lung. NETs may cause specific hormonal symptoms (eg, carcinoid syndrome) or appear nonfunctional. Blood or urine concentrations of tumor-secreted amines and peptides have been used as biomarkers in the diagnosis and management of NETs. This article focuses on currently available biochemical testing of blood or urine for gastroenteropancreatic and lung NETs and discusses the limitations of these tests and the potential role of newer multianalyte markers for NET management.

One of the limiting factors of fertility testing is the relative inefficiency of human reproduction. A careful history and physical examination must be performed on each patient to inform the particular diagnostic tests that are chosen and to create a meaningful treatment plan. Testing parameters, such as sensitivity, specificity, positive predictive value, and negative predictive value, can help to interpret test results, although there is no perfect screening test for the various causes of infertility. This article describes the 4 major categories of testing for infertility: ovarian reserve, ovulatory status, gamete transport, and male factor.

Ultrasound imaging is critical in the detection, diagnosis, and management of thyroid nodules. Ultrasound detection of regional nodal metastatic disease is based on abnormal nodal morphology rather than size and is critical to initial surgical and long-term management of thyroid cancer. Fine-needle aspiration biopsy is the gold standard for malignancy diagnosis in thyroid cancer. Thyroglobulin assay of nodal aspirates improves accuracy in diagnosis of metastases. Reporting lexicons assign risk levels to thyroid nodules with the goal of improving and standardizing patient management. Surveillance ultrasound imaging in papillary microcarcinomas is being evaluated and compared with surgical management.

Modern pituitary imaging is MRI. However, computed tomography (CT) still has limited usefulness. In addition, because CT offers much better bone detail and calcium detection, there are some cases in which such additional information is necessary. Before the advent of CT, plain radiography, pneumoencephalography, and angiography were used to diagnose pituitary masses. More recently, CT, and then especially MRI, made it possible to primarily delineate lesions within and around the pituitary gland rather than depend on secondary information that could only suggest their presence.

Cross-sectional imaging can make a specific diagnosis in lesions, such as myelolipomas, cysts, and hemorrhage, and is often sufficient to distinguish benign from malignant adrenal processes. Computed tomography and MRI are useful studies to identify pheochromocytomas and cortisol-secreting or androgen-secreting tumors. In patients with primary aldosteronism, adrenal venous sampling remains the most accurate localizing study and should be performed in all patients older than 35 years. Radiolabeled isotope studies serve as second-line diagnostic tests for malignant adrenal tumors, primary or metastatic, as well as for pheochromocytoma. Nuclear imaging studies should follow a robust hormonal diagnosis and be correlated with findings on cross-sectional imaging.

Imaging of the endocrine pancreas is dominated by neuroendocrine tumors, a diverse category of neoplasms that may or may not cause symptoms from hormone hypersecretion. These tumors may also be evidence of several different genetic syndromes. Understanding the usefulness of different imaging modalities and entities that simulate neuroendocrine tumors is key for both radiologists and referring physicians.

This article discusses the more controversial areas of the management of differentiated thyroid cancer, namely, the utility of pretherapy staging radioiodine scans; the prescribed activity for iodine-131 remnant ablation, adjuvant treatment, and distant metastases; preparation with thyroid hormone withdrawal versus recombinant human thyroid-stimulating hormone; and the classification of radioiodine refractory differentiated thyroid cancer. The author reviews various aspects of the controversies, such as the recommendations of the 2015 guidelines of the American Thyroid Association, arguments for and against the various controversies, and selected references.

Imaging is critical in the diagnosis, prognosis, and management of neuro-endocrine tumors (NETs). NETs share common imaging features, but each type exhibits unique features. Computed tomography scans or MRI of the abdomen is used to assess tumor burden routinely. Functional imaging with octreotide scan or gallium-68 somatostatin analog PET is used selectively to confirm diagnosis and guide therapy. Clinicians and radiologists should be familiar with the indications and interpretations of imaging modalities. Novel functional imaging modalities likely will be developed to detect small NETs, predict prognosis, guide therapeutic choices, and design novel therapies.

# ENDOCRINOLOGY AND METABOLISM CLINICS OF NORTH AMERICA

**VISIT THE CLINICS ONLINE!**
Access your subscription at:
www.theclinics.com

# Foreword

# Latest Innovations in Biochemical and Imaging Diagnostics in Endocrinology

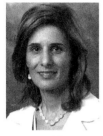 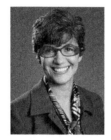

Anat Ben-Shlomo, MD    Maria Fleseriu, MD, FACE
*Consulting Editors*

This issue of Biochemical and Imaging Diagnostics in Endocrinology, from the *Endocrinology and Metabolism Clinics of North America*, summarizes key highlights in the field and provides important and timely updates on biochemical and imaging diagnosis of various endocrine disorders. Our distinguished guest editors, Drs Richard J. Auchus, MD, PhD, FACE, Barry D. Pressman, MD, FACE, Adina F. Turcu, MD, and Alan D. Waxman, MD, are international experts on this topic, in both clinical and laboratory settings. The contributing authors discuss multiple biochemical and imaging techniques as well as their applications, and offer expert opinion on how advances in this field will change clinical practice, both for diagnosis and for follow-up treatment.

In the article, "Role of Mass Spectrometry in Clinical Endocrinology," Drs Ketha, Singh, and Ketha describe the increasingly important role that mass spectrometry, particularly liquid chromatography tandem mass spectrometry and liquid chromatography high-resolution accurate mass spectrometry, play in the diagnosis and management of endocrine diseases. Mass spectrometry measurement of adrenal and sex steroids, vitamin D and its metabolites, metametanephrines and normetanephrines, insulin-like growth factor-1, and plasma renin activity levels are discussed in detail, with an emphasis on the increased sensitivity and specificity it provides over high-performance liquid chromatography and immunoassays.

In "Biochemical Testing in Thyroid Disorders," Drs Esfandiari and Papaleontiou summarize laboratory methodology and appropriate clinical utilization of thyrotropin, thyroid hormones and antibodies, and calcitonin in the diagnosis and management of thyroid disorders.

"Biochemical Testing Relevant to Bone" by Drs Clark and Chaw details the clinical utilization and interpretation of tests used in the diagnosis and follow-up of bone

Endocrinol Metab Clin N Am 46 (2017) xiii–xv
http://dx.doi.org/10.1016/j.ecl.2017.06.002
0889-8529/17/© 2017 Published by Elsevier Inc.

disorders. Measurement of total and ionized calcium phosphorous, vitamin D, parathyroid hormone, and parathyroid hormone–related protein and bone turnover markers is emphasized.

In "Biochemical and Imaging Diagnostics in Endocrinology: Predictors of Fertility," Drs Mahany and Randolph discuss the appropriate diagnostic approach for infertility, with an emphasis on the female factor. Cycle-timed ovarian and pituitary hormones in addition to ovarian reserve assessment with anti-Müllerian hormone and transvaginal ultrasound for antral follicle pool are discussed. The authors also provide case reports for further clarification on clinical applications.

In "Biochemical Testing in Neuroendocrine Tumors," Drs Aluri and Dillon discuss the different biomarkers utilized in the diagnosis and posttreatment follow-up of patients with neuroendocrine tumors. Inaccuracies, advantages, and disadvantages of available markers are described, highlighting the need for new, more predictive markers, and the potential role of emerging multianalyte assays.

Medical imaging plays an indispensable role in the management of endocrine disorders. The article, "Thyroid Cancer: Ultrasound Imaging and Fine Needle Aspiration Biopsy," by Drs Melany and Chen emphasizes the importance of detailed morphology in thyroid ultrasound, and particularly its role in diagnosis, treatment selection, and follow-up of thyroid nodules and suspicious cervical lymph nodes. The authors also discuss the utility of fine needle aspiration biopsy, tissue thyroglobulin assay, and genomic testing for the evaluation of thyroid malignancies.

Dr Pressman discusses the latest pituitary imaging techniques in "Pituitary Imaging." The article explores the critical role of MRI as well as the lesser role of computed tomography in the assessment and treatment of lesions in the pituitary gland and in and around the sella turcica.

"Pancreatic Imaging" by Dr Masciocchi reviews imaging approaches for the evaluation of pancreatic neuroendocrine tumors. The authors provide imaging tips that can assist in differentiating from among these lesions.

In "Selected Controversies of Radioiodine Imaging and Therapy in Differentiated Thyroid Cancer," Dr Van Nostrand reviews the role of radioiodine isotopes I-123 and I-131 in the diagnosis of and I-131 in the treatment and follow-up of differentiated thyroid cancer (DTC). Using the 2015 American Thyroid Association guidelines as a backdrop, the author considers controversies and challenges in the field, including radioiodine isotope dosage for remnant ablation or adjuvant treatment, treatment of distant metastases, and the role of radioiodine in refractory DTC.

Drs Yu and Wachsman focus on the critical role of the anatomical and functional imaging modalities used for diagnosis, prognosis, and management of neuroendocrine tumors in "Imaging of Neuroendocrine Tumors." Indications, interpretations, limitations, and pitfalls of the different imaging techniques are described.

In "Adrenal Imaging," Dr Dunnick reviews imaging modalities used for the evaluation of adrenal lesions, with a focus on their advantages and limitations for clinical practice. Both anatomical and functional imaging techniques as well as adrenal venous sampling are discussed.

The issue concludes with "Point-of-Care Endocrine Diagnostics," by Dr Ehrenkranz. The author looks at the efficiency and affordability of point-of-care endocrine diagnostics and considers the impact of shifting from centralized laboratory testing to point-of-care with a lower cost and a substantially more rapid turnaround time.

We hope you will find this issue on Biochemical and Imaging Diagnostics in Endocrinology in *Endocrinology and Metabolism Clinics of North America* useful in your practice. We thank our guest editors and the authors for the excellent articles and the Elsevier editorial staff for their invaluable help.

Anat Ben-Shlomo, MD
Pituitary Center
Division of Endocrinology, Diabetes, & Metabolism
Cedars Sinai Medical Center
8700 Beverly Boulevard
Los Angeles, CA 90048, USA

Maria Fleseriu, MD, FACE
Northwest Pituitary Center
Departments of Medicine and Neurological Surgery
Oregon Health & Science University
3138 SW Sam Jackson Park Road
Portland, OR 97239, USA

*E-mail addresses:*
benshlomoa@cshs.org (A. Ben-Shlomo)
fleseriu@ohsu.edu (M. Fleseriu)

# Preface

# The Current Status and Evolution of Hormone Testing in the Digital Age

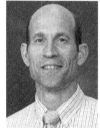
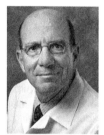
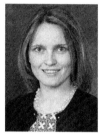
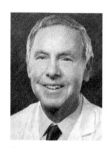

Richard J. Auchus, MD, PhD, FACE     Barry D. Pressman, MD, FACR     Adina F. Turcu, MD     Alan D. Waxman, MD

*Editors*

Among the memorable aphorisms from the great philosopher Yogi Berra are the two paradoxical quips, "The future ain't what it used to be" and "It's like déjà vu all over again." Paradoxically as well, those two quotes fit well with this issue of *Endocrinology and Metabolism Clinics of North America*. Hormone testing arose from humble beginnings with simple bioassays in the field and later expanded to include more cumbersome testing performed in the laboratory. The advent of radioimmunoassays for proteins, peptides, and later conjugated small molecules revolutionized endocrinology starting in the 1960s. Application of mass spectrometry techniques to endocrinology followed soon afterward, and the advances in methodology and instrumentation, which have accelerated in recent years, have cemented its place in endocrine testing. Yet the landscape continues to evolve, and in some ways the pendulum is swinging back in the other direction. In the United States, government regulations and third-party payer demands limit the implementation of new assay methods from research laboratory to clinical practice. Providers of laboratory services face external pressures to offer high-assay quality (sensitivity and accuracy), yet consumer demands also stress ease and convenience. If you have ever collected a 24-hour urine specimen yourself, you understand why no patient is excited about this exercise.

This issue begins with a review of mass spectrometry and its application to endocrine testing. Every endocrinologist today needs to understand the advantages and limitations of mass spectrometry–based assays, particularly for elusive analytes as measured in reference laboratories. We then make a 180° turn and explore the laboratories, liquid chromatography tandem mass spectrometry (LC-MS/MS), which relies on a collision-induced dissociation reaction that occurs in the collision cell in the mass spectrometer, was the prominent LC-MS methodology used. More recently, LC high-resolution accurate mass spectrometry (HRAMS), capable of achieving mass-to-charge analysis with mass error in the low part-per-million range has enabled multisteroid profiling and intact protein biomarker quantitation. This article highlights areas of clinical endocrinology that have witnessed an advent of LC-MS and LC-HRAMS into routine clinical practice.

## ADVENT OF MASS SPECTROMETRY INTO CLINICAL LABORATORIES—A HISTORICAL PERSPECTIVE

Since its inception about 100 hundred years ago, the principle of mass to charge ratio measurement as an analytical tool has found numerous applications in modern science. Sir Joseph J. Thompson, whose work on cathode rays laid the foundation of MS as a field, has been widely considered the inventor of MS.[1] His students F.W. Aston and A.J. Dempster further improved his work and produced more sophisticated versions of mass spectrometers, used to measure atomic weights of elements in early 1900s. MS found an extensive use in the World War II era for enrichment of nuclear material in the Manhattan Project. In the post–World War II era, the petroleum industry used MS for characterizing oil components and for developing oil-based products. Industrial applications of MS fueled advancements in gas-phase ionization and fragmentation techniques. The 1950s witnessed the development of quadrupoles, and work on improving ionization sources intensified. The first system that combined a chromatographic and a mass spectrometric system was performed in late 1950s by Fred McLafferty and Roland Gohlke at Dow Chemical with Bill Wiley and Ian McLaren at Bendix Research Laboratories. By the end of 1980s, introduction of electrospray ionization (ESI; Nobel Prize 2002) allowed interfacing a liquid chromatograph with a mass spectrometer, which marked an important milestone in the field.[2,3] The capability to introduce chromatographed sample extract into the mass spectrometer opened up avenues for clinical applications.[4] Use of high-pressure liquid chromatography (HPLC) was already pervasive in clinical and pharmaceutical laboratories that used traditional detection methods, including ultraviolet, fluorometric, and electrochemical methods. Operating the mass spectrometer in the multiple reaction monitoring mode empowered the laboratories to perform LC-MS/MS analyses with high analytical specificity and sensitivity while achieving relatively short chromatographic separation times. It is not surprising that both pharmaceutical and clinical laboratories dealing with drug analysis, steroid hormone quantitation, and biochemical genetic laboratories (to assess in-born errors of metabolism) have adopted LC-MS/MS platforms widely. In 2010, the Mayo Clinic reference laboratory reported that the number of clinical samples analyzed by LC-MS/MS had exceeded 2,000,000.[4]

With any great application intended to transform the current landscape of clinical laboratories, come great challenges. Several barriers exist toward introduction of LC-MS/MS in the clinical laboratory. LC-MS/MS platforms are expensive enough to deter leadership groups in small- to large-scale hospital laboratories from making a large capital investment. Once purchased, LC-MS/MS instruments need constant upkeep, may suffer from significant down time, and need expensive service contracts for yearly maintenance. Clinical assays have to be optimized and validated on the instrument for which highly trained personnel are needed. Medical technologists do not receive specific training in LC-MS/MS method development. Therefore, highly trained personnel are needed to develop and implement LC-MS/MS clinical assays.

Additionally, LC-MS/MS assays are laboratory-developed tests whose performance characteristics have to be developed and validated for clinical use by the performing laboratory. Laboratory developed tests have come under the US Food and Drug Administration radar recently, and how these are regulated may change in the future.

Despite the aforementioned challenges, clinical laboratories around the globe are using LC-MS/MS and LC-HRAMS successfully for clinical care. It is now well understood that although the initial capital and technical investment with mass spectrometers can be high, the valuable output can be envisioned in terms of high efficacy workflows, result accuracy, and improved analytical specificity and sensitivity offered by mass spectrometers. The US Food and Drug Administration and Clinical Laboratory and Standards Institute have developed guidelines for clinical laboratory scientists to use for successful implementation and functioning of LC-MS/MS clinical assays.[5] In this review, we highlight the areas in clinical endocrinology in which MS has made a significant impact.

## CONGENITAL ADRENAL HYPERPLASIA

CAH encompasses a wide spectrum of autosomal recessive disorders caused by a deficiency of enzymes responsible for cortisol biosynthesis (**Fig. 1**).[6] Some forms of CAH can be fatal when not recognized, with mortality rates in patients with severe forms (salt wasting) between 4% and 10%.[7] Deficiency of each 1 of the 4 specific P-450 cytochrome enzymes (CYP), namely CYP11A1 (cholesterol desmolase), CYP21 (21-hydroxylase), CYP11B1 (11β-hydroxylase), CYP17 (17α-hydroxylase), or of the steroidogenic acute regulatory protein (STAR), 3-β-hydroxysteroid dehydrogenase type 2 (3β-HSD2) or P450-oxidoreductase deficiency is related to some degree of deficiency in cortisol synthesis. Mutations in the CYP21 gene account for more than 90% of CAH cases. Clinical manifestations of classic CYP21 deficiency have been classified as salt wasting or simple virilizing, depending on whether the mutation can lead to spontaneous hypotensive crises in the infant. A mild nonclassic form of CYP21 deficiency has also been described in which patients are asymptomatic with signs of postnatal androgen excess. Approximately 1 in 16,000 births in most populations are affected by classic CAH, whereas the non-lassic forms occur in approximately 0.2% of the general population. Certain in-bred populations such as Ashkenazi Jews (Eastern European) have a higher disease prevalence (1%–2%). More than 100 mutations in the gene encoding for the 21-hydroxylase enzyme, *CYP21A2,* are known, and disease severity is related to the allelic variation. Compound heterozygosity for 2 or more different mutant *CYP21A2* alleles, observed in many CAH patients, leads to a wide spectrum of phenotypes.[6,8]

Diagnosis of CYP21 deficiency is most commonly achieved by measurement of 17-hydroxyprogesterone (17OHP) in infants. In CAH patients, a loss in CYP21 activity results in cortisol deficiency leading to a compensatory production of excess cortisol precursors by the adrenal cortex. CYP21 facilitates the conversion of 17OHP to 11-deoxycortisol (cortisol precursor) and progesterone to deoxycorticosterone (aldosterone precursor). Newborn screening programs for CAH measure 17OHP in dried blood spots collected on filter paper cards, also called *Guthrie* cards after Robert Guthrie, who implemented the first test for phenylketonuria diagnosis.[9] The Endocrine Society Guidelines recommend that screening for 21-hydroxylase deficiency should be included in all newborn screening protocols because early diagnosis and treatment can prevent CAH-associated morbidity and mortality.[8] Newborn screening programs in all 50 states in the United States now include CAH testing. A false-positive CAH result can cause significant psychological distress and unnecessary physician time

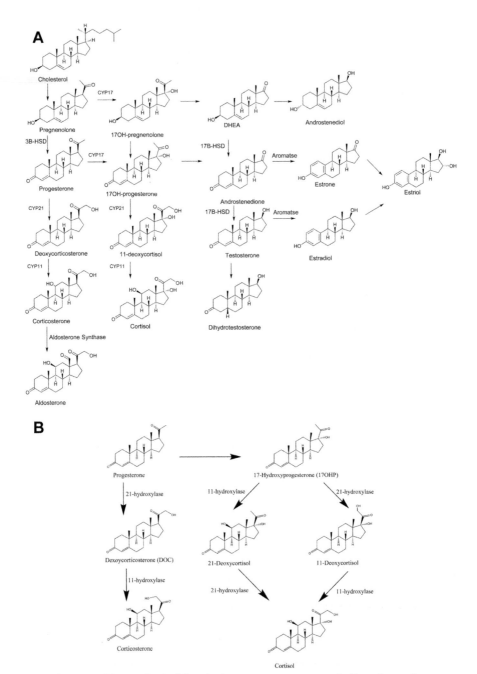

**Fig. 1.** (*A*) Steroid biosynthesis; (*B*) 17-hydroxyprogesterone metabolic pathway shows conversion to 21-deoxycortisol and 11-deoxycortisol and finally to cortisol.

spent counseling parents. Therefore, screening methods with low false-positive rates are recommended. A 2-tiered screening protocol with first-tier screen with immunoassay and a second-tier evaluation of positive cases of LC-MS/MS is used. First-tier screens for CAH are performed on dried blood spots on filter paper cards using immunoassays. Radioimmunoassay (RIA) and enzyme-linked immunosorbent assay formats have been used, but many centers in the United States have transitioned to an automated time-resolved dissociation-enhanced lanthanide flouroimmunoassay.[10] Immunoassays measuring 17OHP for first-tier CAH screening have analytical (lack of antibody specificity)[11] and clinical (true elevations in premature, stressed or sick infants)[12] limitations.

A particularly useful approach in improving positive predictive value of CAH screening is to use steroid ratios. Three large studies showing improvement in positive predictive value of CAH screening by using steroid ratios instead of single analytes have been published.[9,13,14] In one approach adopted by Matern and colleagues[9] the false-positive rate for CAH testing was reduced from 0.64% to 0.06% using a ratio of (17OHP + androstenedione)/cortisol instead of only 17OHP. The idea that a true enzyme deficiency will cause an increase in the concentration of its substrate and a concomitant decrease in the concentration of product is the rationale for using steroid ratio rather than a single analyte as a positive predictor of disease.[9] In another study, use of this ratio resulted in a decrease in false-positive rates from 2.6% to 0.09% in which results from 64,615 infants screened over a 13-month period were used. Another marker that has been used as a sensitive marker to detect CAH is 21-deoxycortisol. Janzen and colleagues[14] found that calculating the (17OHP+21-deoxycortisol)/cortisol ratio can improve the sensitivity of CAH diagnosis.

LC-MS/MS assays for 17OHP measurement circumvent the lack of analytical specificity seen in first-tier immunoassays. Several laboratories reported LC-MS/MS methods for measurement of 17OHP.[15–19] Many 17OHP LC-MS/MS clinical assays use an organic solvent or solid-phase extraction (SPE) step, which helps eliminate most nonspecific analytes. Kushnir and colleagues[19] used the oxime product of 17OHP, 11-deoxycortisol, 17-hydroxypregnenolone, and pregnenolone after SPE for achieving a desirable functional sensitivity in a multisteroid LC-MS/MS assay. Another key feature in developing an LC-MS/MS steroid profile for CAH is that 11-deoxycortisol and 21-deoxycortisol (see **Fig. 1B**) are of the same molecular mass and therefore must be separated by chromatography because of similarity in fragmentation patterns. Newly emerging LC-HRAMS instruments are allowing high-resolution accurate mass measurement and generate steroid profiles in a single-sample injection. Steroid profile assays can be challenging to develop, but steroid profiling might offer a diagnostic use as the utility of multisteroid ratio becomes more prevalent for the evaluation of patients with suspected CAH.

## VITAMIN D METABOLITE QUANTITATION

Vitamin D and the parathyroid hormone endocrine system concomitantly regulate the calcium homeostasis in humans.[20,21] Vitamin $D_3$ (cholecalciferol) is the mammalian form, whereas vitamin $D_2$ (ergocalciferol) is derived from plants, and both have similar physiologic effects on calcium homeostasis. They differ structurally only in the side chain composition wherein vitamin $D_2$ has an extra double bond and a methyl group. This article refers to vitamin $D_3$ or vitamin $D_2$ when a distinction is needed, otherwise the term vitamin D will refer to the total vitamin D ($D_3+D_2$).

We owe our understanding the role of the vitamin D metabolic pathway (**Fig. 2**) in calcium homeostasis to work accomplished by experts in the last few decades.[21–25] It is now well understood that vitamin D, formed in the skin, is transported to the liver by vitamin D–binding protein and converted to 25-hydroxyvitamin D (25(OH)D) by CYP2R1. Conversion of 25(OH)D, the most abundant circulatory form, to its active dihydroxylated metabolite 1,25-dihydroxyvitamin D (1,25(OH)$_2$D) by

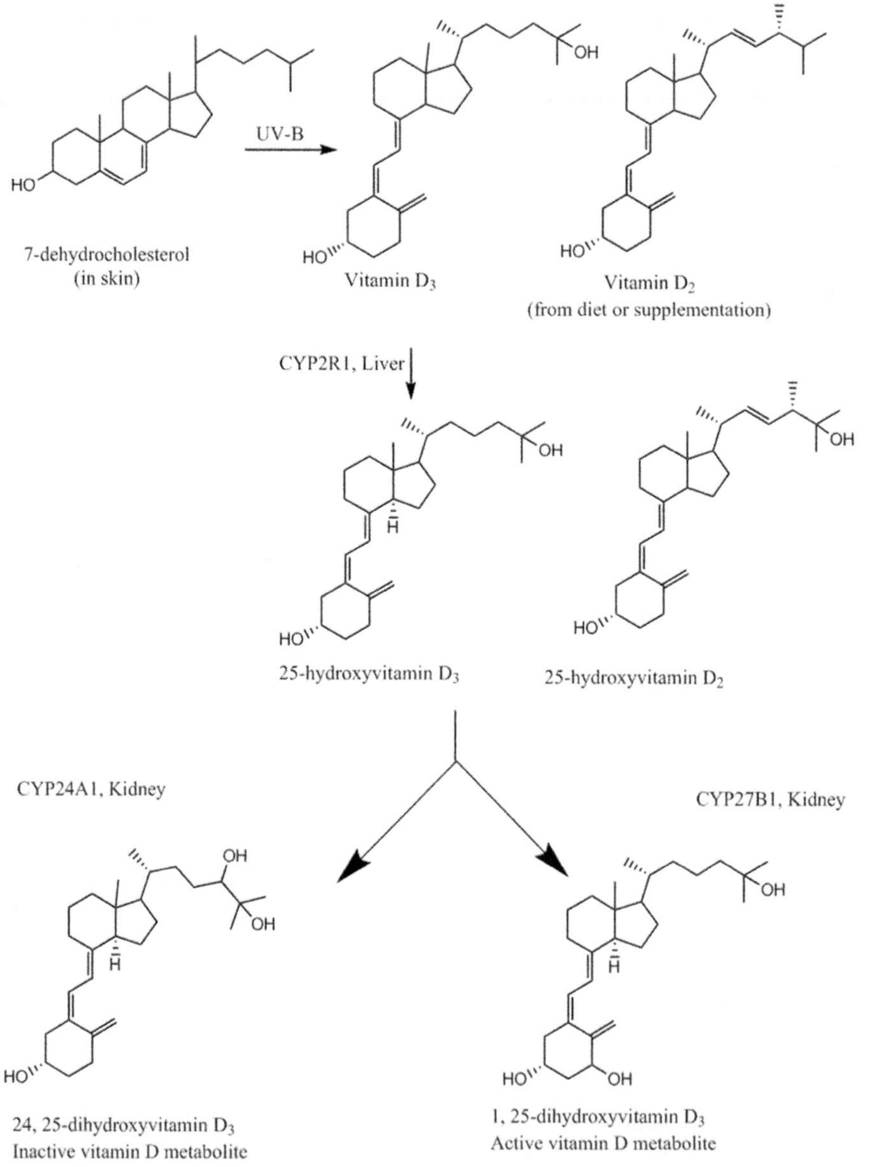

**Fig. 2.** Vitamin D metabolic pathway. (*Adapted from* Ketha H, Singh RJ. Chapter 9 - Vitamin D metabolite quantitation by LC-MS/MS. In: Nair H, Clarke W, editors. Mass spectrometry for the clinical laboratory. San Diego: Academic Press; 2017. p. 181–204; with permission.)

25-hydroxyvitamin $D_3$ 1-$\alpha$-hydroxylase (CYP27B1) is triggered by calcium demand, whereas during low calcium demand 25(OH)D is converted to its inactive metabolite, 24,25-dyhydroxyvitamin D (24,25(OH)$_2$D) by 25-hydroxyvitamin $D_3$ 24-hydroxylase (CYP24A1). Clinically relevant vitamin D metabolites include 25-(OH)D, 1,25(OH)$_2$D, and 24,25(OH)$_2$D.[20,21,24] Biochemical profiles observed in vitamin D deficiency or excess or vitamin D–related genetic diseases are shown in **Table 1**.

**Table 1**
Clinical utility of vitamin D metabolite quantitation and biochemical effect on parathyroid hormone and serum calcium in various pathologic states

| Vitamin D Metabolite | Reference Interval | Used in the Differential Diagnosis of | Effect on Vitamin D Metabolite[a] | PTH | Serum Calcium |
|---|---|---|---|---|---|
| 25(OH)D | 10–65 ng/mL<br>25–162 nmol/L | • Nutritional rickets<br>• Vitamin D deficiency<br>• Vitamin D toxicity<br>• Monitoring vitamin D supplementation<br>• VDDR type I<br>• VDDR type II; 1,25(OH)2D is low<br>• CYP24A1 mutations; has to be measured in conjunction with 24,25(OH)2D | ↓<br>↓<br>↑<br>Variable<br>Normal<br>Normal | ↑<br>↑[a]<br>↓<br>Normal<br>↑<br>↑<br>↓ | ↓<br>↓[a]<br>↑<br>Normal<br>↓<br>↓<br>↑ |
| C3-epi-25(OH)D | Variable percentage; dependent on 25(OH)D | • To accurately determine the "native" 25(OH)D present, as the 2 forms may have differential downstream calcemic effects | Variable | Variable | Variable |
| 1,25(OH)2D | 15–60 pg/mL<br>36–144 pmol/L | • Vitamin D deficiency<br>• Iatrogenic vitamin D toxicity<br>• Hypercalcemia caused by malignancy, primary hyperparathyroidism, recurrent kidney stones, hypercalciuria<br>• Hypocalcemia in end-stage renal disease | ↑<br>↑ or normal<br>↑<br>↓ | ↑<br>↓<br>↓<br>↑ | ↓<br>↑<br>↑<br>↓ |
| 24,25(OH)2D and 25(OH) (25(OH)D/24,25(OH)2D) | 7–35 | • CYP24A1 mutations; has to be measured in conjunction with 24,25(OH)2D; elevated 1,25(OH)2D, recurrent hypercalcemia and kidney stones are common | ↑ | ↓ | ↑ |

*Abbreviation:* PTH, parathyroid hormone; VDDR, Vitamin D-dependent rickets.

[a] Refers to the change in vitamin D metabolite mentioned in column 1.

*Adapted from* Ketha H, Singh RJ. Chapter 9 - Vitamin D metabolite quantitation by LC-MS/MS. In: Nair H, Clarke W, editors. Mass spectrometry for the clinical laboratory. San Diego: Academic Press; 2017. p. 181–204; with permission.

In the last decade, clinical laboratories witnessed an unprecedented increase in 25(OH)D testing.[26,27] This trend could, in part, be attributed to the numerous clinical studies undertaken to explore the role of vitamin D metabolic pathway in various aspects of health and disease. This trend has raised some questions regarding the clinical utility of populationwide screening for vitamin D deficiency. In fact, as a part of the Choosing Wisely initiative by the American Board of Internal Medicine, the American Society of Clinical Pathology recommends not to perform population-based screening for 25(OH)D deficiency. However, laboratory testing is recommended for higher-risk patients (eg, osteoporosis, chronic kidney disease, malabsorption, some infections, obese individuals) and when results case be used to start more aggressive therapy.

Parallel to clinical demand, vitamin D assays witnessed a surge in technologic advances in the last decade. Several immunoassays and LC-MS/MS assays are currently used in hospital and reference clinical laboratories. LC-MS/MS assays for cholecalciferol,[28] ergocalciferol,[28] 25(OH)D,[29–36] $1,25(OH)_2D$,[37,38] and $24,25(OH)_2D$[39–41] are available in many clinical laboratories.

25(OH)D is the most commonly measured vitamin D metabolite. It is the only metabolite that should be tested when a nutritional deficiency of vitamin D is suspected. The key technical consideration in developing an LC-MS/MS assay for vitamin D metabolites is the separation of 25(OH)D from vitamin D–binding protein, which is conveniently achieved by liquid-liquid extraction (LLE) or SPE based methods. Numerous methods have been published for 25(OH)D quantitation by LC-MS/MS, and many are reproducible in the clinical laboratory. Online SPE for sample clean-up and improved sensitivity have been used to simplify clinical workflow.[42] Derivatization of the 1,3-diene system, common to all vitamin D metabolites, using a Diels-Alder adduct formation with 4-phenyl-1,2,4-triazole-3,5-dione (PTAD) or related compounds has been used to improve sensitivity and throughput.[29,34] In one approach, 5 different patient samples were derivatized, each with a unique PTAD. Then the 5 derivatized patient samples were pooled and analyzed in a single injection using mass-to-charge ion pairs corresponding to the uniquely mass-tagged PTAD–vitamin D derivative allowing improved throughput by 5-fold.[29]

$1,25(OH)_2D$ LC-MS/MS assays, on the other hand, can be challenging to develop. $1,25(OH)_2D$ circulates in picomolar quantities in normal humans. Measurement of serum $1,25(OH)_2D$ is useful for diagnosis or management of patients with chronic kidney disease or oncogenic osteomalacia, to investigate abnormalities in phosphate metabolism, and in patients with suspected CYP24A1 mutations.[22,23,25,43,44] In one approach, the serum is first subjected to an SPE followed by an immunoenrichment of the SPE eluate with a solid-phase bound $1,25(OH)_2D$-specific antibody followed by an elution and a derivatization step using a PTAD reagent. This method is long and labor intensive, and implementing it in a clinical laboratory requires specialized expertise. One method circumventing the use of the immunoenrichment step has been described that uses a cationic derivatization reagent to gain the sensitivity needed to accurately quantitate serum $1,25(OH)_2D$.[38]

$24,25(OH)_2D$ is the marker of 24-hydroxalse function.[45] Measurement of $24,25(OH)_2D$ is useful for identifying the cause of persistent hypercalcemia and recurrent kidney stones in patients with CYP24A1 gene mutations.[46–51] The metabolic product of CYP24A1 enzyme is undetectable in patients with homozygous mutations in the corresponding gene. These patients have persistent hypercalcemia, suppressed parathyroid hormone, elevated serum $1,25(OH)_2D$, and, in many cases, recurrent nephrolithiasis. Of note, measurement of $24,25(OH)_2D$ alone will not provide clinically useful information, as there is a significant linear correlation between

24,25(OH)$_2$D and its precursor 25(OH)D. Therefore, use of the 25(OH)D/24,25(OH)$_2$D ratio is recommended to diagnose patients with CYP24A1 mutations. In patients with an elevated 25(OH)D/24,25(OH)$_2$D (>99), a CYP24A1 mutation is highly likely. 24,25(OH)$_2$D circulates at concentrations that are 7% to 35% of 25(OH)D in normal adults.[40] Sample preparation steps amenable to 25(OH)D quantitation can be used to optimize the LC-MS/MS method for 24,25(OH)$_2$D. Methods with or without derivatization with PTAD have been published and clinically used.[39]

## PHEOCHROMOCYTOMA

Pheochromocytoma and extra-adrenal paraganglioma are rare catecholamine-producing (epinephrine, norepinephrine, and dopamine) tumors resulting in poorly managed hypertension in affected patients. A schematic of catecholamine metabolism is shown in **Fig. 3**. Although used interchangeably, pheochromocytoma and paraganglioma are distinct in their risk for malignancy and the need for follow-up genetic testing. Pheochromocytomas are rare, occurring in 0.2% patients with hypertension.[52] Although most occur sporadically, approximately 30% catecholamine-secreting tumors have a familial cause. Several autosomal-dominant genetic disorders are associated with high frequency (up to 10%–20%) of pheochromocytoma occurrence in affected patients, including von Hippel-Lindau syndrome, multiple endocrine neoplasia type 2, neurofibromatosis 1, and succinate dehydrogenase gene familial syndromes.[53,54] Diagnosis of a catecholamine-secreting tumor is often based on history of a symptomatic patient, an incidental adrenal mass, or presence of familial disease.[55–57] Tumors secreting only dopamine are rare but, when they do occur, lead to a poorer prognosis than other catecholamine-producing tumors, as they tend to be asymptomatic, are detected later, and are likely to be malignant at the time of diagnosis.[58] Biochemical diagnosis using screening tests in a symptomatic patient should be used as the basis for further radiologic imaging studies rather than the other way around.[59] In the First International Symposium on Pheochromocytoma, a group of experts recommended the use of plasma or urinary-fractionated metanephrine (META) and normetanephrine (NMETA) as the most accurate screening approach.[60,61]

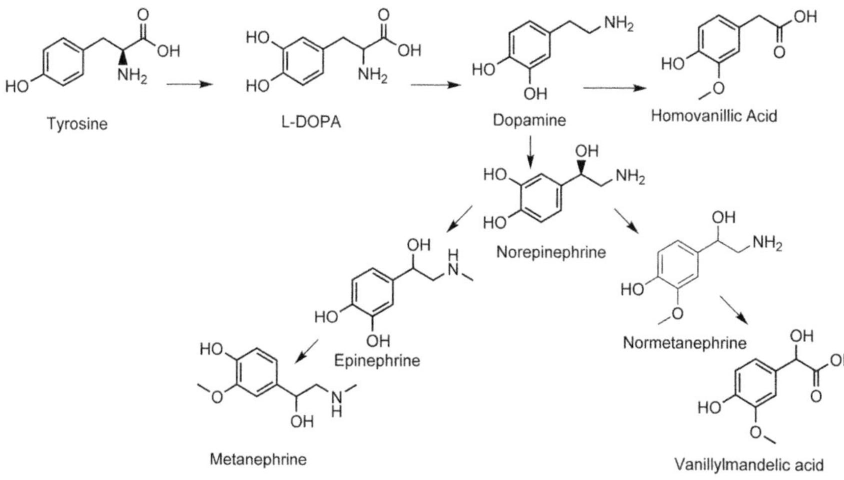

**Fig. 3.** Catecholamine metabolism.

Biochemical diagnosis of catecholamine-producing tumor is commonly made by a combination of 24-hour urinary catecholamine or META quantitation.[62] HPLC-based quantitation of epinephrine, norepinephrine, META, NMETA, and dopamine in urine has been used for decades for diagnosis of catecholamine-secreting tumors. Catecholamine quantitation by HPLC in urine is extremely tedious and is prone to several limitations. Most clinical laboratories use an ion exchange resin to extract and concentrate the analytes before introduction onto the LC system for separation and quantitation. HPLC-based assays for catecholamines (and META) are prone to interferences by commonly used drugs like acetaminophen.[63] Sample preparation steps for catecholamine quantitation are labor intensive and time consuming. In one method, the alumina has to be acid washed and dried before use in the clinical assay. More-efficient 96-well format alumina plates have been prepared but are not commercially available.[64] Additionally, 24-hour urine collections can be erroneous, and incomplete collections can result in false-negative results. Appropriate additives (most of them acidic) have to be added before the urine collection begins,[65] but lack of adherence to proper collection methods for 24-hour urine catecholamine quantitation remains a problem. Plasma catecholamine determination is also challenging, as secretion is subject to wide biological variation. Several common stimuli like smoking and mild exercise (eg, taking a flight of stairs) can affect plasma catecholamine levels.[66] The sample collection process for plasma catecholamine quantitation from a patient with suspected pheochromocytoma requires that a catheter be placed in the patient's arm followed by at least a 15-minute period during which the patient remains seated in a dark quiet room. Needless to say, adherence to this procedure can be challenging. To circumvent the challenges associated with catecholamine quantitation, many clinical laboratorians now recommend the use of META and NMETA for pheochromocytoma screening and diagnosis. META and NMETA are more stable compared with catecholamines in urine, and plasma and sample collection procedures are not different from other routine analytes. Even though many groups have published and reviewed methods for urine and plasma catecholamine quantitation by LC-MS/MS,[67–70] their adoption into the clinical laboratories has been slow. Tedious sample extraction process, variability in ionization efficiency, and poorly shaped chromatographic peaks (on standard reverse phase or hydrophobic interaction chromatography columns) are some of the challenging aspects of catecholamine analysis by LC-MS/MS (Hemamalini Ketha, MD, unpublished data, 2016).

META and NMETA are more amenable to detection by LC-MS/MS compared with catecholamines. Gas chromatography mass spectrometry (GC-MS) has also been used for META and NMETA quantitation.[71] Several clinical laboratories have already implemented clinical LC-MS/MS assays for META and NMETA quantitation on plasma and urine.[72–76] For quantitation of urine META and NMETA, the sample is treated with a strong acid at 60°C to 70°C for approximately 60 minutes to hydrolyze the META and NMETA conjugates.[72] The pH of the resulting solution is then adjusted to 6.5 ± 0.5 so that a weak cation exchange SPE can be used for analyte extraction. This step is followed by separation of the SPE eluate on a C-18 (or equivalent) reverse phase column and MS/MS analysis.[72] For quantitation of plasma META and NMETA, the hydrolysis step is not needed, but the sensitivity of the method can be demanding, as normal levels of META and NMETA are approximately several-fold lower (in picomole per milliliter range) in plasma compared with a 24-hour urine sample. Ion pairing agents have been also used successfully with LC-MS/MS assays for METAs.[76] To automate the sample preparation process, the plasma sample was subject to protein precipitation using 10% (wt/vol) trichloroacetic acid followed by cooling and centrifugation. The supernatant was then subject to an online mixed-mode cation exchange extraction using a turbulent flow chromatography column assisted with ion-pairing reagent, and a porous graphitic column was used for chromatographic separation.[76] Ion-pairing reagents are mobile-phase additives that facilitate separation of ionic and highly polar substances on reversed phase HPLC columns. Ion-pairing agents are commonly used in HPLC methods for catecholamine and META quantitation. It is important to use highly pure mobile-phase additives, as they can affect assay performance.[67]

Catecholamines and their metabolites are biomarkers useful for diagnosis of a catecholamine-secreting tumor. There is now a consensus that use of catecholamine quantitation for pheochromocytoma screening or diagnosis was most often based on institutional preference rather that clinical evidence. Quantitation of fractionated META and NMETA in urine or plasma offer diagnostic sensitivity that is superior to that achieved by measuring the precursor catecholamines.[55,56,60] Additionally, improvement in analytical methods and the need for simpler clinical laboratory workflows led to a transition to LC-MS/MS for META and NMETA quantitation. Algorithms recommending the use of fractionated plasma META and NMETA assay to screen and urine META and NMETA as a confirmatory test for patients with suspected pheochromocytoma have also been developed.

## TESTOSTERONE AND ESTRADIOL

Quantitation of testosterone and estradiol is important for the diagnosis or management of disorders of puberty, hypogonadism, polycystic ovary syndrome, amenorrhea, and tumors of ovary, testes, breast, and prostate. Before direct quantitation of testosterone and estradiol was feasible, ketosteroids in urine were measured as the key metabolites of testosterone and estradiol. Ketosteroid measurement was performed using colorimetric assays that lacked sensitivity and specificity because of endogenous and exogenous interferences.[77] Manual RIAs that relied on extensive organic extractions offered increased sensitivity yet suboptimal specificity. Because of increased demand to improve turnaround time and on sample throughput, automated immunoassays mostly replaced manual RIAs. These offered better throughput and precision but suffered worse specificity problems. Moreover, agreement between different immunoassays has often been poor, and they are all compromised by a limited dynamic measurement range.

Approximately 60% serum testosterone is bound to sex hormone–binding globulin, whereas approximately 40% is bound to albumin, and only about 1% to 2% is present as free testosterone. Albumin-bound testosterone is loosely bound compared with sex hormone–binding globulin–bound testosterone fraction, and the combination of free testosterone and albumin-bound testosterone is called the *bioavailable testosterone*. Clinical practice guidelines recommend the use of early morning total testosterone measurement for facilitating the diagnosis of primary hypogonadism. Endocrine Society and Urology Society guidelines have highlighted the limitations of the immunoassays for sex steroids and have provided convincing evidence that MS methods are preferable for measurement of sex steroid hormones.[78] There is also a lack of consensus related to the appropriate testosterone type (total, bioavailable, or free) to monitor patients receiving testosterone therapy.[79,80]

The use of testosterone assays is growing in clinical laboratories, especially for monitoring patients who are receiving testosterone supplements. In adult men, the correlation between certain immunoassays and LC-MS/MS assays for testosterone is acceptable. **Fig. 4** shows comparison of total testosterone measured by an automated immunoassay (ADIVA Centaur; Siemens Diagnostics) and an LC-MS/MS method ($r^2 = 0.92$; slope = 0.91). But the correlation in women and pediatric patients

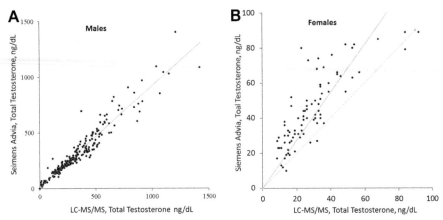

**Fig. 4.** Comparison of total testosterone measurement by LC-MS/MS with Siemens Advia Centaur Assay in (*A*) men (N = 243) and (*B*) women (N = 88).

between the same assays reveals a positive bias by the immunoassay method ($r^2$ = 0.65; slope = 1.37). LC-MS/MS methods for measurement of all 3 types of testosterone have been described. Total testosterone can be measured by subjecting the supernatant resulting from LLE of serum or the eluate from SPE of serum to LC-MS/MS analysis. When an LLE is used as a sample preparation method, an online SPE may need to be performed on the LC system before MS analysis.[81] Quantitation of free testosterone requires a laborious equilibrium dialysis step followed by derivatization of the dialysate extract with hydroxylamine before LC-MS/MS analysis. Bioavailable testosterone measurement requires a selective precipitation step to remove only the sex hormone–binding globulin–bound fraction before LC-MS/MS analysis.[82–84]

An Endocrine Society position statement highlighted the problems with accurate and specific quantitation of estradiol over the wide range of physiologically relevant levels in diverse populations.[85] A single estradiol assay that can measure estradiol accurately in clinical situations including in vitro fertilization and ovulation induction and in patients receiving aromatase inhibitor therapy must have a broad dynamic range (0.2–5000 pg/mL). Most of the direct automated immunoassay methods are optimized to measure estradiol concentrations between 40 and 2000 pg/mL. Wide intermethod variability has been shown in many studies.[86–88] In an analysis of data reported in a College of American Pathologists (CAP) proficiency testing survey showing an estradiol concentration of 29 pg/mL (LC-MS/MS), all 14 participating immunoassay platforms overestimated the estradiol concentration—some by up to 300%.[89] Estradiol measurement at low levels by LC-MS/MS has also proven to be more difficult compared with testosterone.[85,90] Common LC-MS/MS methods use an LLE of serum followed by a dansyl chloride derivatization to improve sensitivity.[81,91–95] In another method, a combination of LLE, derivatization with dansyl chloride, and 2-dimensional chromatography helped achieve a functional sensitivity of 0.3 pg/mL for serum estradiol measurement.[89]

Serum testosterone and estradiol measurements are important for diagnosing and monitoring many diseases. The sensitivity, specificity, and wide dynamic range that are needed to accurately measure these hormones in all clinical situations and in diverse populations (eg, testosterone in men and women or estradiol measurement during in vitro fertilization treatment vs postmenopausal women) are not available in current immunoassays. LC-MS/MS assays for testosterone and estradiol are used in many clinical laboratories, are robust, circumvent the limitations of automated immunoassays, and can be used in situations in which immunoassays are known to be problematic.

## INSULINLIKE GROWTH FACTOR 1

IGF-1, an 84-amino-acid peptide hormone plays a critical role in human growth. Most of the physiologic effects of growth hormone (GH) on somatic growth are mediated via IGF-1. Measurement of IGF-1 is used as the first step in the diagnosis of acromegaly (GH excess) or conditions related to GH deficiency like short stature. IGF-1 is a more reliable biomarker compared with GH to investigate GH excess caused by wide biological variability in GH levels. GH levels fluctuate broadly during the day because of its pulsatile release every 60 to 90 minutes and based on stimuli such as exercise, meals, and sleep. Additionally, GH has a short plasma half-life (~20 min). On the other hand, serum IGF-1, which is indicative of circulating GH levels, shows significantly lower variability toward the same physiologic stimuli. Therefore, serum IGF-1 measurement is commonly used as a first step for the diagnosis of GH deficiency or excess.[96–99]

IGF-1 is produced mainly in the liver, and its production is regulated by GH. Greater than 99% IGF-1 in circulation is protein bound and exists as a ternary complex bound to IGF binding protein 3 (IGFBP-3) and acid labile subunit. Although there are overall 6 binding proteins in the IGFBP family (IGFBP1-6), IGF-1 has the highest affinity toward IGFBP-3. IGF-1 immunoassays are commercially available and used commonly in clinical laboratories. Because IGF-1 is highly protein bound in circulation, it has to be dissociated from its ternary complex with IGFBP-3 and acid labile subunit before quantitation. Most IGF-1 immunoassay formats use a dissociation buffer to dissociate IGF-1 from its ternary complex. But IGFBPs are known to be a source of interference in immunoassays. Additionally, standardization of assays from different vendors is lacking.[100–102] These challenges led to the development of MS assays for IGF-1 quantitation.[103]

IGF-1 quantitation by LC-MS/MS has been achieved using trypsinized and methylated peptides from IGF-1.[104] In another approach, IGF1 was enriched using an immunoaffinity method followed by matrix-assisted laser desorption ionization time-of-flight MS.[105] Specifically designed pipette tips conjugated to IGF-1–specific antibody that allows microscale immunoaffinity purification of IGF-1 has also been developed.[103,105,106] The eluate is then subject to trypsin digestion, and the resulting IGF-1–specific peptides are analyzed by LC-MS/MS. Lack of availability of isotopically labeled proteins to be used as internal standards can be an impediment toward implementing mass spectrometric quantitative protein assays amenable for clinical use. The microscale immunoaffinity purification IGF-1 assay uses a long arginine 3 (LR3–IGF-1) as an internal standard. LR3–IGF-1 has 13 extra amino acids at the N-terminus and an arginine at position 3 instead of glutamic acid. The antibody used in the microscale immunoaffinity purification IGF-1 assay displays similar binding affinity to wild-type IGF-1 and LR3–IGF-1. The N-terminal modification reduces binding of LR3–IGF-1 to IGFBPs.

Being a small peptide (MW: 7467 Da), IGF-1 is also amenable to quantification by LC-high-resolution MS (HRMS) as an intact protein. Bystrom and colleagues[107,108] described an LC-HRMS method for IGF-1 quantitation as an intact protein. They used the dissociation buffer used in the Nichols Advantage immunoassay (considered the gold standard for IGF-1 quantitation until its discontinuation) as the sample preparation method. The acidic ethanoic buffer dissociates IGF-1 from its ternary complex effectively while allowing large proteins (like albumin) to precipitate leaving IGF-1 in the supernatant. The advantages of this method are (1) no antibody reagents are used enabling assay standardization across different laboratories, (2) dissociation buffer is inexpensive, and (3) IGF-1 remains in the supernatant allowing an easy determination by LC-HRMS. The supernatant is analyzed by an HRAM instrument. IGF-1 is quantified in a +7 charge state at a mass accuracy of approximately 10 ppm. LC-HRMS analysis of IGF-1 has allowed discovery of IGF-1 polymorphisms observed in approximately 0. 5% of the general population. Intact protein quantitation enables screening for a range of mass-to-charge changes in the protein that may be missed by immunoassays.[109]

## PLASMA RENIN ACTIVITY

Renin mediates its effect on blood pressure by converting angiotensinogen to AngI, which is converted to AngII, the active metabolite in mediating renin's effects on blood pressure. AngII increases blood pressure by vasoconstriction and stimulates aldosterone production, which promotes potassium excretion and sodium retention.[110] PRA assay measures the rate of production of AngI from angiotensinogen. Aldosterone/PRA ratio is useful for monitoring mineralocorticoid activity and aides the diagnosis of primary aldosteronism in hypertensive subjects. AngII is the active peptide involved in regulating blood pressure control in humans. However, an accurate measurement of the circulating concentration of AngII is challenging. AngII is unstable in blood samples, and anti-AngII antibodies have high cross-reactivity to degradation products.[111] Therefore, the production rate of AngI (expressed in nanograms per milliliter per hour) is used as a surrogate for PRA. The first study exemplifying the utility of AngI measurement as a reflection of the ability of the renin-angiotensin system to generate AngII was published in the 1970s.[112,113] Several hospital clinical laboratories use a version of this RIA method. Although the RIA for PRA is known to be robust and reliable, it is laborious to perform and offers a limited dynamic range.

Several groups have developed LC-MS/MS PRA assays amenable to clinical use.[111,114–116] One method used 2 parallel AngI generation reactions (6.5 h and 24 h) so that longer reaction times can be used for low AngI samples. Additionally, this method used an online anion exchange SPE before separation of the SPE eluate on a C-18 reverse-phase chromatographic column.[114] Another method used an SPE cartridge containing a reverse-phase cartridge capable of retaining hydrophilic and lipophilic analytes.[111] Therefore, the LC-MS/MS assay for PRA uses steps or the AngI generation used in a traditional RIA, except the use of radioactivity is eliminated. Purified AngI and the corresponding isotopically labeled internal standards are commercially available for use as calibrators and internal standards.[117] Of note, calibrators and controls may need to be prepared in an artificial serum matrix, as residual PRA has been observed in commercial stripped serum products. Therefore, PRA measurement by LC-MS/MS offers an alternative to using a laborious RIA, helps eliminate the use of radioactivity, and provides a wider analytical measurement range.

## SUMMARY

MS has found numerous uses in the clinical laboratory. Although MS as a field is not new, its applications are beginning to see new frontiers in the clinical space. MS offers improved sensitivity and specificity over HPLC and in many cases over automated immunoassays. Most small-molecule drug candidates and endocrine analytes are highly amenable to analysis by LC-MS/MS. A new era in MS is emerging with the use of LC-HRMS in clinical laboratories in which even analysis of large proteins like immunoglobulins is being performed on mass spectrometers. LC-HRMS offers the possibility of multisteroid profiling, which may be a useful modality in diagnosing and treating endocrine diseases that require the clinician to have information about several metabolites at once. Currently, sample processing is an impediment toward expansion of MS in the clinical laboratory. But it is not too farfetched to envision a completely automated system capable of handling sample processing, analysis, and result reporting, all in the form of a "magic black box."

## REFERENCES

1. Thompson JJ. On the cathode rays. Proc Camb Philos Soc 1897;9:243–4.
2. Hites RA. Development of gas chromatographic mass spectrometry. Anal Chem 2016;88(14):6955–61.
3. Yates JR III. A century of mass spectrometry: from atoms to proteomes. Nat Methods 2011;8(8):633.
4. Grebe SK, Singh RJ. LC-MS/MS in the clinical laboratory - where to from here? Clin Biochem Rev 2011;32(1):5–31.
5. González O, Blanco ME, Iriarte G, et al. Bioanalytical chromatographic method validation according to current regulations, with a special focus on the non-well defined parameters limit of quantification, robustness and matrix effect. J Chromatogr A 2014;1353:10–27.
6. Speiser PW, White PC. Congenital adrenal hyperplasia. N Engl J Med 2003; 349(8):776–88.
7. Grosse SD, Van Vliet G. How many deaths can be prevented by newborn screening for congenital adrenal hyperplasia? Horm Res 2007;67(6):284–91.
8. Speiser PW, Azziz R, Baskin LS, et al. Congenital adrenal hyperplasia due to steroid 21-hydroxylase deficiency: an endocrine society clinical practice guideline. J Clin Endocrinol Metab 2010;95(9):4133–60.
9. Matern D, Tortorelli S, Oglesbee D, et al. Reduction of the false-positive rate in newborn screening by implementation of MS/MS-based second-tier tests: the Mayo Clinic experience (2004-2007). J Inherit Metab Dis 2007;30(4):585–92.
10. Gonzalez RR, Maentausta O, Solyom J, et al. Direct solid-phase time-resolved fluoroimmunoassay of 17 alpha-hydroxyprogesterone in serum and dried blood spots on filter paper. Clin Chem 1990;36(9):1667–72.
11. Makela SK, Ellis G. Nonspecificity of a direct 17 alpha-hydroxyprogesterone radioimmunoassay kit when used with samples from neonates. Clin Chem 1988;34(10):2070–5.
12. al Saedi S, Dean H, Dent W, et al. Reference ranges for serum cortisol and 17-hydroxyprogesterone levels in preterm infants. J Pediatr 1995;126(6):985–7.
13. Schwarz E, Liu A, Randall H, et al. Use of steroid profiling by UPLC-MS/MS as a second tier test in newborn screening for congenital adrenal hyperplasia: the Utah experience. Pediatr Res 2009;66(2):230–5.
14. Janzen N, Peter M, Sander S, et al. Newborn screening for congenital adrenal hyperplasia: additional steroid profile using liquid chromatography-tandem mass spectrometry. J Clin Endocrinol Metab 2007;92(7):2581–9.
15. Etter ML, Eichhorst J, Lehotay DC. Clinical determination of 17-hydroxyprogesterone in serum by LC-MS/MS: comparison to Coat-A-Count RIA method. J Chromatogr B Analyt Technol Biomed Life Sci 2006;840(1):69–74.
16. Lai CC, Tsai CH, Tsai FJ, et al. Rapid screening assay of congenital adrenal hyperplasia by measuring 17 alpha-hydroxyprogesterone with high-performance

liquid chromatography/electrospray ionization tandem mass spectrometry from dried blood spots. J Clin Lab Anal 2002;16(1):20–5.

17. Lacey JM, Minutti CZ, Magera MJ, et al. Improved specificity of newborn screening for congenital adrenal hyperplasia by second-tier steroid profiling using tandem mass spectrometry. Clin Chem 2004;50(3):621–5.

18. Cristoni S, Cuccato D, Sciannamblo M, et al. Analysis of 21-deoxycortisol, a marker of congenital adrenal hyperplasia, in blood by atmospheric pressure chemical ionization and electrospray ionization using multiple reaction monitoring. Rapid Commun Mass Spectrom 2004;18(1):77–82.

19. Kushnir MM, Rockwood AL, Roberts WL, et al. Development and performance evaluation of a tandem mass spectrometry assay for 4 adrenal steroids. Clin Chem 2006;52(8):1559–67.

20. Audran M, Gross M, Kumar R. The physiology of the vitamin D endocrine system. Semin Nephrol 1986;6(1):4–20.

21. Kumar R. The metabolism and mechanism of action of 1,25-dihydroxyvitamin D3. Kidney Int 1986;30(6):793–803.

22. Audran M, Kumar R. The physiology and pathophysiology of vitamin D. Mayo Clin Proc 1985;60(12):851–66.

23. Berndt T, Kumar R. Phosphatonins and the regulation of phosphate homeostasis. Annu Rev Physiol 2007;69:341–59.

24. deLuca HF. The metabolism, physiology and funciton of vitamin D. Leiden, Boston: Martinus Nijhoff Publishing; 1984.

25. Kumar R, Tebben PJ, Thompson JR. Vitamin D and the kidney. Arch Biochem Biophys 2012;523(1):77–86.

26. Farrell CJ, Martin S, McWhinney B, et al. State-of-the-art vitamin D assays: a comparison of automated immunoassays with liquid chromatography-tandem mass spectrometry methods. Clin Chem 2012;58(3):531–42.

27. Shahangian S, Alspach TD, Astles JR, et al. Trends in laboratory test volumes for Medicare Part B reimbursements, 2000-2010. Arch Pathol Lab Med 2014; 138(2):189–203.

28. Adamec J, Jannasch A, Huang J, et al. Development and optimization of an LC-MS/MS-based method for simultaneous quantification of vitamin D2, vitamin D3, 25-hydroxyvitamin D2 and 25-hydroxyvitamin D3. J Separat Sci 2011;34(1): 11–20.

29. Netzel BC, Cradic KW, Bro ET, et al. Increasing liquid chromatography-tandem mass spectrometry throughput by mass tagging: a sample-multiplexed high-throughput assay for 25-hydroxyvitamin D2 and D3. Clin Chem 2011;57(3): 431–40.

30. Hoofnagle AN, Laha TJ, Donaldson TF. A rubber transfer gasket to improve the throughput of liquid-liquid extraction in 96-well plates: application to vitamin D testing. J Chromatogr B Analyt Technol Biomed Life Sci 2010;878(19):1639–42.

31. Saenger AK, Laha TJ, Bremner DE, et al. Quantification of serum 25-hydroxyvitamin D(2) and D(3) using HPLC-tandem mass spectrometry and examination of reference intervals for diagnosis of vitamin D deficiency. Am J Clin Pathol 2006; 125(6):914–20.

32. Vogeser M. Quantification of circulating 25-hydroxyvitamin D by liquid chromatography–tandem mass spectrometry. J Steroid Biochem Mol Biol 2010; 121(3–5):565–73.

33. Vogeser M, Kyriatsoulis A, Huber E, et al. Candidate reference method for the quantification of circulating 25-hydroxyvitamin D3 by liquid chromatography-tandem mass spectrometry. Clin Chem 2004;50(8):1415–7.

34. Tsugawa N, Suhara Y, Kamao M, et al. Determination of 25-hydroxyvitamin D in human plasma using high-performance liquid chromatography–tandem mass spectrometry. Anal Chem 2005;77(9):3001–7.

35. Maunsell Z, Wright DJ, Rainbow SJ. Routine isotope-dilution liquid chromatography-tandem mass spectrometry assay for simultaneous measurement of the 25-hydroxy metabolites of vitamins D2 and D3. Clin Chem 2005; 51(9):1683–90.

36. Chen H, McCoy LF, Schleicher RL, et al. Measurement of 25-hydroxyvitamin D3 (25OHD3) and 25-hydroxyvitamin D2 (25OHD2) in human serum using liquid chromatography-tandem mass spectrometry and its comparison to a radioimmunoassay method. Clin Chim Acta 2008;391(1–2):6–12.

37. Strathmann FG, Laha TJ, Hoofnagle AN. Quantification of 1alpha,25-dihydroxy vitamin D by immunoextraction and liquid chromatography-tandem mass spectrometry. Clin Chem 2011;57(9):1279–85.

38. Chan N, Kaleta EJ. Quantitation of 1alpha,25-dihydroxyvitamin D by LC-MS/MS using solid-phase extraction and fixed-charge derivitization in comparison to immunoextraction. Clin Chem Lab Med 2015;53(9):1399–407.

39. Wagner D, Hanwell HE, Schnabl K, et al. The ratio of serum 24,25-dihydroxyvitamin D(3) to 25-hydroxyvitamin D(3) is predictive of 25-hydroxyvitamin D(3) response to vitamin D(3) supplementation. J Steroid Biochem Mol Biol 2011; 126(3–5):72–7.

40. Ketha H, Kumar R, Singh RJ. LC-MS/MS for identifying patients with CYP24A1 mutations. Clin Chem 2016;62(1):236–42.

41. Ketha H, Singh RJ. Chapter 9 - Vitamin D metabolite quantitation by LC-MS/MS. In: Nair H, Clarke W, editors. Mass spectrometry for the clinical laboratory. San Diego: Academic Press; 2017. p. 181–204.

42. Singh RJ, Taylor RL, Reddy GS, et al. C-3 epimers can account for a significant proportion of total circulating 25-hydroxyvitamin D in infants, complicating accurate measurement and interpretation of vitamin D status. J Clin Endocrinol Metab 2006;91(8):3055–61.

43. Wiesner RH, Kumar R, Seeman E, et al. Enterohepatic physiology of 1,25-dihydroxyvitamin D3 metabolites in normal man. J Lab Clin Med 1980;96(6): 1094–100.

44. Reinhardt TA, Napoli JL, Beitz DC, et al. 1,24,25-Trihydroxyvitamin D3: a circulating metabolite in vitamin D2-treated bovine. Arch Biochem Biophys 1982; 213(1):163–8.

45. Beckman MJ, Tadikonda P, Werner E, et al. Human 25-hydroxyvitamin D3-24-hydroxylase, a multicatalytic enzyme. Biochemistry 1996;35(25):8465–72.

46. Jacobs TP, Kaufman M, Jones G, et al. A lifetime of hypercalcemia and hypercalciuria, finally explained. J Clin Endocrinol Metab 2014;99(3):708–12.

47. Kaufmann M, Gallagher JC, Peacock M, et al. Clinical utility of simultaneous quantitation of 25-Hydroxyvitamin D and 24,25-Dihydroxyvitamin D by LC-MS/MS Involving Derivatization With DMEQ-TAD. J Clin Endocrinol Metab 2014; 99(7):2567–74.

48. Schlingmann KP, Kaufmann M, Weber S, et al. Mutations in CYP24A1 and idiopathic infantile hypercalcemia. N Engl J Med 2011;365(5):410–21.

49. Dauber A, Nguyen TT, Sochett E, et al. Genetic defect in CYP24A1, the vitamin D 24-hydroxylase gene, in a patient with severe infantile hypercalcemia. J Clin Endocrinol Metab 2012;97(2):E268–74.

50. O'Keeffe DT, Tebben PJ, Kumar R, et al. Clinical and biochemical phenotypes of adults with monoallelic and biallelic CYP24A1 mutations: evidence of gene dose effect. Osteoporos Int 2016;27(10):3121–5.

51. Tebben PJ, Milliner DS, Horst RL, et al. Hypercalcemia, hypercalciuria, and elevated calcitriol concentrations with autosomal dominant transmission due to CYP24A1 mutations: effects of ketoconazole therapy. J Clin Endocrinol Metab 2012;97(3):E423–7.

52. Stein PP, Black HR. A simplified diagnostic approach to pheochromocytoma. A review of the literature and report of one institution's experience. Medicine 1991; 70(1):46–66.

53. Walther MM, Herring J, Enquist E, et al. von Recklinghausen's disease and pheochromocytomas. J Urol 1999;162(5):1582–6.

54. Neumann HP, Berger DP, Sigmund G, et al. Pheochromocytomas, multiple endocrine neoplasia type 2, and von Hippel-Lindau disease. N Engl J Med 1993;329(21):1531–8.

55. Lenders JW, Pacak K, Eisenhofer G. New advances in the biochemical diagnosis of pheochromocytoma: moving beyond catecholamines. Ann N Y Acad Sci 2002;970:29–40.

56. Lenders JW, Pacak K, Walther MM, et al. Biochemical diagnosis of pheochromocytoma: which test is best? JAMA 2002;287(11):1427–34.

57. Guller U, Turek J, Eubanks S, et al. Detecting pheochromocytoma: defining the most sensitive test. Ann Surg 2006;243(1):102–7.

58. Dubois LA, Gray DK. Dopamine-secreting pheochromocytomas: in search of a syndrome. World J Surg 2005;29(7):909–13.

59. Sawka AM, Jaeschke R, Singh RJ, et al. A comparison of biochemical tests for pheochromocytoma: measurement of fractionated plasma metanephrines compared with the combination of 24-hour urinary metanephrines and catecholamines. J Clin Endocrinol Metab 2003;88(2):553–8.

60. Pacak K, Eisenhofer G, Ahlman H, et al. Pheochromocytoma: recommendations for clinical practice from the First International Symposium. Nat Clin Pract End Met 2007;3(2):92–102.

61. Perry CG, Sawka AM, Singh R, et al. The diagnostic efficacy of urinary fractionated metanephrines measured by tandem mass spectrometry in detection of pheochromocytoma. Clin Endocrinol (Oxf) 2007;66(5):703–8.

62. Young WF Jr. Adrenal causes of hypertension: pheochromocytoma and primary aldosteronism. Rev Endocr Metab Disord 2007;8(4):309–20.

63. Davidson FD. Paracetamol-associated interference in an HPLC-ECD assay for urinary free metadrenalines and catecholamines. Ann Clin Biochem 2004; 41(4):316–20.

64. Dunand M, Gubian D, Stauffer M, et al. High-throughput and sensitive quantitation of plasma catecholamines by Ultraperformance Liquid Chromatography–Tandem Mass Spectrometry using a solid phase microwell extraction plate. Anal Chem 2013;85(7):3539–44.

65. Willemsen JJ, Ross HA, Lenders JWM, et al. Stability of urinary fractionated metanephrines and catecholamines during collection, shipment, and storage of samples. Clin Chem 2007;53(2):268–72.

66. Bravo EL, Tarazi RC, Gifford RW, et al. Circulating and urinary catecholamines in pheochromocytoma. Diagnostic and pathophysiologic implications. N Engl J Med 1979;301(13):682–6.

67. Kushnir MM, Urry FM, Frank EL, et al. Analysis of catecholamines in urine by positive-ion electrospray tandem mass spectrometry. Clin Chem 2002;48(2): 323–31.

68. Eisenhofer G, Kopin IJ, Goldstein DS. Catecholamine metabolism: a contemporary view with implications for physiology and medicine. Pharmacol Rev 2004; 56(3):331–49.

69. Hasegawa T, Wada K, Hiyama E, et al. Pretreatment and one-shot separating analysis of whole catecholamine metabolites in plasma by using LC/MS. Anal Bioanal Chem 2006;385(5):814–20.

70. Thomas A, Geyer H, Mester HJ, et al. Quantitative determination of adrenaline and noradrenaline in urine using liquid chromatography-tandem mass spectrometry. Chroma 2006;64(9–10):587–91.

71. Canfell C, Binder SR, Khayam-Bashi H. Quantitation of urinary normetanephrine and metanephrine by reversed-phase extraction and mass-fragmentographic analysis. Clin Chem 1982;28(1):25–8.

72. Taylor RL, Singh RJ. Validation of liquid chromatography-tandem mass spectrometry method for analysis of urinary conjugated metanephrine and normetanephrine for screening of pheochromocytoma. Clin Chem 2002;48(3):533–9.

73. Lagerstedt SA, O'Kane DJ, Singh RJ. Measurement of plasma free metanephrine and normetanephrine by liquid chromatography-tandem mass spectrometry for diagnosis of pheochromocytoma. Clin Chem 2004;50(3):603–11.

74. Crockett DK, Frank EL, Roberts WL. Rapid analysis of metanephrine and normetanephrine in urine by gas chromatography-mass spectrometry. Clin Chem 2002;48(2):332–7.

75. Chan EC, Ho PC. High-performance liquid chromatography/atmospheric pressure chemical ionization mass spectrometric method for the analysis of catecholamines and metanephrines in human urine. Rapid Commun Mass Spectrom 2000;14(21):1959–64.

76. He X, Kozak M. Development of a liquid chromatography–tandem mass spectrometry method for plasma-free metanephrines with ion-pairing turbulent flow online extraction. Anal Bioanal Chem 2012;402(9):3003–10.

77. Vogeser M, Seger C. LC-MS/MS in clinical chemistry. J Chromatogr B Analyt Technol Biomed Life Sci 2012;883-884:1–2.

78. Bhasin S, Cunningham GR, Hayes FJ, et al. Testosterone therapy in men with androgen deficiency syndromes: an Endocrine Society Clinical Practice Guideline. J Clin Endocrinol Metab 2010;95(6):2536–59.

79. Diver MJ. Analytical and physiological factors affecting the interpretation of serum testosterone concentration in men. Ann Clin Biochem 2006;43(Pt 1):3–12.

80. Morley JE, Patrick P, Perry HM 3rd. Evaluation of assays available to measure free testosterone. Metabolism 2002;51(5):554–9.

81. Nelson RE, Grebe SK, Okane DJ, et al. Liquid chromatography-tandem mass spectrometry assay for simultaneous measurement of estradiol and estrone in human plasma. Clin Chem 2004;50(2):373–84.

82. de Ronde W, van der Schouw YT, Pols HA, et al. Calculation of bioavailable and free testosterone in men: a comparison of 5 published algorithms. Clin Chem 2006;52(9):1777–84.

83. Giton F, Guéchot J, Fiet J. Comparative determinations of non SHBG-bound serum testosterone, using ammonium sulfate precipitation, Concanavalin A binding or calculation in men. Steroids 2012;77(12):1306–11.

84. Morris PD, Malkin CJ, Channer KS, et al. A mathematical comparison of techniques to predict biologically available testosterone in a cohort of 1072 men. Eur J Endocrinol 2004;151(2):241–9.

85. Rosner W, Hankinson SE, Sluss PM, et al. Challenges to the measurement of estradiol: an endocrine society position statement. J Clin Endocrinol Metab 2013;98(4):1376–87.

86. Handelsman DJ, Newman JD, Jimenez M, et al. Performance of direct estradiol immunoassays with human male serum samples. Clin Chem 2014;60(3):510–7.

87. Hsing AW, Stanczyk FZ, Belanger A, et al. Reproducibility of serum sex steroid assays in men by RIA and mass spectrometry. Cancer Epidemiol Biomarkers Prev 2007;16(5):1004–8.

88. Jaque J, Macdonald H, Brueggmann D, et al. Deficiencies in immunoassay methods used to monitor serum Estradiol levels during aromatase inhibitor treatment in postmenopausal breast cancer patients. Springerplus 2013;2(1):5.

89. Ketha H, Girtman A, Singh RJ. Estradiol assays - The path ahead. Steroids 2015;99(Pt A):39–44.

90. Koal T, Schmiederer D, Pham-Tuan H, et al. Standardized LC-MS/MS based steroid hormone profile-analysis. J Steroid Biochem Mol Biol 2012;129(3–5):129–38.

91. Eliassen AH, Spiegelman D, Xu X, et al. Urinary estrogens and estrogen metabolites and subsequent risk of breast cancer among premenopausal women. Cancer Res 2012;72(3):696–706.

92. Geisler J, Ekse D, Helle H, et al. An optimised, highly sensitive radioimmunoassay for the simultaneous measurement of estrone, estradiol and estrone sulfate in the ultra-low range in human plasma samples. J Steroid Biochem Mol Biol 2008;109(1–2):90–5.

93. Guo T, Gu J, Soldin OP, et al. Rapid measurement of estrogens and their metabolites in human serum by liquid chromatography-tandem mass spectrometry without derivatization. Clin Biochem 2008;41(9):736–41.

94. Kushnir MM, Rockwood AL, Bergquist J, et al. High-sensitivity tandem mass spectrometry assay for serum estrone and estradiol. Am J Clin Pathol 2008;129(4):530–9.

95. Santen RJ, Demers L, Ohorodnik S, et al. Superiority of gas chromatography/tandem mass spectrometry assay (GC/MS/MS) for estradiol for monitoring of aromatase inhibitor therapy. Steroids 2007;72(8):666–71.

96. Giustina A, Barkan A, Chanson P, et al. Guidelines for the treatment of growth hormone excess and growth hormone deficiency in adults. J Endocrinol Invest 2008;31(9):820–38.

97. Melmed S, Casanueva FF, Cavagnini F, et al. Guidelines for acromegaly management. J Clin Endocrinol Metab 2002;87(9):4054–8.

98. Melmed S, Vance ML, Barkan AL, et al. Current status and future opportunities for controlling acromegaly. Pituitary 2002;5(3):185–96.

99. Clemmons DR. Modifying IGF1 activity: an approach to treat endocrine disorders, atherosclerosis and cancer. Nat Rev Drug Discov 2007;6(10):821–33.

100. Clemmons DR. IGF-I assays: current assay methodologies and their limitations. Pituitary 2007;10(2):121–8.

101. Clemmons DR. Value of insulin-like growth factor system markers in the assessment of growth hormone status. Endocrinol Metab Clin North Am 2007;36(1):109–29.

102. Frystyk J, Freda P, Clemmons DR. The current status of IGF-I assays–a 2009 update. Growth Horm IGF Res 2010;20(1):8–18.

103. Ketha H, Singh RJ. Clinical assays for quantitation of insulin-like-growth-factor-1 (IGF1). Methods 2015;81:93–8.

104. Kirsch S, Widart J, Louette J, et al. Development of an absolute quantification method targeting growth hormone biomarkers using liquid chromatography coupled to isotope dilution mass spectrometry. J Chromatogr A 2007; 1153(1–2):300–6.

105. Nelson RW, Nedelkov D, Tubbs KA, et al. Quantitative mass spectrometric immunoassay of insulin like growth factor 1. J Proteome Res 2004;3(4):851–5.

106. Niederkofler EE, Phillips DA, Krastins B, et al. Targeted selected reaction monitoring mass spectrometric immunoassay for insulin-like growth factor 1. PLoS One 2013;8(11):e81125.

107. Bystrom C, Sheng S, Zhang K, et al. Clinical utility of insulin-like growth factor 1 and 2; determination by high resolution mass spectrometry. PLoS One 2012; 7(9):e43457.

108. Bystrom CE, Sheng S, Clarke NJ. Narrow mass extraction of time-of-flight data for quantitative analysis of proteins: determination of insulin-like growth factor-1. Anal Chem 2011;83(23):9005–10.

109. Hines J, Milosevic D, Ketha H, et al. Detection of IGF-1 protein variants by use of LC-MS with high-resolution accurate mass in routine clinical analysis. Clin Chem 2015;61(7):990–1.

110. Burtis CA, Ashwood ER, Bruns DE. Tietz textbook of clinical chemistry and molecular diagnostics. Elsevier Health Sciences; 2012.

111. Bystrom CE, Salameh W, Reitz R, et al. Plasma renin activity by Liquid Chromatography–Tandem Mass Spectrometry (LC-MS/MS): development of a prototypical clinical assay reveals a subpopulation of human plasma samples with substantial peptidase activity. Clin Chem 2010;56(10):1561–9.

112. Sealey JE, Laragh JH. Radioimmunoassay of plasma renin activity. Semin Nucl Med 1975;5(2):189–202.

113. Fyhrquist F, Soveri P, Puutula L, et al. Radioimmunoassay of plasma renin activity. Clin Chem 1976;22(2):250–6.

114. Carter S, Owen L, Kerstens M, et al. A liquid chromatography tandem mass spectrometry assay for plasma renin activity using online solid-phase extraction. Ann Clin Biochem 2012;49(6):570–9.

115. Chappell DL, McAvoy T, Weiss B, et al. Development and validation of an ultra-sensitive method for the measurement of plasma renin activity in human plasma via LC-MS/MS. Bioanalysis 2012;4(23):2843–50.

116. Fredline VF, Kovacs EM, Taylor PJ, et al. Measurement of plasma renin activity with use of HPLC-Electrospray-Tandem Mass Spectrometry. Clin Chem 1999; 45(5):659–64.

117. Owen LJ, Adaway J, Morris K, et al. A widely applicable plasma renin activity assay by LC-MS/MS with offline solid phase extraction. Ann Clin Biochem 2014;51(Pt 3):409–11.

# Point-of-Care Endocrine Diagnostics

Joel Ehrenkranz, MD[a,b],*

## KEYWORDS

- Point-of-care • Diagnostics • Endocrinology • Hormones • Smartphones

## KEY POINTS

- Point-of-care endocrine diagnostics are replacing centralized laboratory testing.
- Point-of-care endocrine diagnostics can be used to screen for endocrine disease and for the diagnosis and management of endocrine disorders.
- Point-of-care endocrine diagnostics streamlines endocrine care and increases the accessibility, availability, and affordability of endocrine laboratory testing.

*There are three things you need to know before you treat a patient.*
*The diagnosis.*
*The diagnosis.*
*And the diagnosis.*

—D. Lynn Loriaux, MD, PhD, 1979

## INTRODUCTION, HISTORICAL REVIEW, AND DEFINITIONS

Measuring and monitoring the concentration of a metabolic product, such as glucose, or a marker of endocrine gland function, a hormone, represents the metric by which endocrine function is assessed. Analytes can be measured using bioassays in which a biological response correlates with the concentration of an analyte or using chemical assays in which specific chemical reactions are used to produce a signal that corresponds to analyte concentration; both methods are in use today. Conducting biochemical monitoring represents a core skill that is used to identify a physician, demonstrate professional competence, and distinguish a physician from a surgeon.[1]

The earliest known biochemical test dates to around 4000 BCE; by this time Near East physicians used the color change that occurs when copper sulfate is added to

Disclosure Information: J. Ehrenkranz is the inventor of several point-of-care diagnostic technologies, receives royalties from these technologies, and owns equity in a company that manufactures and markets point-of-care diagnostics.
[a] i-calQ LLC, 466 North Wall Street, Salt Lake City, UT 84103, USA; [b] Division of Endocrinology, Department of Medicine, University of Colorado School of Medicine, 13001 East 17th Place, Aurora, CO 80045, USA
* i-calQ LLC, 466 North Wall Street, Salt Lake City, UT 84103.
*E-mail address:* Joel.ehrenkranz@i-calQ.com

glucose-containing urine to detect glycosuria. Around 1500 BCE, 2500 years later, Indian physicians described a bioassay for detecting glycosuria (madhumeha—honey urine) based on ants congregating around puddles of urine from a diabetic individual.[2] The earliest known solid phase (ie, dipstick), diagnostic dates to Avicenna's description in 1000 AD of using linen to detect bilirubin in jaundiced individuals.[3] The modern era of endocrine diagnostics can be traced to 1956 when Berson and Yalow described the first immunoassay.[4]

Methods for measuring analytes in body fluids antedated understanding the clinical pathologic condition that accounted for the presence of these analytes in body fluids. For example, methods to detect glycosuria preceded by centuries the understanding of the pathophysiology of diabetes mellitus. Pregnancy diagnostics, in contrast, used the clinical condition as the starting point for identifying a biochemical marker of a gravid female. The first bioassay for pregnancy dates to 1350 BCE.[5]

Point-of-care (POC) endocrine diagnostics with integrated rules-based decision support algorithms for interpreting test results were in widespread use during medieval times (**Fig. 1**). The earliest clinical chemists provided a clinical prognosis by inspecting a patient's urine sample at the point of care and were termed piss prophets (**Fig. 2**). In 1957, Free and colleagues replaced chemical methods developed by Egyptian physicians 6 millennia earlier to detect glycosuria with a solid phase enzymatic glucose assay.[6] This product was successfully commercialized as the first urine dipstick, launching the business of POC biochemical diagnostics and, in so doing, transformed physicians, piss prophets, into economic centers, or piss profits.

Rapid turn-around time, low cost, use outside of the clinical laboratory, and minimal technical skills for test performance and results interpretation characterize POC diagnostics.[7] POC is not synonymous with single-use or disposable. Many laboratory instruments use single-use and disposable reagent cartridges and cuvettes. POC diagnostics has been a standard medical care practice provided by physicians until very recently (**Fig. 3**). The development of a centralized facility for the high throughput

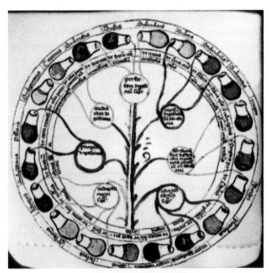

**Fig. 1.** Medieval urine color wheel with integrated decision support. (Ulrich Pinder. Epiphanie Medicorum. Speculum videndi urinas hominum. Clavis aperiendi portas pulsuum. Berillus discernendi causas & differentias febrium. Nuremberg: 1506. Rosenwald Collection. Rare Book and Special Collections Division; Library of Congress (128.2).)

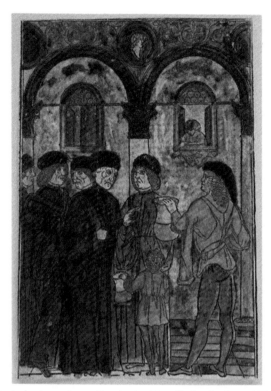

**Fig. 2.** Petrus, his students, and an attendant with a flask of urine, c1500. From Fasciculus Medicinae, Venice, C. Arrivabenus, 1522. Harvard Art Museums, Fogg Museum, Gray Collection of Engravings Fund, G5121.2. (Harvard Art Museums/Fogg Museum, Gray Collection of Engravings Fund.)

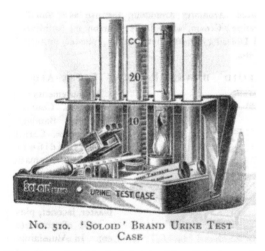

No. 510.   'SOLOID' BRAND URINE TEST CASE

**Fig. 3.** POC urinalysis kit. (*From* An historical sketch of the clinical examination of urine. Lecture Memoranda, American Medical Association, Los Angeles. London: Burroughs Wellcome; 1911. p. 147; with permission.)

of diagnostic tests, the clinical laboratory, is a recent innovation that can be traced to the introduction of the first chemistry autoanalyzers in the 1950s.[8] These instruments require large numbers of specimens to operate efficiently, substantial infrastructure, trained technical personnel for instrument operation and maintenance, and a centralized facility, now termed the clinical laboratory, evolved.

The earliest clinical laboratory instrument, the Duboscq colorimeter (**Fig. 4**) appeared in 1870. In 1939, experts predicted "the future does seem to be in the direction of the photoelectric types, for there is no inherent limit in the attainable sensitivity and objectivity of the measurement."[9] Clinical laboratory equipment akin to mainframe computers has driven the development of a centralized laboratory model for diagnostics that currently dominates laboratory medicine in the industrialized world. In the same way that personal computers replaced mainframes, POC testing using smartphones and tablets is replacing centralized laboratory testing. The ongoing transformation of centralized industrial clinical laboratory facilities to POC testing, a process in part triggered by rapidly evolving consumer electronics, represents a return of diagnostics to its roots as an integrated part of clinical practice. Health care applications of consumer electronics hardware are changing the way medicine is practiced. Nowhere is this more apparent than in POC diagnostics.

This comprehensive review of POC testing in endocrinology, written from a clinical perspective, covers the use of in vitro endocrine POC diagnostics in public health

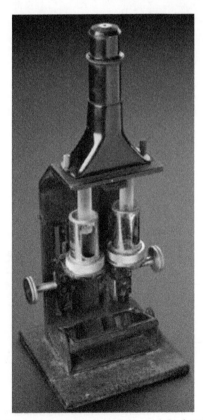

**Fig. 4.** Duboscq colorimeter. (© Science Museum/Science & Society Picture Library–All rights reserved.)

screening for endocrine diseases and in the clinical decision-making process for endocrine disease diagnosis and management.

## THE REGULATION OF POINT-OF-CARE TESTING

POC tests are regulated medical devices. In the United States, the Food and Drug Administration (FDA) is responsible for approving medical devices before marketing. FDA approval is based on a review of data provided to the FDA to confirm that test performance complies with industry guidelines and substantiates the test's labeling and claims. The standard path to market for a POC endocrine in vitro diagnostic is to show equivalence to a predicate (ie, approved) test. Section 510(k) of the Food and Drug Act describes this regulatory pathway for obtaining FDA premarket approval and, as a result, POC endocrine diagnostics in the United States are said to be 510(k) approved. Each country has its own medical device regulatory authority and approval in a jurisdiction (eg, country or region) does not automatically carry over to others. The use of the term POC is considered by the FDA to be a labeling claim and validation of the test in a POC environment by the intended user is required to label a test as POC.[10]

The Clinical Laboratory Improvement Act of 1988 (CLIA) represents legislation that categorizes the environment in which a specific test can be performed. Tests that do not require manual sample preparation (eg, centrifugation) or formal performance monitoring (eg, external quality assurance) can be performed outside of a clinical laboratory environment and are termed CLIA-waived. **Table 1** provides a list of endocrine POC tests by analyte, regulatory status, intended user, and indication.

## THE CLINICAL UTILITY OF POINT-OF-CARE TESTING

The concentration of several endocrine analytes changes ex vivo. Erythrocytes, leukocytes, platelets, and bacteria metabolize glucose. Proteolytic enzymes degrade vasopressin. Thyroxine is physically unstable when exposed to ambient temperature and humidity.[11] These preanalytic sources of error are time and temperature dependent. By minimizing the time from specimen collection to analysis, POC testing decreases preanalytic variability and makes POC testing especially useful for the measurement of unstable analytes. A second benefit that accrues from decreased specimen transport time is a decrease in the elapsed time from specimen collection to results reporting. For this reason, POC tests are commonly referred to as rapid tests. There are several endocrine emergencies, such as hypoglycemia, acute adrenal insufficiency, and congenital hypothyroidism, in which the clinical outcome depends on prompt diagnosis and treatment. POC tests can be life-saving in these circumstances. For example, an infant with untreated congenital hypothyroidism will lose up to half of their intelligence quotient (I.Q.) points a day during the first month of life. A POC thyroid-stimulating hormone (TSH) assay minimizes the delay in diagnosis associated with dried blood spot–based newborn screening. Before the advent of POC cortisol assays, patients in shock in whom acute adrenal insufficiency is a diagnostic consideration were presumptively given stress doses of glucocorticoids because of the delayed turn-around time for cortisol measurement. This practice exposes patients to unnecessary risks, such as hyperglycemia, and creates additional costs. Other examples of the benefits of decreased turnaround time with POC test use include rapid cortisol assays to confirm catheter location during adrenal vein catheterization and rapid parathyroid hormone (PTH) assays used during parathyroid surgery to confirm removal of the offending parathyroid adenoma.

Another categorical advantage of POC tests is their simplicity. POC tests do not require specialized equipment, temperature, and humidity-controlled laboratory

**Table 1**
**Point-of-care endocrine in vitro diagnostics**

| Analyte by Gland and Disease | US FDA 510(k) | Regulatory Status | User | Indication |
|---|---|---|---|---|
| Pancreas (diabetes mellitus) | | | | |
| Glucose | Yes | CLIA-waived | Consumer, professional | Diagnosis, monitoring |
| Insulin | No | | Professional | Diagnosis, monitoring |
| Hemoglobin A1C | Yes | CLIA-waived | Consumer, professional | Diagnosis, monitoring |
| Fructosamine | Yes | CLIA-waived | Professional | Diagnosis, monitoring |
| Beta hydroxy butyrate | Yes | CLIA-waived | Consumer, professional | Diagnosis, monitoring |
| Urinary microalbumin | Yes | CLIA-waived | Professional | Diagnosis, monitoring |
| Creatinine | Yes | CLIA-waived | Professional | Diagnosis, monitoring |
| Lipids (hyperlipidemia) | | | | |
| Total cholesterol | Yes | CLIA-waived | Consumer | Monitoring |
| Triglycerides | Yes | CLIA-waived | Consumer | Monitoring |
| Anterior pituitary | | | | |
| LH | Yes | CLIA-waived | Consumer | Monitoring |
| FSH | Yes | CLIA-waived | Consumer | Monitoring |
| TSH | Yes | CLIA-waived | Professional | Screening |
| Prolactin | | | Professional | Diagnosis, monitoring |
| Posterior pituitary | | | | |
| Tear osmolarity | Yes | CLIA-waived | Professional | Diagnosis |
| Urine-specific gravity | Yes | CLIA-waived | Professional | Diagnosis, monitoring |
| Serum electrolytes | Yes | CLIA-waived | Professional | Diagnosis, monitoring |
| Thyroid | | | | |
| TSH | Yes | CLIA-waived | Professional | Screening |
| T4 | No | | Professional | Diagnosis |
| T3 | No | | Professional | Diagnosis |
| Parathyroid | | | | |
| Parathyroid hormone | Yes | | Professional | Monitoring |
| Calcium | Yes | CLIA-waived | Professional | Diagnosis, monitoring |
| Magnesium | Yes | CLIA-waived | Professional | Diagnosis, monitoring |
| 25-hydroxy vitamin D | No | | Professional | Screening |
| Urinary N-telopeptides | Yes | CLIA-waived | Professional | Monitoring |

(*continued on next page*)

| Table 1 (continued) | | | | |
|---|---|---|---|---|
| Analyte by Gland and Disease | US FDA 510(k) | Regulatory Status | User | Indication |
| Adrenal cortex | | | | |
| Cortisol | No | | Professional | Diagnosis |
| Testes | No | | | |
| Testosterone | | | Professional | Diagnosis |
| Sperm count or function | Yes | CLIA-waived | Consumer | Monitoring |
| PSA | No | | Professional | Screening |
| Ovary | | | | |
| Estrone 3-glucouronide | Yes | CLIA-waived | Consumer | Monitoring |
| Progesterone bioassay | Yes | CLIA-waived | Consumer | Monitoring |
| hCG | Yes | CLIA-waived | Consumer, professional | Diagnosis, monitoring |

environments, calibrators or standards, or technical personnel for test performance and instrument maintenance. As a result, POC testing increases the accessibility, availability, and affordability of endocrine diagnostic testing. In resource-limited environments, patients have no access to diagnostics other than POC tests. With the exception of a handful of major cities, almost all of sub-Saharan Africa lacks access to any endocrine diagnostics. Cretinism and myxedema persist; thyrotoxicosis usually presents as a cardiac arrhythmia; and patients with pituitary, adrenal, parathyroid disease, dyslipidemia, and secondary hypertension go undiagnosed.[12] The diagnosis of diabetes and monitoring of glycemic control are based exclusively on POC glucose measurement. POC endocrine diagnostics provide a solution to this lack of essential health care resources.

POC tests do have limitations. The throughput (ie, the number of tests performed per hour) using a POC test is a fraction of the number of tests that an automated instrument can perform. Because trained technical personnel do not necessarily perform POC tests, user error is not uncommon. Many POC hormone assays are colorimetric, semiquantitative (yes or no) tests, immunochromatographic assays that are read by eye. This feature introduces subjective variability in test interpretation. POC test results are manually recorded; this step increases the likelihood of transcription error. Finally, there is no statutory requirement for stat reporting of critical results because it is assumed that POC tests obviate expedient reporting of clinically urgent results.

## POINT-OF-CARE TESTING BY DISEASE AND ANALYTE
### Diabetes Mellitus

POC glucose tests use electrochemical methods to measure capillary glucose concentration. Test strips are impregnated with enzymes that generate a small electric current that is proportional to the amount of glucose present. A glucometer is essentially a voltmeter that measures the amount of current generated by glucose oxidation and is able to convert the voltage generated into a glucose concentration.[13] Because glucose is measured in serum and capillary glucose test strips are designed to measure glucose in whole blood, glucose meters need to correct for hematocrit. This adjustment is done by measuring the hemoglobin concentration in a capillary blood sample and then using the hemoglobin concentration to calculate the volume of the blood sample that is serum. Capillary glucose measurement is plus or minus 20%. This analytical imprecision makes POC capillary glucose measurement for the diagnosis of hypoglycemic disorders, such as insulinoma, unreliable. Electrochemical glucose measurement uses a smaller sample volume and has less analytical variability than optical glucometry, such as hydrogen peroxide generation by glucose oxidase, that are used by older capillary glucose and urine glucose methods.

Acetoacetate and β-hydroxybutyrate are the 2 ketone bodies produced during diabetic ketoacidosis (DKA). Serum measurement of β-hydroxybutyrate is more reliable than urine or serum acetoacetate measurement for the diagnosis and monitoring of DKA.[14] POC ketone meters are widely used in a variety of POC settings to detect DKA and to monitor the efficacy of DKA therapy.[15] These devices are similar to glucometers because the test strip contains reagents that generate a voltage that is proportional to the amount of β-hydroxybutyrate present in serum. Ketone meters have rendered measurement of acetoacetate in urine or serum obsolete.

Microfluidic POC methods for measuring glycohemoglobin are widely available. The current generation of POC glycohemoglobin tests uses a noncompetitive immunochromatographic assay format to measure glycohemoglobin in lysed capillary erythrocytes. Because glycohemoglobin is expressed as a percentage of total hemoglobin, these tests also measure capillary blood hemoglobin. Like all glycohemoglobin assays, POC glycohemoglobin assays are affected by red blood cell turnover, hemoglobinopathies, and duration and amplitude of hyperglycemia.[16,17] The clinical significance of variant hemoglobins on the measurement of glycohemoglobin is significant. All POC methods for measuring glycohemoglobin, as well as laboratory methods for measuring glycohemoglobin that do not incorporate hemoglobin electrophoresis, are inappropriate for use in patients with labile hemoglobin A1c; carbamylated hemoglobin; hemoglobin F, S, C, SC, D, or E; erythrocyte disorders, such as beta thalassemia and hemolytic anemias; and transfusion recipients.[18]

Rapid immunochromatographic insulin assays are commercially available outside the United States. A POC insulin assay has been used to guide surgical therapy in patients undergoing insulinoma resection.[19] Algorithms for closed loop insulin administration, which use rapid serum insulin measurement, are another use for a POC insulin assay. However, assay specificity, the cross-reactivity of antibodies used to measure endogenous insulin with insulin analogues that are used in artificial pancreas systems, needs to be determined.[20]

### Lipid Disorders

POC methods and devices for measuring total cholesterol and triglycerides from capillary blood are commercially available in the United States. These devices use colorimetric chemical reactions and a hand-held reflectance meter to quantify cholesterol and triglyceride concentrations and, using this information, calculate low-density lipoprotein, high-density lipoprotein, and very low-density lipoprotein cholesterol. Their use increases patient compliance in achieving target lipid levels.[21]

### Diseases of the Anterior Pituitary

Although urinary luteinizing hormone (LH) and follicle-stimulating hormone (FSH) immunoassays have been available in the United States as consumer products for decades, quantitative POC serum gonadotropin assays are not approved for use in North America. In addition to serum LH and FSH, serum prolactin can be measured with a quantitative POC immunoassay. LH, FSH, and prolactin POC tests are approved for sale in the European Union. A semiquantitative capillary TSH assay to screen for primary hypothyroidism was approved for use as a screening test for primary hypothyroidism by the US FDA in 1998. This CLIA-waived test is designed to detect serum TSH greater than 5 mIU/L. A quantitative POC TSH assay that uses a smartphone to read an immunochromatographic TSH cassette (**Fig. 5**) is used in Thailand, India, and Uganda for newborn thyroid screening and for the monitoring of iodine nutrition. Proof of concept has been shown for a POC intraoperative growth hormone assay in patients with acromegaly[22] and a rapid adrenocorticotropin (ACTH) assay in patients with Cushing disease who are undergoing pituitary surgery.[23]

### Posterior Pituitary

Disorders of water metabolism can be diagnosed and monitored using urine-specific gravity measurements. Colorimetric methods for estimating urine specific gravity are approved for use. Urine specific gravity is essentially a bioassay of vasopressin activity and can, under tightly controlled conditions, be used to aid in the diagnosis and management of diabetes insipidus. A CLIA-waived POC technology for measuring tear osmolarity based on impedance is commercially available. Adapting this technology to measure urine and serum osmolarity would provide a more reliable method to diagnose diabetes insipidus and the syndrome of inappropriate antidiuresis (SIADH).

### Thyroid

POC technologies are available for measuring T4 and T3 as well as TSH. These technologies use an immunochromatographic format in which the amount of analyte present corresponds to an optical signal (**Fig. 6**).[24] Smartphones, tablets, or desktop instruments can be used to quantify the optical signal intensity and thus provide a measure of the amount of analyte present. Integrated rules-based decision support algorithms, termed mobile medical apps, interpret results and provide treatment and follow-up recommendations.

### Parathyroid or Diseases of Calcium Metabolism

Several analytes involved in calcium metabolism and markers of metabolic bone disease can be measured at the point of care. Instrument-based ionized calcium assays are available on several POC platforms for professional use. PTH immunoassays with a rapid turnaround time are widely used for the intraoperative monitoring of parathyroidectomy. A decrease of greater than 50% in circulating PTH levels is a reliable

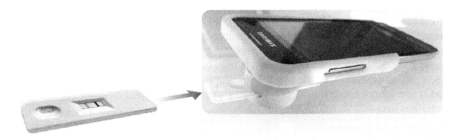

**Fig. 5.** Smartphone POC TSH immunochromatic assay. (*Courtesy of* i-calQ LLC, Salt Lake City, Utah, USA, 2016.)

endocrine disease that would benefit from a POC method for treatment monitoring is Addison disease. Endocrinologists essentially guess the dose of glucocorticoid replacement that the patient must take because there is no objective method for a patient to use for self-monitoring to adjust the dose of hydrocortisone. A POC salivary cortisol assay would aid the management of this disorder.[41]

As closed-loop systems for endocrine disease management, such as an indwelling glucose sensor that provides data to an insulin pump, become available, the need for additional POC endocrine diagnostics to provide the afferent limb for a closed loop endocrine disease management system, will grow. Hypoparathyroidism, hypertension, and circadian rhythm disturbances are examples of endocrine diseases that will benefit from POC diagnostics-based closed-loop systems.

Because endocrine disease presentation can be subtle and insidious and laboratory testing protocols are complex, time-consuming, and expensive, the diagnosis of an endocrine disease is often overlooked. POC methods can assist in the diagnosis of several endocrine diseases. POC screening for congenital hypothyroidism has dramatically increased access to this basic component of newborn care and represents a major public health achievement. Hyperaldosteronism is a common cause of treatment-resistant hypertension; however, the diagnosis is often overlooked because diagnostic algorithms rely on laboratory-based hormone measurement methods using blood samples collected under controlled circumstances.[42] A POC aldosterone assay would simplify screening for this curable cause of secondary hypertension. Because POC testing minimizes preanalytic variability, POC tests are a useful and reliable first-line diagnostic for endocrine diseases. The diagnosis of pheochromocytoma is complicated by the chemical instability of catecholamines ex vivo. POC catecholamine assays minimize preanalytic variability and obviate 24-hour urine collection or dynamic testing.[43] Several hormones, such as ACTH and vasopressin, have a half-life of minutes, and laboratory methods for measuring these hormones must take special measures to maintain analyte integrity. A POC vasopressin or copeptin assay would aid in the diagnosis of both SIADH and diabetes insipidus.[44]

## GET READY FOR THE FUTURE: MULTIPLEXED MICROFLUIDICS AND SMARTPHONE POCKET MINILABS

The differential diagnosis of hormonal causes of secondary amenorrhea consists of pregnancy, hypothyroidism, hyperprolactinemia, primary gonadal failure, and hypothalamic amenorrhea. POC tests for hCG, TSH, prolactin, LH, and FSH are commercially available. Performing these 5 tests at once, a process known as multiplexing, uses 100 µL of serum, provides results in minutes, and substantially simplifies an infertility workup. The technology for measuring analyte concentrations in small volumes of biologic fluids is already in use. Examples of this include capillary glucose and hemoglobin measurement, each of which uses a 3 µL sample volume. Next-generation POC laboratory-on-a chip diagnostics interface POC immunoassays with smartphones or tablets. Because visual acuity, ambient lighting, and test orientation make reading POC tests by eye unreliable, charge-coupled devices and complementary metaloxide semiconductor cameras used in smartphones and tablets eliminate the subjective variability that occurs when tests are read by visual inspection.[45] Smartphones and tablets provide imaging, computation, and communications functionality to objectively read tests, interpret and archive each result, and wirelessly upload data to an electronic medical record. In Thailand, a smartphone POC quantitative TSH immunoassay is replacing central laboratory dried blood spot newborn thyroid screening (see **Fig. 6**). Test results are automatically uploaded from the newborn nursery or home

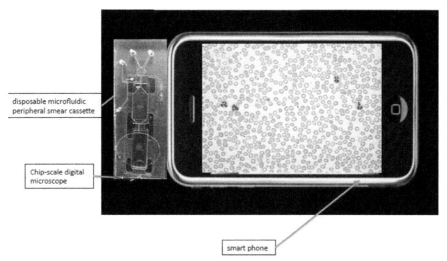

disposable microfluidic
peripheral smear cassette

Chip-scale digital
microscope

smart phone

**Fig. 7.** Microfluidic smartphone digital microscope. (*Courtesy of* i-calQ LLC, Salt Lake City, Utah, 2015.)

where the tests are performed to the Thailand Ministry of Public Health database to provide real-time monitoring of a population's iodine nutrition.

Microfluidic devices that that use minute sample volumes, on-board reagent dispensing, miniature pumps and valving systems, laminar flow, and integrated spectroscopy to perform cytometry, immunoassay, and enzymatic assays have been developed. **Fig. 7** shows a prototype smartphone microfluidic device for performing a complete blood count. The laboratory-on-a-chip component uses a drop of capillary blood to create a monolayer of circulating blood cells; then fixes, stains, and rinses the peripheral blood smear; and uses a digital chip-scale microscopic that interfaces with a smartphone equipped with image analysis software to measure hemoglobin and provide a cell count and differential. In the not-too-distant future, endocrine diagnostics that now require dedicated instrumentation, complex sample preparation, controlled reagent storage dispensing, and extensive infrastructure support will be replaced by portable, single-use, disposable, credit card–sized devices. Smartphones and tablets will provide power, analysis of test results, and seamless cloud-based electronic medical record archiving.

## SUMMARY

POC endocrine diagnostics have their limitations and understanding these limitations will result in the appropriate use of POC in endocrinology. Appropriate use optimizes efficiency. Inappropriate use leads to adverse clinical consequences. The precision and repeatability of POC endocrine tests is not equivalent to laboratory instrument-based endocrine tests; however, the clinical relevance of this discrepancy is often trivial. For example, third-generation TSH assays measure TSH to 4 decimal points but this level of accuracy is clinically irrelevant.[46] In the case of glucose measurement, the analytical imprecision of glucometers means that POC glucose measurement cannot be used to diagnose hypoglycemia. Smartphone POC TSH measurement, in contrast, provides quantitative results that can be used to diagnose hypothyroidism, titrate thyroxine therapy, and screen for hyperthyroidism because physiologic variation in circulating TSH concentrations exceeds the TSH immunoassay's coefficient of variation. Commercially available POC diagnostics that avoid regulatory oversight, such as a 25-hydroxyvitamin D lateral flow assay, underscore the need to verify that POC tests are approved for use at the point of care and that the device's performance under actual use conditions corresponds to the test's specifications and meets the clinical needs for which it is intended. Independent of a test's performance in a laboratory environment, the proficiency of the person performing the test is critical to the accuracy of the results. The US FDA requires documentation that intended users of a test (eg, physician's assistants) are able to correctly perform a test before allowing a test to claim that it is a POC test.

Advances in assay development, microfluidics, and consumer electronics have made hormone and metabolite measurement, the hallmark of endocrinology, a POC process. As a result, POC endocrine diagnostics are replacing centralized laboratory testing. POC endocrine diagnostics can be used for endocrine disease screening, diagnosis, and management. POC endocrine diagnostics streamline endocrine care and increase the accessibility, availability, and affordability of endocrine laboratory testing.

## REFERENCES

1. Osler W. Discussion. JAMA 1900;35:230.
2. Wellcome HS. The evolution of urine analysis. London: Burroughs Wellcome; 1911. p. 16.
3. Gruner OC. A treatise on the canon of medicine of Avicenna. London: Luzac; 1930. p. 326.
4. Roth J. A tribute to Rosalyn S. Yalow. J Clin Invest 2011;121:2949–51.
5. Ehrenkranz J. Home and point of care pregnancy tests: a review of the technology. Epidemiology 2000;13(3 Suppl):SW15–8.
6. Free AH, Adams EC, Kercher ML, et al. Simple specific test for urine glucose. Clin Chem 1957;3:163–8.
7. Kost GJ. Goals, guidelines, and principles for point-of-care testing. In: Kost JG, editor. Principles and practice of point-of-care testing. Philadelphia: Lippincott Williams and Wilkins; 2002. p. 3–12.
8. Alpert NL. Automated instruments for clinical chemistry: review and preview. Clin Chem 1969;15:1198–209.
9. Muller R. Instrumental methods of chemical analysis. Ind Eng Chem Anal Ed 1941;13:667–754.
10. Kramer DB, Xu S, Kesselheim AS. Regulation of medical devices in the United States and European Union. N Engl J Med 2012;366:848–55.
11. Bourdoux PP, Van Thi HV, Courtois PA, et al. Superiority of thyrotropin to thyroxine as a tool in the screening for congenital hypothyroidism by the filter paper spot technique. Clin Chim Acta 1991;195:97–105.
12. Fualal J, Ehrenkranz J. Access, availability, and infrastructure deficiency: the current management of thyroid disease in the developing world. Rev Endocr Metab Disord 2016;17(4):583–9.
13. Moodley N, Ngxamngxa U, Turzyniecka MJ, et al. Historical perspectives in clinical pathology; a history of glucose measurement. J Clin Pathol 2015;68:258–64.
14. Wolfsdorf J, Glaser N, Sperling MA. Diabetic ketoacidosis in infants, children, and adolescents: a consensus statement from the American Diabetes Association. Diabetes care 2006;29:1150–9.

15. Noyes KJ, Crofton P, Bath LE, et al. Hydroxybutyrate near-patient testing to evaluate a new end-point for intravenous insulin therapy in the treatment of diabetic ketoacidosis in children. Pediatr Diabetes 2007;8:150–6.
16. Lenters-Westra E, Slingerland RJ. Six of eight hemoglobin A1c point-of-care instruments do not meet the general accepted analytical performance criteria. Clin Chem 2010;56:44–52.
17. Ehrenkranz J. Cheers and jeers for a pancreas tonic. Metabolism 2005;54: 1407–8.
18. Little RR, Roberts WL. A review of variant hemoglobins interfering with hemoglobin A1c measurement. J Diabetes Sci Technol 2009;3(3):446–51.
19. Nakamura Y, Matsushita A, Katsuno A, et al. Clinical outcomes of 15 consecutive patients who underwent laparoscopic insulinoma resection: the usefulness of monitoring intraoperative blood insulin during laparoscopic pancreatectomy. Asian J Endosc Surg 2015;8:303–9.
20. Van Uytfanghe K, Rodríguez-Cabaleiro D, Stöckl D, et al. New liquid chromatography/electrospray ionisation tandem mass spectrometry measurement procedure for quantitative analysis of human insulin in serum. Rapid Commun Mass Spectrom 2007;21:819–21.
21. Taylor JR, Lopez LM. Cholesterol: point-of-care testing. Ann Pharmacother 2004; 38:1252–7.
22. Van Den Berg G, Van Dulken H, Frölich M, et al. Can intra-operative GH measurement in acromegalic subjects predict completeness of surgery? Clin Endocrinol 1998;49:45–51.
23. Fahlbusch R, Buchfelder M, Müller OA. Transsphenoidal surgery for Cushing disease. J R Soc Med 1986;79:262–9.
24. Ehrenkranz J, Fualal J, Ndizihiwe A, et al. Neonatal age and point of care TSH testing in the monitoring of iodine deficiency disorders: findings from western Uganda. Thyroid 2012;21:183–8.
25. Wilhelm SM, Wang TS, Ruan DT, et al. The American Association of Endocrine Surgeons guidelines for definitive management of primary hyperparathyroidism. JAMA Surg 2016;151(10):959–68.
26. Greenspan SL, Cheng S, Miller PD, et al, QUS-2 PMA Trials Group. Clinical performance of a highly portable, scanning calcaneal ultrasonometer. Osteoporos Int 2001;12:391–8.
27. Genant HK, Li J, Wu CY, et al. Vertebral fractures in osteoporosis: a new method for clinical assessment. J Clin Densitom 2000;3:281–90.
28. Choi S, Kim S, Yang JS, et al. Real-time measurement of human salivary cortisol for the assessment of psychological stress using a smartphone. Sensing Bio-Sensing Res 2014;2:8–11.
29. Yoneda T, Karashima S, Kometani M, et al. Impact of new quick gold nanoparticle-based cortisol assay during adrenal vein sampling for primary aldosteronism. J Clin Endo Metab 2016;101:2554–61.
30. Kaushik A, Vasudev A, Arya SK, et al. Recent advances in cortisol sensing technologies for point-of-care application. Biosens Bioelectron 2014;53:499–512.
31. Findling JW. Evolution, global warming, smart phones, and Lat3-night salivary cortisol. Endocr Pract 2015;21(2):205–7.
32. Bjorndahl L, Kirkman-Brown J, Hart G, et al. Development of a novel home sperm test. Hum Reprod 2006;21:145–9.
33. Reddy KVR, Kedar NG, Vadigoppula AD, et al. Evaluation of resazurin reduction test results and their correlation with conventional semen parameters: a large scale study. Journal of Endocrinology and Reproduction 1998;2(1&2):1–11.

34. Coppola MA, Klotz KL, Kim KA, et al. SpermCheck® Fertility, an immunodiagnostic home test that detects normozoospermia and severe oligozoospermia. Hum Reprod 2010;25:853–61.
35. Nerenz RD, Gronowski AM. Point-of-care and over-the-counter qualitative human chorionic gonadotropin (hCG) devices remain susceptible to false-negative results caused by excess hCG β core fragment. Clin Chem 2013;59:1672–4.
36. Brezina PR, Haberl E, Wallach E. At home testing: optimizing management for the infertility physician. Fertil Sterility 2011;95:1867–78.
37. Ehrenkranz J. A new method for measuring body temperature. N J Med 1986; 83:93–6.
38. Klinefelter HF Jr, Albright F, Griswold GC. Experience with a quantitative test for normal or decreased amounts of follicle stimulating hormone in the urine in endocrinological diagnosis. J Clin Endo Metab 1943;3:529–44.
39. Hovorka R. Closed-loop insulin delivery: from bench to clinical practice. Nat Rev Endocrinol 2011;7:385–95.
40. Ly TT, Breton MD, Keith-Hynes P, et al. Overnight glucose control with an automated, unified safety system in children and adolescents with type 1 diabetes at diabetes camp. Diabetes Care 2014;37:2310–6.
41. Raff H. Measurement of salivary cortisone to assess the adequacy of hydrocortisone replacement. J Clin Endo Metab 2016;101:1350–2.
42. Käyser SC, Dekkers T, Groenewoud HJ, et al. Study heterogeneity and estimation of prevalence of primary aldosteronism: a systematic review and meta-regression analysis. J Clin Endocrinol Metab 2016;101:2826–35.
43. Li XS, Li S, Kellermann G. Pre-analytical and analytical validations and clinical applications of a miniaturized, simple and cost-effective solid phase extraction combined with LC- MS/MS for the simultaneous determination of catecholamines and metanephrines in spot urine samples. Talanta 2016;159:238–47.
44. Lewandowski KC, Brabant G. Potential clinical utility of Copeptin (C-terminal pro-vasopressin) measurements in clinical medicine. Exp Clin Endocrinol Diabetes 2016;124:173–7.
45. You DJ, Prak TS, Yoon JY. Cell-phone-based measurement of TSH using Mie scatter optimized lateral flow assays. Biosens Bioelectron 2013;40:180–5.
46. Ehrenkranz J, Bach P, Snow G, et al. Circadian and circannual rhythms in thyroid hormones: determining the TSH and Free T4 reference intervals based upon time of day, age, and sex. Thyroid 2015;25:954–60.

# Biochemical Testing in Thyroid Disorders

Nazanene H. Esfandiari, MD[a], Maria Papaleontiou, MD[b],*

## KEYWORDS

- Biochemical testing • Thyroid • TSH • Thyroglobulin • Calcitonin

## KEY POINTS

- Serum thyroid-stimulating hormone (TSH) remains the primary screening test for thyroid dysfunction. Current guidelines recommend that serum TSH is used as the first-line test for detecting thyroid dysfunction.
- Thyroid autoantibodies are present in autoimmune thyroid disorders. Measurement is recommended in evaluating subclinical hypothyroidism; antibodies directed against the TSH receptor can be used in Graves' disease.
- Thyroglobulin (Tg) is primarily used as a tumor marker to evaluate the effectiveness of treatment and to monitor for recurrence of well-differentiated thyroid cancers.
- When measuring a Tg level, Tg antibodies should always be measured concurrently to allow for accurate interpretation of the Tg level.
- Calcitonin is mainly used as a tumor marker to monitor for the recurrence of medullary thyroid cancer.

## INTRODUCTION

This review summarizes the main principles for the appropriate use of laboratory testing in the diagnosis and management of thyroid disorders, as well as controversies that have arisen in association with some of these biochemical tests. To place a test in perspective, the sensitivity and accuracy of the test should be taken into account. Ordering the correct laboratory tests facilitates the early diagnosis of a thyroid disorder and institutes timely and appropriate treatment. This review will focus on a comprehensive update regarding thyroid-stimulating hormone (TSH),

The authors have nothing to disclose.
[a] Division of Metabolism, Endocrinology and Diabetes, Department of Internal Medicine, University of Michigan, Domino's Farms Lobby C, Suite 1300, 24 Frank Lloyd Wright Drive, Ann Arbor, MI 48106, USA; [b] Division of Metabolism, Endocrinology and Diabetes, Department of Internal Medicine, University of Michigan, Domino's Farms Lobby G, Room 1649, 24 Frank Lloyd Wright Drive, Ann Arbor, MI 48106, USA
* Corresponding author.
E-mail address: mpapaleo@med.umich.edu

Endocrinol Metab Clin N Am 46 (2017) 631–648
http://dx.doi.org/10.1016/j.ecl.2017.04.002
0889-8529/17/© 2017 Elsevier Inc. All rights reserved.

thyroxine (T4)/triiodothyronine (T3), thyroid autoantibodies, thyroglobulin (Tg), and calcitonin. The clinical uses of these biochemical tests are outlined in **Table 1**.

## THYROID-STIMULATING HORMONE
*Overview*

TSH or thyrotropin is a glycoprotein secreted by the anterior pituitary gland and is regulated by negative feedback from the serum free thyroid hormones (T4 and T3). TSH exhibits diurnal variation, with the lowest value in the late afternoon and highest value between midnight and 4 AM.[1–3] Therefore, variations of serum TSH values within the normal range of up to 50% do not necessarily reflect a change in thyroid status.[3] TSH secretion is extremely sensitive to minor changes in serum free T4, and abnormal TSH levels occur while developing hypothyroidism and hyperthyroidism before free T4 abnormalities are detectable.[4]

*Available Assays and Functional Sensitivity*

Several advances have been made in the last few decades in the development of sensitive assays for TSH measurement. The first-generation of TSH assays were based on radioimmunoassay methodology that had limited functional sensitivity ($\sim 1.0$ mIU/L).[5–7] Second-generation assays were developed in the 1970s by using modified radioimmunoassay procedures and had a functional sensitivity of 0.1 mIU/L.[8–11]

Currently, the most widely used assays are third-generation immunometric assays (also called "sandwich" or "noncompetitive" assays), which became available in the

| Table 1 | |
|---|---|
| **Clinical uses of biochemical tests for thyroid disorders** | |
| **Biochemical Test** | **Clinical Uses** |
| TSH | • Primary screening test for thyroid dysfunction<br>• Evaluation of thyroid hormone replacement therapy in patients with primary hypothyroidism<br>• Evaluation of suppressive therapy in patients with follicular cell-derived thyroid cancer |
| T4 | • Detection of thyroid dysfunction in conjunction with TSH<br>• Evaluation of thyroid hormone replacement therapy in patients with secondary hypothyroidism (free T4)<br>• Evaluation of thyroid dysfunction in pregnancy (total T4) |
| T3 | • Detection of hyperthyroidism<br>• No usefulness in the management of hypothyroidism<br>• May be useful in diagnosis of nonthyroidal illness |
| Thyroid autoantibodies | • Positive in autoimmune thyroid disease<br>• TPOAb – evaluation of patients with subclinical hypothyroidism and women with recurrent miscarriages<br>• TRAb – diagnosis of Graves' disease; help to predict which Graves' patients can be weaned from antithyroid medications |
| Thyroglobulin | • Evaluation of effectiveness of treatment for differentiated thyroid cancer and monitoring for residual or recurrent disease<br>• Diagnosis of thyrotoxicosis factitia |
| Calcitonin | • To diagnose medullary thyroid cancer and monitor for recurrence, progression, and response to treatment |

*Abbreviations:* T3, triiodothyronine; T4, thyroxine; TPOAb, antibodies to thyroid peroxidase; TRAb, antibodies directed against the thyroid-stimulating hormone receptor; TSH, thyroid-stimulating hormone.

mid 1980s.[4] Mechanistically, these assays use an excess of TSH monoclonal antibody bound to a solid support ("capture antibody") that captures TSH from the serum specimen during an incubation period. Different polyclonal or monoclonal TSH antibodies, targeted at different TSH epitopes, and labeled with a signal (most recently chemiluminescent and fluorescent) are then added and, after further incubation, the unbound constituents are removed by washing. The signal bound to the solid support is quantified as being directly proportional to the serum TSH concentration in the test sample. More recent modifications to this concept include the use of chimeric monoclonal antibodies to reduce interference by heterophilic antibodies (defined as human antibodies with a broad reactivity with antibodies of other animal species), and the use of avidin–biotin and magnetic particle separation techniques.[12–14] These assays have resulted in inherently better sensitivity and specificity, with a functional sensitivity at 0.01 mIU/L.

### Reference Range

There continues to be ongoing debate regarding the upper limit of normal for serum TSH. According to the National Health and Nutrition Examination Survey III survey, the upper limit of normal for serum TSH level was found to be 4.5 mIU/L based on a disease-free population, excluding those on thyroid medications.[15] When looking at a "reference population" taken from this disease-free population composed of nonpregnant adults, without laboratory evidence of thyroid dysfunction, undetectable thyroid autoantibodies and not on estrogens, androgens, or lithium, the upper normal TSH value of 4.12 mIU/L was found. The Hanford Thyroid Disease Study further supported this upper limit.[16] However, the National Academy of Clinical Biochemists proposed that 95% of individuals without evidence of thyroid disease have TSH concentrations of less than 2.5 mIU/L, and it has been advocated by some investigators that the upper limit of the TSH reference range be lowered to 2.5 mIU/L.[17,18]

The National Health and Nutrition Examination Survey III reference population was also further analyzed to determine normal TSH ranges based on age, race and ethnicity, and sex.[19] This study showed that the 97.5th percentile TSH values were as low as 3.24 mIU/L for African-Americans between the ages of 30 and 39 years, and as high as 7.84 mIU/L for Mexican Americans 80 years of age or older. For every 10-year age increase after 30 to 39 years, the 97.5th percentile of serum TSH was shown to increase by 0.3 mIU/L.[19] Additionally, in adults without evidence of thyroid autoantibodies, TSH values higher than 3.0 mIU/L occur with increasing frequency with age, with individuals greater than 80 years of age having a 24% prevalence of TSH values ranging between 2.5 and 4.5 mIU/L and a 12% prevalence of TSH values that are greater than 4.5 mIU/L.[20] These data suggest an age-related shift toward higher TSH concentrations in older patients and may indicate that mild increases in TSH in the elderly may not reflect thyroid dysfunction but rather be a normal manifestation of aging.[21] Despite current guidelines not advocating for specific TSH goals for different age groups with hypothyroidism, clinical practice patterns reflect an impact of age in the management of hypothyroidism.[22]

### Clinical Usefulness and Test Interpretation

Serum TSH remains the primary screening test for thyroid dysfunction. Current guidelines recommend that serum TSH is used as the first-line test for detecting both overt and subclinical thyroid dysfunction in ambulatory patients who have intact hypothalamic and pituitary function.[3,23] Furthermore, TSH is used to evaluate thyroid hormone replacement therapy in patients with primary hypothyroidism, and suppressive therapy in patients with follicular cell–derived thyroid cancer.[3]

### Challenges in the interpretation of serum thyroid-stimulating hormone

**Nonthyroidal illness** Nonthyroidal illness can often alter thyroid hormone peripheral metabolism and hypothalamic/pituitary function, and can lead to a range of thyroid test abnormalities, including both decreased and increased serum TSH levels.[24–26] In hospitalized patients with acute illness, serum TSH level may be suppressed to less than 0.1 mIU/L, in combination with a subnormal free T4. This can especially be seen in patients receiving dopamine infusions[27] or high doses of glucocorticoids.[28] In addition, during the recovery phase from nonthyroidal illness, TSH levels may increase above normal, but usually are less than 20 mIU/L.[29] Therefore, in critically ill or hospitalized patients, a serum TSH measurement should only be obtained if there is high suspicion for thyroid dysfunction.[3,30]

**Pregnancy** Variations in serum TSH can occur physiologically in pregnancy. During the first trimester, serum TSH usually becomes lower, but rarely decreases to less than 0.1 mU/L, owing to the stimulatory effects of human chorionic gonadotropin on the thyroid. Serum TSH subsequently returns to normal in the second trimester.[3,31] Trimester-specific ranges for serum TSH as set by each different laboratory should be used in pregnancy. If not available, the following upper limits of normal range are recommended: TSH 2.5 mIU/L for the first trimester, 3.0 mIU/L for the second trimester, and 3.5 mIU/L for the third trimester.[3]

**Medication interference** Several medications may interfere with the measurement of serum TSH via a variety of mechanisms and therefore impact its interpretation. These mechanisms include interference with T4 absorption (eg, calcium, iron supplements), interference with thyroid gland hormone production and secretion (eg, amiodarone, lithium, tyrosine kinase inhibitors), direct and indirect effects on the hypothalamic–pituitary–thyroid axis (eg, bexarotene, dopamine, octreotide, ipilimumab), increased clearance (eg, phenytoin, carbamazepine), and interference with peripheral metabolism (eg, glucocorticoids, beta-blockers).[3]

In recent years, the effect of biotin on TSH measurement has received considerable attention. Biotin (vitamin $B_7$) is a cofactor for carboxylases involved in fatty acid synthesis, gluconeogenesis, and energy production. Biotin is a common component of multivitamins with the daily recommended dose ranging from 30 to 70 μg.[32] It has also been shown that biotin improves clinical outcomes and quality of life in patients with progressive multiple sclerosis at very high doses.[33] However, in moderate doses, biotin can cause interference in some TSH immunoassays, resulting in abnormal thyroid function tests.[34,35] Many immunoassays use the biotin–streptavidin interaction as an immobilizing system. Streptavidin binds biotin with high affinity and high specificity, making it useful as a general bridge system.[36] Ingestion of high doses of biotin may cause spurious results in these assays. Mechanisms to remove biotin, such as a streptavidin agarose column in nonbiotinated assays, minimize the impact of assay interference and improve the accurate measurement of TSH. In immunometric assays, excess biotin displaces the biotinylated antibodies and causes spuriously low results, whereas in competitive assays, excess biotin competes with biotinylated analogue and results in falsely high results.[34,37] There have been cases of factitious Graves' disease reported in the literature owing to high doses of biotin.[37,38] Physicians must be aware of immunoassay interference by biotin to avoid misdiagnosis and unnecessary treatment. If patients taking high doses of biotin are found to have suppressed TSH and elevated T4, they should stop taking biotin and have repeat measurements at least 2 days later before making the diagnosis of hyperthyroidism.[23]

**Other considerations** Patients with anorexia nervosa may have low TSH levels in combination with low levels of free T4,[39] mimicking laboratory results seen in critically ill patients and in patients with central hypothyroidism owing to pituitary and hypothalamic disorders. Patients with central hypothyroidism, for example, owing to nonfunctioning pituitary adenomas, may have mildly elevated serum TSH levels that are explained by the secretion of bioinactive isoforms of TSH.[40] Increased TSH levels with elevated serum thyroid hormone levels are seen in patients with resistance to thyroid hormone.[41] Adrenal insufficiency may also be associated with TSH elevations that are corrected with glucocorticoid replacement.[42,43]

Heterophilic or interfering antibodies including human anti-animal (most commonly mouse) antibodies, rheumatoid factor, and autoimmune anti-TSH antibodies may cause falsely elevated serum TSH values by interfering with the assays.[44,45]

## THYROXINE AND TRIIODOTHYRONINE
### Overview and Available Assays

Approximately 99.97% of serum T4 and 99.7% of T3 are bound to T4-binding globulin, transthyretin, prealbumin, or albumin.[3,46,47] Therefore, only a small amount of T4 and T3 are unbound and act on the hypothalamus–pituitary–thyroid axis as the metabolically available moieties. Assessment of serum free T4 has now largely replaced serum total T4 as a measure of thyroid status. Methods for assessing serum free T4 include a direct immunoassay of free T4 after ultrafiltration or equilibrium dialysis of serum or after addition of anti-T4 antibody to serum.[48,49] Additionally, measurement of the serum free T4 index can be derived as the product of total T4 and a thyroid hormone binding ratio.[48] Methods for assessing free T3 concentration by direct immunoassay have also been developed and are currently used.[49] However, assays for estimating free T3 are not as widely validated as those for free T4, and measurement of total T3 may be preferred in clinical practice.

### Clinical Usefulness and Test Interpretation

A low serum free T4 indicates hypothyroidism, either primary when TSH is elevated, or central, when TSH is normal or low.[6,40] Serum free T4 is also the test of choice for detecting hypothyroidism in patients with treated hyperthyroidism (either by antithyroid drugs, radioiodine ablation, or surgery), because serum TSH may remain low for many weeks to months. In pregnancy, serum total T4 measurement is recommended instead of serum free T4 measurement.[31] This is recommended because changes in serum proteins in pregnancy may lead to lower values of free T4 by direct immunoassay based on reference ranges that were established with normal nonpregnant sera. Total T4 increases during the first trimester of pregnancy and the reference range is approximately 1.5-fold that of the nonpregnant range throughout the pregnancy.[50,51]

Serum T3 measurement, whether total or free, has limited usefulness in hypothyroidism because levels are often normal owing to hyperstimulation of the remaining functioning thyroid tissue by elevated TSH, and also because of upregulation of type 2 iodothyronine deiodinase.[52] Additionally, T3 levels are low in the absence of thyroid disease in patients with severe illness because of reduced peripheral conversion of T4 to T3 and increased inactivation of thyroid hormone.[3,30,53] In contrast, free or total T3 should be measured in patients who are suspected to have hyperthyroidism.[23]

## THYROID AUTOANTIBODIES
### Overview

Thyroid autoantibodies are circulating antibodies against several thyroid antigens, which are present in most patients with autoimmune thyroid disorders, such as Hashimoto's thyroiditis and Graves' disease.[54] The thyroid autoantibodies discussed here are widely available in clinical diagnostic laboratories and commonly used, and these include antibodies to thyroid peroxidase (TPOAb), antibodies to Tg (TgAb) and antibodies directed against the TSH receptor (TRAb).

### Available Assays

Modern assays for thyroid autoantibodies depend on direct measurement of the interaction between the autoantibody (patient's serum) and the labeled thyroid antigen. Despite improvement of these assays in recent years, specificity remains an issue, because many euthyroid individuals exhibit low levels of these autoantibodies. The higher the concentration of the autoantibody, the greater is its clinical specificity.[15] Attempts have been made to standardize these assays to allow for comparisons of thyroid autoantibody concentrations from one office visit to the next, among different patients, and among laboratories. However, owing to autoantibodies differing considerably in their affinity and epitope recognition of antigen, results from different commercial assays may still vary significantly.[55]

### Clinical Usefulness and Test Interpretation

#### Autoantibodies to thyroid peroxidase and to thyroglobulin

Both TPO and Tg autoantibodies are polyclonal antibodies and are thought to occur owing to a secondary response to thyroid injury, and may contribute to the development and chronicity of disease. Almost 100% of patients with Hashimoto's thyroiditis have elevated TgAb and TPOAb, but TPOAb have higher affinity and occur in higher concentrations. TgAb and TPOAb are also detectable in 50% to 90% of patients with Graves' disease. These antibodies are also frequently seen in the general population and are 5-fold more common in women than in men.[15] However, their significance in individuals with normal thyroid function remains uncertain, except that they confer a risk factor in families with autoimmune thyroid disorders.[56]

In patients with known overt hypothyroidism, measurement of these antibodies is not required, because it does not alter management. However, current guidelines recommend measurement of TPOAb when evaluating patients with subclinical hypothyroidism, because their presence may influence the decision to treat.[3] If positive, progression to overt hypothyroidism occurs at a rate of 4.3% per year versus 2.6% per year when TPOAb are negative. Additionally, measurement of TPOAb should be considered when evaluating patients with recurrent miscarriage, with or without infertility.[3] This is because women with positive TPOAb may have an increased risk of miscarriage in the first trimester,[57] for preterm delivery,[58] and for offspring with impaired cognitive development.[59] It is hypothesized that these increased risks may be owing to decreased thyroid functional reserve from chronic autoimmune thyroiditis leading to subtle hypothyroidism.[60]

#### Autoantibodies to the thyroid-stimulating hormone receptor

TRAb are directed against the TSH receptor. In hyperthyroid patients with Graves' disease, these autoantibodies behave as thyroid-stimulating antibodies (thyroid-stimulating immunoglobulin), because they compete with TSH for binding to its specific receptor site in the cell membrane.[61] This stimulation induces thyroid growth, increases gland vascularity, and leads to an increased rate of thyroid hormone production and secretion. Other types of TRAbs exist, including antibodies that act as TSH antagonists and are referred to as blocking TRAbs (thyrotropin-binding inhibitor immunoglobulin) and neutral antibodies, which do not influence TSH binding but may act as weak agonists.[61] Blocking TRAbs can be found in 15% of patients with autoimmune thyroiditis, especially in patients without a goiter.[62] However, TRAbs are not detectable in the normal population with the use of currently available assays, and thus are disease specific.

Measurement of TRAbs can be used to diagnose Graves' disease. Most TRAb assays are specific for Graves' disease, but thyroid-stimulating immunoglobulin and first-generation thyrotropin-binding inhibitor immunoglobulin assays are less sensitive.[63–65] Measurement of TRAb levels before stopping antithyroid drug therapy is recommended, because it helps in predicting which patients can be weaned from the medication, with normal levels indicating a greater chance for remission.[63] Persistently high levels of TRAb along with high thyroid blood flow identified by color Doppler ultrasound imaging are associated with higher relapse rates,[66–69] and these patients should be assessed more frequently and at shorter intervals after antithyroid drugs are discontinued. In contrast, patients with mild disease, small goiters, and negative TRAb have remission rates of greater than 50%, making the use of antithyroid medications potentially more favorable in this group of patients.[70]

TRAb levels should be measured in pregnant women with hyperthyroidism when the etiology is unclear. If Graves' disease is confirmed with elevated TRAbs, then these antibodies should be measured again at 22 to 26 weeks of gestation. In hypothyroid pregnant patients who were treated for Graves' disease with radioactive iodine or thyroidectomy before pregnancy, TRAb levels should be measured using a sensitive assay either initially at 20 to 26 weeks of gestation, or initially during the first trimester, and if elevated, again at 22 to 26 weeks of gestation.[63] This recommendation is based on the strong correlation between a high titer of TRAbs and the development of fetal or neonatal Graves' disease, because TRAbs can cross the placenta and affect the fetal thyroid gland. Thus, TRAb levels measured at 22 to 26 weeks of gestation should be used to guide decisions regarding neonatal monitoring.[63]

## THYROGLOBULIN
### Overview

Tg is a large, homodimeric glycoprotein (660 KDa) that is produced by thyroid follicular cells. It contains 8% to 10% carbohydrates and iodine. T4 and T3 are synthesized on Tg within the lumen of thyroid follicles. Most Tg is reabsorbed into thyrocytes and proteolytically degraded during T4 and T3 secretion. However, small amounts of intact Tg are secreted with T4 and T3 and are detectable in the serum of healthy individuals, with levels roughly paralleling thyroid gland size (0.5–1.0 ng/mL Tg per gram of thyroid tissue, depending on the TSH level).[71] TgAb are present in approximately 10% of the general population and an estimated 25% of patients with differentiated thyroid cancer.[15,72,73]

### Available Assays

Several assays are available for Tg measurement. Even though significant improvements have been made in standardizing Tg assays, marked variability still exists between some assays.[74,75] Because of this, the current recommendation is that measurements in individual patients be performed with the same method for reliable interpretation.[72] If a change in the assay method is necessary, it is recommended that a baseline level is reestablished, which can be used to interpret change over time.[76]

### Immunometric assays

Immunometric assays are the most commonly used assays to measure serum Tg in clinical laboratories. Guidelines recommend that these assays be calibrated against the CRM-457 international standard.[72] In addition to their limited dynamic range, immunometric assays are prone to interference by TgAb, which often cause falsely low serum Tg measurements. Additionally, heterophile antibodies, if present, can interact with the antibodies used in immunoassays, usually resulting in erroneously high Tg measurements.

### Radioimmunoassays

Tg measurement by radioimmunoassay has been traditionally used for TgAb-positive patients, because it is less prone to antibody interference. Nowadays, these assays are not as widely available as immunometric assays because they require handling and disposal of radioactive materials, often necessitate prolonged incubation times, and may need organic extraction and chromatography before the actual assay procedure to minimize nonspecific and specific interferences (cross-reactivity).[77] Additionally, they may be less sensitive than immunometric assays in detecting small amounts of Tg.[72]

### Liquid chromatography/tandem mass spectrometry

This new methodology has been recently introduced by some laboratories for quantitative Tg measurement in patients with positive TgAb (or heterophile antibodies) and validated as a cost-effective method with acceptable performance characteristics for use in clinical diagnostic applications.[78] This method overcomes the issue of TgAb interference by using tryptic digestion of patient serum with subsequent measurement of Tg-proteotypic peptides by liquid chromatography/tandem mass spectrometry.[78–80] Limitations include the high complexity of the instrumentation's operation and maintenance, as well as sample throughput limits.[77]

### Functional Sensitivity

Although most data arise from studies using methods with a functional sensitivity of 1 ng/mL, many contemporary assays have a functional sensitivity as low as 0.1 ng/mL or less. These sensitive assays may reduce the need to perform TSH-stimulated Tg measurements during the initial and long-term follow-up of follicular cell–derived thyroid cancer patients and allow Tg surveillance measurements without interrupting thyroid hormone therapy instead.[72] In general, the highest degrees of sensitivity for serum Tg occur after thyroid hormone withdrawal or stimulation using recombinant human TSH (rhTSH),[81] and basal serum Tg increases by 5- to 10-fold with TSH stimulation. Patients with an unstimulated serum Tg of greater than 0.2 ng/mL using a highly sensitive assay during T4 suppression therapy are likely to have a TSH-stimulated Tg of greater than 1 ng/mL using a less sensitive assay.[72]

### Clinical Usefulness and Test Interpretation

Tg is primarily used as a tumor marker to evaluate the effectiveness of treatment for differentiated thyroid cancer and to monitor for residual or recurrent disease.[72,82,83] Because it is only produced by thyroid follicular cells, Tg is expected to be undetectable in patients who underwent total or near-total thyroidectomy and 131-I remnant ablation.[81] This is defined as a serum Tg level less than 0.2 ng/mL during TSH suppression or a serum Tg of less than 1 ng/mL after stimulation in the absence of interfering antibodies.[72] However, serum Tg levels should always be interpreted in view of the pretest probability of clinically significant residual disease. Serum Tg measurements obtained during thyroid hormone suppression should be interpreted cautiously because they may fail to identify patients with small amounts of residual disease.[84–87] A neck ultrasound examination is thus invaluable to identify possible residual cancer even when serum Tg is undetectable.[88–90] Additionally, even TSH-stimulated Tg measurement may fail to identify patients with clinically significant thyroid cancer because of either anti-Tg antibodies (which should always be quantitatively assessed with every measurement of serum Tg) or because of decreased or absent production and secretion of immunoreactive Tg by tumor cells, as seen in poorly differentiated thyroid cancers.[72,85,86]

During the initial follow-up of patients with differentiated thyroid cancer who have a low or intermediate risk for recurrence, serum Tg on levothyroxine therapy should be measured every 6 to 12 months. For those patients who achieve an excellent response to therapy, the usefulness of subsequent Tg measurements has not been established, but current recommendations advocate that the time interval between serum Tg measurements can be increased to 12 to 14 months.[72] For patients with differentiated thyroid cancer at high risk for recurrence regardless of response to therapy, and for patients who have biochemical incomplete, structural incomplete, or indeterminate response to therapy, Tg levels should be checked at least every 6 to 12 months for several years.[72] Additionally, all patients should undergo a serum Tg on levothyroxine therapy with a sensitive Tg assay (<0.2 ng/mL) or after rhTSH stimulation at 6 to 18 months to verify excellent response and absence of neoplastic disease. A single rhTSH-stimulated serum Tg of less than 0.5 to 1.0 ng/mL in the absence of interfering antibodies has a 98% to 99.5% likelihood of identifying patients completely free of thyroid cancer on follow-up, indicating excellent response to treatment.[91–95] If excellent response to treatment is not confirmed, subsequent rhTSH-stimulated Tg testing may be considered to monitor and reassess response to additional therapies.[72]

Tg levels can also be increased in patients with goiter (degree of elevation correlates with thyroid size), hyperthyroidism, or inflammatory or physical injury to the thyroid gland.[55] Subnormal or undetectable Tg concentrations are seen in patients with an intact thyroid gland who have thyrotoxicosis factitia owing to suppression of endogenous thyroid function. This aids in differentiating thyrotoxicosis factitia from other causes of thyrotoxicosis with a low thyroid radioiodine uptake.[96]

## CALCITONIN
### Overview

Calcitonin is a polypeptide produced almost exclusively by neuroendocrine C cells of the thyroid gland. It results from cleavage and posttranslational processing of procalcitonin, a precursor peptide derived from pre-procalcitonin.[97]

### Available Assays and Functional Sensitivity

Commercial assays for measuring calcitonin have shifted over the past decade to the immunochemiluminometric assays that are highly sensitive and specific for monomeric calcitonin. With these assays, the cross-reactivity with procalcitonin and other calcitonin-related peptides is essentially eliminated. This is important because inflammatory conditions, such as sepsis, can lead to significant elevations of procalcitonin in tissues.[98,99]

Depending on the assay, 56% to 88% of normal subjects have calcitonin levels below the functional sensitivity, and up to 10% have calcitonin levels of greater than 10 pg/mL. Reference ranges for calcitonin are higher in men as compared with women; this is owing to the larger C-cell mass in men.[100,101] However, the current revised medullary thyroid cancer guidelines do not specify reference ranges of basal or stimulated serum calcitonin levels; rather, individual laboratories may set their own criteria defining these reference ranges.[102] Owing to variability in calcitonin measurements among different commercial assays, individual patient samples should be evaluated using the same assay whenever possible.

Heterophile antibodies can cause falsely elevated (and rarely falsely lower) serum calcitonin levels.[103] It is important to consider the "hook effect" in patients with a large tumor burden from medullary thyroid cancer and unexpectedly low serum calcitonin levels. This condition occurs when very high serum calcitonin levels saturate the binding capacity of the capture antibody, leading to the detection of falsely low analyte levels in the sample.[104] The "hook effect" is less likely to occur with current immunochemiluminometric assays than with some of the older assays, but physicians should still be aware of it.

Last, provocative testing with the use of potent secretagogues, such as intravenous calcium or pentagastrin, has been shown to increase the sensitivity of calcitonin testing.[105–108] However, with the introduction of the sensitive immunochemiluminometric assays, the usefulness of provocative testing has become less widespread.

### Clinical Usefulness and Test Interpretation

Calcitonin is the most specific and sensitive serum marker for medullary thyroid cancer both before and after total thyroidectomy.[109,110] Basal serum calcitonin correlates well with tumor burden and also reflects tumor differentiation.[111] To detect the presence of residual disease, a calcitonin level should be checked 3 to 6 months after the initial operation.[102] If the calcitonin level is undetectable, the patient is considered biochemically cured with excellent prognosis, with a 5-year recurrence rate of only 5%.[112] It is important to remember that calcitonin has a long half-life. Therefore, the rate of decrease in serum calcitonin can be slow in some patients.[113] There has been controversy regarding the length of time needed to reach the nadir of the calcitonin level after total thyroidectomy. In some patients who are surgically cured, the calcitonin level declines rapidly within the first postoperative hour, achieving an undetectable level with the first few days after the operation.[114–116] However, owing to differences in clearance, it has been proposed that 3 months postoperative is the optimal time to determine serum calcitonin levels.[110,114] If calcitonin is undetectable at 3 to 6 months postoperative, it should be measured every 6 months for 1 year and then annually thereafter.[102] Persistently elevated calcitonin levels at 6 months postoperative indicate persistent disease. Additionally, the calcitonin level can also indicate the site of recurrence. When serum calcitonin is less than 150 pg/mL, this usually indicates persistent locoregional disease in the neck.[102,117] If the serum calcitonin is greater than 150 pg/mL, this may point to the possibility of distant metastases.[102] However, many patients with distant metastases often have a serum calcitonin level of greater than 1000 pg/mL.[102]

Persistent hypercalcitoninemia should lead to further workup with several different imaging studies to localize the recurrence or persistent disease. It should be noted that very few patients may develop tumor recurrence without elevated calcitonin.[118]

It is important to recognize that serum calcitonin can be falsely elevated in several conditions other than medullary thyroid cancer, including chronic renal failure, autoimmune thyroiditis, large cell lung cancers, prostate cancer, mastocytosis, gastrointestinal and pulmonary neuroendocrine tumors, and hyperparathyroidism.[119–123]

In parallel with calcitonin, carcinoembryonic antigen (CEA) can be used as another tumor marker to detect persistent or recurrent medullary thyroid cancer, because neoplastic C cells also produce CEA. CEA is a nonspecific tumor marker for medullary thyroid cancer, but it does help to predict outcome.[124–126] Owing to its prolonged half-life, serum levels of CEA may take even longer to reach a nadir. In addition, CEA level can be falsely elevated owing to heterophilic antibodies, smoking, gastrointestinal tract inflammatory disease, benign lung tumors, or several nonthyroid malignancies.[102]

In patients with medullary thyroid cancer, simultaneously increasing serum CEA and calcitonin levels indicate disease progression. If these patients have increased CEA levels but stable or decreasing calcitonin levels, physicians should consider poorly differentiated medullary thyroid cancer.[127] Therefore, it is important that calcitonin and CEA levels are measured concurrently. Finally, assessment of calcitonin and CEA doubling times postoperatively provides a useful tool for assessing the progression and aggressiveness of medullary thyroid cancer.[128,129] In patients with persistent and recurrent disease, serum calcitonin and CEA should be monitored every 6 months to determine doubling times.[130] If the doubling time is less than 6 months, the 5- and 10-year survival rates are 23% and 15%, respectively. If the doubling time is greater than 24 months, the 5- and 10-year survival rates are 100% and 100%, respectively.[128,129] A calculator is available on the American Thyroid Association website to determine doubling times of serial serum calcitonin and CEA measurements.[131]

## REFERENCES

1. Caron PJ, Nieman LK, Rose SR, et al. Deficient nocturnal surge of thyrotropin in central hypothyroidism. J Clin Endocrinol Metab 1986;62(5):960–4.
2. Karmisholt J, Andersen S, Laurberg P. Variation in thyroid function tests in patients with stable untreated subclinical hypothyroidism. Thyroid 2008;18(3): 303–8.
3. Garber JR, Cobin RH, Gharib H, et al, American Association of Clinical Endocrinologists, American Thyroid Association Taskforce on Hypothyroidism in Adults. Clinical practice guidelines for hypothyroidism in adults: cosponsored by the American Association of Clinical Endocrinologists and the American Thyroid Association. Thyroid 2012;22(12):1200–35.
4. Spencer CA, LoPresti JS, Patel A, et al. Applications of a new chemiluminometric thyrotropin assay to subnormal measurement. J Clin Endocrinol Metab 1990; 70(2):453–60.
5. Yalow RS, Berson SA. Immunoassay of endogenous plasma insulin in man. J Clin Invest 1960;39:1157–75.
6. Utiger RD. Radioimmunoassay of human plasma thyrotropin. J Clin Invest 1965; 44:1277–86.
7. Odell WD, Wilber JF, Paul WE. Radioimmunoassay of thyrotropin in human serum. J Clin Endocrinol Metab 1965;25(9):1179–88.
8. Gordin A, Saarinen P. Methodological study of the radioimmunoassay of human thyrotrophin. Acta Endocrinol (Copenh) 1972;71(1):24–36.
9. Spencer CA, Nicoloff JT. Improved radioimmunoassay for human TSH. Clin Chim Acta 1980;108(3):415–24.
10. Mori T, Imura H, Bito S, et al. Clinical usefulness of a highly sensitive enzyme-immunoassay of TSH. Clin Endocrinol (Oxf) 1987;27(1):1–10.
11. Wehmann RE, Rubenstein HA, Nisula BC. A sensitive, convenient radioimmunoassay procedure which demonstrates that serum hTSH is suppressed below the normal range in thyrotoxic patients. Endocr Res Commun 1979;6(3):249–55.
12. Odell WD, Griffin J, Zahradnik R. Two-monoclonal-antibody sandwich-type assay for thyrotropin, with use of an avidin-biotin separation technique. Clin Chem 1986;32(10):1873–8.

13. Wilkins TA, Brouwers G, Mareschal JC, et al. High sensitivity, homogeneous particle-based immunoassay for thyrotropin (Multipact). Clin Chem 1988; 34(9):1749–52.

14. Athey D, Ball M, McNeil CJ. Avidin-biotin based electrochemical immunoassay for thyrotropin. Ann Clin Biochem 1993;30(Pt 6):570–7.

15. Hollowell JG, Staehling NW, Flanders WD, et al. T(4), and thyroid antibodies in the United States population (1988 to 1994): National Health and Nutrition Examination Survey (NHANES III). J Clin Endocrinol Metab 2002;87(2):489–99.

16. Hamilton TE, Davis S, Onstad L, et al. Thyrotropin levels in a population with no clinical, autoantibody, or ultrasonographic evidence of thyroid disease: implications for the diagnosis of subclinical hypothyroidism. J Clin Endocrinol Metab 2008;93(4):1224–30.

17. Baloch Z, Carayon P, Conte-Devolx B, et al, Guidelines Committee, National Academy of Clinical Biochemistry. Laboratory medicine practice guidelines. Laboratory support for the diagnosis and monitoring of thyroid disease. Thyroid 2003;13(1):3–126.

18. Wartofsky L, Dickey RA. The evidence for a narrower thyrotropin reference range is compelling. J Clin Endocrinol Metab 2005;90(9):5483–8.

19. Boucai L, Hollowell JG, Surks MI. An approach for development of age-, gender-, and ethnicity-specific thyrotropin reference limits. Thyroid 2011;21(1): 5–11.

20. Surks MI, Hollowell JG. Age-specific distribution of serum thyrotropin and anti-thyroid antibodies in the US population: implications for the prevalence of subclinical hypothyroidism. J Clin Endocrinol Metab 2007;92(12):4575–82.

21. Papaleontiou M, Cappola AR. Thyroid-stimulating hormone in the evaluation of subclinical hypothyroidism. JAMA 2016;316(15):1592–3.

22. Papaleontiou M, Gay BL, Esfandiari NH, et al. The impact of age in the management of hypothyroidism: results of a nationwide survey. Endocr Pract 2016; 22(6):708–15.

23. Ross DS, Burch HB, Cooper DS, et al. 2016 American thyroid association guidelines for diagnosis and management of hyperthyroidism and other causes of thyrotoxicosis. Thyroid 2016;26(10):1343–421.

24. Lamb EJ, Martin J. Thyroid function tests: often justified in the acutely ill. Ann Clin Biochem 2000;37(Pt 2):158–64.

25. Mebis L, van den Berghe G. The hypothalamus-pituitary-thyroid axis in critical illness. Neth J Med 2009;67(10):332–40.

26. Mebis L, Paletta D, Debaveye Y, et al. Expression of thyroid hormone transporters during critical illness. Eur J Endocrinol 2009;161(2):243–50.

27. Kaptein EM, Spencer CA, Kamiel MB, et al. Prolonged dopamine administration and thyroid hormone economy in normal and critically ill subjects. J Clin Endocrinol Metab 1980;51(2):387–93.

28. Sowers JR, Carlson HE, Brautbar N, et al. Effect of dexamethasone on prolactin and TSH responses to TRH and metoclopramide in man. J Clin Endocrinol Metab 1977;44(2):237–41.

29. Wong ET, Bradley SG, Schultz AL. Elevations of thyroid-stimulating hormone during acute nonthyroidal illness. Arch Intern Med 1981;141(7):873–5.

30. Kaplan MM, Larsen PR, Crantz FR, et al. Prevalence of abnormal thyroid function test results in patients with acute medical illnesses. Am J Med 1982;72(1): 9–16.

31. Stagnaro-Green A, Abalovich M, Alexander E, et al, American Thyroid Association Taskforce on Thyroid Disease During Pregnancy and Postpartum.

Guidelines of the American Thyroid Association for the diagnosis and management of thyroid disease during pregnancy and postpartum. Thyroid 2011; 21(10):1081–125.

32. Report of the standing committee on the scientific evaluation of dietary reference intakes and its panel on folate, other B vitamins, and choline, and subcommittee on upper reference levels of nutrients, food and nutrition board, Institute of Medicine. Dietary reference intakes for thiamine, riboflavin, niacin, vitamin B6, folate, vitamin B12, pantothenic acid, biotin, and choline. Washington, DC: National Academies Press; 1998. Available at: https://www.ncbi.nlm.nih.gov/books/NBK114310/.

33. Sedel F, Bernard D, Mock DM, et al. Targeting demyelination and virtual hypoxia with high-dose biotin as a treatment for progressive multiple sclerosis. Neuropharmacology 2016;110(Pt B):644–53.

34. Kwok JS, Chan IH, Chan MH. Biotin interference on TSH and free thyroid hormone measurement. Pathology 2012;44(3):278–80.

35. Wang KS, Kearns GL, Mock DM. The clearance and metabolism of biotin administered intravenously to pigs in tracer and physiologic amounts is much more rapid than previously appreciated. J Nutr 2001;131(4):1271–8.

36. Diamandis EP, Christopoulos TK. The biotin-(strept)avidin system: principles and applications in biotechnology. Clin Chem 1991;37(5):625–36.

37. Barbesino G. Misdiagnosis of Graves' disease with apparent severe hyperthyroidism in a patient taking biotin megadoses. Thyroid 2016;26(6):860–3.

38. Elston MS, Sehgal S, Du Toit S, et al. Factitious Graves' disease due to biotin immunoassay interference-a case and review of the literature. J Clin Endocrinol Metab 2016;101(9):3251–5.

39. Lawson EA, Klibanski A. Endocrine abnormalities in anorexia nervosa. Nat Clin Pract Endocrinol Metab 2008;4(7):407–14.

40. Beck-Peccoz P, Amr S, Menezes-Ferreira MM, et al. Decreased receptor binding of biologically inactive thyrotropin in central hypothyroidism. Effect of treatment with thyrotropin-releasing hormone. N Engl J Med 1985;312(17):1085–90.

41. Gershengorn MC, Weintraub BD. Thyrotropin-induced hyperthyroidism caused by selective pituitary resistance to thyroid hormone. A new syndrome of "inappropriate secretion of TSH". J Clin Invest 1975;56(3):633–42.

42. Stryker TD, Molitch ME. Reversible hyperthyrotropinemia, hyperthyroxinemia, and hyperprolactinemia due to adrenal insufficiency. Am J Med 1985;79(2): 271–6.

43. Abdullatif HD, Ashraf AP. Reversible subclinical hypothyroidism in the presence of adrenal insufficiency. Endocr Pract 2006;12(5):572.

44. Halsall DJ, English E, Chatterjee VK. Interference from heterophilic antibodies in TSH assays. Ann Clin Biochem 2009;46(Pt 4):345–6.

45. Ross HA, Menheere PP, Endocrinology Section of SKML (Dutch Foundation for Quality Assessment in Clinical Laboratories), et al. Interference from heterophilic antibodies in seven current TSH assays. Ann Clin Biochem 2008;45(Pt 6):616.

46. Surks MI, Sievert R. Drugs and thyroid function. N Engl J Med 1995;333(25): 1688–94.

47. Oppenheimer JH, Squef R, Surks MI, et al. Binding of thyroxine by serum proteins evaluated by equilibrium dialysis and electrophoretic techniques. Alterations in nonthyroidal illness. J Clin Invest 1963;42:1769–82.

48. Mendel CM. The free hormone hypothesis: a physiologically based mathematical model. Endocr Rev 1989;10(3):232–74.

49. Stockigt JR. Free thyroid hormone measurement. A critical appraisal. Endocrinol Metab Clin North Am 2001;30(2):265–89.

50. Lee RH, Spencer CA, Mestman JH, et al. Free T4 immunoassays are flawed during pregnancy. Am J Obstet Gynecol 2009;200(3):260.e1–6.
51. Mandel SJ, Spencer CA, Hollowell JG. Are detection and treatment of thyroid insufficiency in pregnancy feasible? Thyroid 2005;15(1):44–53.
52. Lum SM, Nicoloff JT, Spencer CA, et al. Peripheral tissue mechanism for maintenance of serum triiodothyronine values in a thyroxine-deficient state in man. J Clin Invest 1984;73(2):570–5.
53. Peeters RP, Wouters PJ, Kaptein E, et al. Reduced activation and increased inactivation of thyroid hormone in tissues of critically ill patients. J Clin Endocrinol Metab 2003;88(7):3202–11.
54. Rapoport B, McLachlan SM. Thyroid autoimmunity. J Clin Invest 2001;108(9): 1253–9.
55. Melmed S, Polonsky K, Larsen PR, et al. Williams textbook of endocrinology. 12th edition. Philadelphia: Saunders; 2012.
56. Vanderpump MP, Tunbridge WM, French JM, et al. The incidence of thyroid disorders in the community: a twenty-year follow-up of the Whickham Survey. Clin Endocrinol (Oxf) 1995;43(1):55–68.
57. Stagnaro-Green A, Roman SH, Cobin RH, et al. Detection of at-risk pregnancy by means of highly sensitive assays for thyroid autoantibodies. JAMA 1990; 264(11):1422–5.
58. Negro R, Schwartz A, Gismondi R, et al. Thyroid antibody positivity in the first trimester of pregnancy is associated with negative pregnancy outcomes. J Clin Endocrinol Metab 2011;96(6):E920–4.
59. Pop VJ, de Vries E, van Baar AL, et al. Maternal thyroid peroxidase antibodies during pregnancy: a marker of impaired child development? J Clin Endocrinol Metab 1995;80(12):3561–6.
60. Glinoer D, Riahi M, Grun JP, et al. Risk of subclinical hypothyroidism in pregnant women with asymptomatic autoimmune thyroid disorders. J Clin Endocrinol Metab 1994;79(1):197–204.
61. Davies TF, Ando T, Lin RY, et al. Thyrotropin receptor-associated diseases: from adenomata to Graves' disease. J Clin Invest 2005;115(8):1972–83.
62. Kraiem Z, Lahat N, Glaser B, et al. Thyrotrophin receptor blocking antibodies: incidence, characterization and in-vitro synthesis. Clin Endocrinol (Oxf) 1987; 27(4):409–21.
63. Bahn RS, Burch HB, Cooper DS, et al, American Thyroid Association, American Association of Clinical Endocrinologists. Hyperthyroidism and other causes of thyrotoxicosis: management guidelines of the American Thyroid Association and American Association of Clinical Endocrinologists. Endocr Pract 2011; 17(3):456–520.
64. Costagliola S, Morgenthaler NG, Hoermann R, et al. Second generation assay for thyrotropin receptor antibodies has superior diagnostic sensitivity for Graves' disease. J Clin Endocrinol Metab 1999;84(1):90–7.
65. Paunkovic J, Paunkovic N. Does autoantibody-negative Graves' disease exist? A second evaluation of the clinical diagnosis. Horm Metab Res 2006;38(1):53–6.
66. Orunesu E, Bagnasco M, Salmaso C, et al. Use of an artificial neural network to predict Graves' disease outcome within 2 years of drug withdrawal. Eur J Clin Invest 2004;34(3):210–7.
67. Orgiazzi J, Madec AM. Reduction of the risk of relapse after withdrawal of medical therapy for Graves' disease. Thyroid 2002;12(10):849–53.
68. Glinoer D, de Nayer P, Bex M, Belgian Collaborative Study Group on Graves Disease. Effects of l-thyroxine administration, TSH-receptor antibodies and

smoking on the risk of recurrence in Graves' hyperthyroidism treated with anti-thyroid drugs: a double-blind prospective randomized study. Eur J Endocrinol 2001;144(5):475–83.

69. Takasu N, Yamashiro K, Komiya I, et al. Remission of Graves' hyperthyroidism pre-dicted by smooth decreases of thyroid-stimulating antibody and thyrotropin-binding inhibitor immunoglobulin during antithyroid drug treatment. Thyroid 2000;10(10):891–6.

70. Laurberg P, Buchholtz Hansen PE, Iversen E, et al. Goitre size and outcome of med-ical treatment of Graves' disease. Acta Endocrinol (Copenh) 1986;111(1):39–43.

71. Rasmussen LB, Ovesen L, Bulow I, et al. Relations between various measures of iodine intake and thyroid volume, thyroid nodularity, and serum thyroglobulin. Am J Clin Nutr 2002;76(5):1069–76.

72. Haugen BR, Alexander EK, Bible KC, et al. 2015 American Thyroid Association Management guidelines for adult patients with thyroid nodules and differenti-ated thyroid cancer: the American Thyroid Association guidelines task force on thyroid nodules and differentiated thyroid cancer. Thyroid 2016;26(1):1–133.

73. Spencer CA, LoPresti JS, Fatemi S, et al. Detection of residual and recurrent differentiated thyroid carcinoma by serum thyroglobulin measurement. Thyroid 1999;9(5):435–41.

74. Spencer CA, Bergoglio LM, Kazarosyan M, et al. Clinical impact of thyroglobulin (Tg) and Tg autoantibody method differences on the management of patients with differentiated thyroid carcinomas. J Clin Endocrinol Metab 2005;90(10): 5566–75.

75. Schlumberger M, Hitzel A, Toubert ME, et al. Comparison of seven serum thyro-globulin assays in the follow-up of papillary and follicular thyroid cancer pa-tients. J Clin Endocrinol Metab 2007;92(7):2487–95.

76. Access immunoassay systems thyroglobulin [package insert]. Brea, CA: Beck-man Coulter, inc; 2010.

77. Grebe SK, Singh RJ. LC-MS/MS in the clinical laboratory - where to from here? Clin Biochem Rev 2011;32(1):5–31.

78. Kushnir MM, Rockwood AL, Roberts WL, et al. Measurement of thyroglobulin by liquid chromatography-tandem mass spectrometry in serum and plasma in the presence of antithyroglobulin autoantibodies. Clin Chem 2013;59(6):982–90.

79. Netzel BC, Grebe SK, Carranza Leon BG, et al. Thyroglobulin (Tg) testing revis-ited: Tg assays, TgAb assays, and correlation of results with clinical outcomes. J Clin Endocrinol Metab 2015;100(8):E1074–83.

80. Hoofnagle AN, Becker JO, Wener MH, et al. Quantification of thyroglobulin, a low-abundance serum protein, by immunoaffinity peptide enrichment and tan-dem mass spectrometry. Clin Chem 2008;54(11):1796–804.

81. Eustatia-Rutten CF, Smit JW, Romijn JA, et al. Diagnostic value of serum thyro-globulin measurements in the follow-up of differentiated thyroid carcinoma, a structured meta-analysis. Clin Endocrinol (Oxf) 2004;61(1):61–74.

82. Mazzaferri EL, Robbins RJ, Spencer CA, et al. A consensus report of the role of serum thyroglobulin as a monitoring method for low-risk patients with papillary thyroid carcinoma. J Clin Endocrinol Metab 2003;88(4):1433–41.

83. Spencer CA, Lopresti JS. Measuring thyroglobulin and thyroglobulin autoanti-body in patients with differentiated thyroid cancer. Nat Clin Pract Endocrinol Metab 2008;4(4):223–33.

84. Schlumberger M, Berg G, Cohen O, et al. Follow-up of low-risk patients with differentiated thyroid carcinoma: a European perspective. Eur J Endocrinol 2004;150(2):105–12.

85. Giovanella L, Suriano S, Ceriani L, et al. Undetectable thyroglobulin in patients with differentiated thyroid carcinoma and residual radioiodine uptake on a post-ablation whole-body scan. Clin Nucl Med 2011;36(2):109–12.

86. Bachelot A, Leboulleux S, Baudin E, et al. Neck recurrence from thyroid carcinoma: serum thyroglobulin and high-dose total body scan are not reliable criteria for cure after radioiodine treatment. Clin Endocrinol (Oxf) 2005;62(3): 376–9.

87. Cherk MH, Francis P, Topliss DJ, et al. Incidence and implications of negative serum thyroglobulin but positive I-131 whole-body scans in patients with well-differentiated thyroid cancer prepared with rhTSH or thyroid hormone withdrawal. Clin Endocrinol (Oxf) 2012;76(5):734–40.

88. Frasoldati A, Pesenti M, Gallo M, et al. Diagnosis of neck recurrences in patients with differentiated thyroid carcinoma. Cancer 2003;97(1):90–6.

89. Pacini F, Agate L, Elisei R, et al. Outcome of differentiated thyroid cancer with detectable serum Tg and negative diagnostic (131)I whole body scan: comparison of patients treated with high (131)I activities versus untreated patients. J Clin Endocrinol Metab 2001;86(9):4092–7.

90. Torlontano M, Crocetti U, Augello G, et al. Comparative evaluation of recombinant human thyrotropin-stimulated thyroglobulin levels, 131I whole-body scintigraphy, and neck ultrasonography in the follow-up of patients with papillary thyroid microcarcinoma who have not undergone radioiodine therapy. J Clin Endocrinol Metab 2006;91(1):60–3.

91. Castagna MG, Brilli L, Pilli T, et al. Limited value of repeat recombinant human thyrotropin (rhTSH)-stimulated thyroglobulin testing in differentiated thyroid carcinoma patients with previous negative rhTSH-stimulated thyroglobulin and undetectable basal serum thyroglobulin levels. J Clin Endocrinol Metab 2008; 93(1):76–81.

92. Kloos RT, Mazzaferri EL. A single recombinant human thyrotropin-stimulated serum thyroglobulin measurement predicts differentiated thyroid carcinoma metastases three to five years later. J Clin Endocrinol Metab 2005;90(9):5047–57.

93. Han JM, Kim WB, Yim JH, et al. Long-term clinical outcome of differentiated thyroid cancer patients with undetectable stimulated thyroglobulin level one year after initial treatment. Thyroid 2012;22(8):784–90.

94. Klubo-Gwiezdzinska J, Burman KD, Van Nostrand D, et al. Does an undetectable rhTSH-stimulated Tg level 12 months after initial treatment of thyroid cancer indicate remission? Clin Endocrinol (Oxf) 2011;74(1):111–7.

95. Diaz-Soto G, Puig-Domingo M, Martinez-Pino I, et al. Do thyroid cancer patients with basal undetectable Tg measured by current immunoassays require rhTSH testing? Exp Clin Endocrinol Diabetes 2011;119(6):348–52.

96. Chow E, Siddique F, Gama R. Thyrotoxicosis factitia: role of thyroglobulin. Ann Clin Biochem 2008;45(Pt 4):447–8 [author reply: 448].

97. Costante G, Durante C, Francis Z, et al. Determination of calcitonin levels in C-cell disease: clinical interest and potential pitfalls. Nat Clin Pract Endocrinol Metab 2009;5(1):35–44.

98. Becker KL, Nylen ES, White JC, et al. Clinical review 167: procalcitonin and the calcitonin gene family of peptides in inflammation, infection, and sepsis: a journey from calcitonin back to its precursors. J Clin Endocrinol Metab 2004; 89(4):1512–25.

99. Whang KT, Steinwald PM, White JC, et al. Serum calcitonin precursors in sepsis and systemic inflammation. J Clin Endocrinol Metab 1998;83(9):3296–301.

100. Basuyau JP, Mallet E, Leroy M, et al. Reference intervals for serum calcitonin in men, women, and children. Clin Chem 2004;50(10):1828–30.
101. Guyetant S, Rousselet MC, Durigon M, et al. Sex-related C cell hyperplasia in the normal human thyroid: a quantitative autopsy study. J Clin Endocrinol Metab 1997;82(1):42–7.
102. Wells SA Jr, Asa SL, Dralle H, et al, American Thyroid Association Guidelines Task Force on Medullary Thyroid Carcinoma. Revised American Thyroid Association guidelines for the management of medullary thyroid carcinoma. Thyroid 2015;25(6):567–610.
103. Preissner CM, Dodge LA, O'Kane DJ, et al. Prevalence of heterophilic antibody interference in eight automated tumor marker immunoassays. Clin Chem 2005; 51(1):208–10.
104. Leboeuf R, Langlois MF, Martin M, et al. "Hook effect" in calcitonin immunoradiometric assay in patients with metastatic medullary thyroid carcinoma: case report and review of the literature. J Clin Endocrinol Metab 2006;91(2):361–4.
105. Lorenz K, Elwerr M, Machens A, et al. Hypercalcitoninemia in thyroid conditions other than medullary thyroid carcinoma: a comparative analysis of calcium and pentagastrin stimulation of serum calcitonin. Langenbecks Arch Surg 2013; 398(3):403–9.
106. Trimboli P, Giovanella L, Crescenzi A, et al. Medullary thyroid cancer diagnosis: an appraisal. Head Neck 2014;36(8):1216–23.
107. Colombo C, Verga U, Mian C, et al. Comparison of calcium and pentagastrin tests for the diagnosis and follow-up of medullary thyroid cancer. J Clin Endocrinol Metab 2012;97(3):905–13.
108. Mian C, Perrino M, Colombo C, et al. Refining calcium test for the diagnosis of medullary thyroid cancer: cutoffs, procedures, and safety. J Clin Endocrinol Metab 2014;99(5):1656–64.
109. Melvin KE, Tashjian AH Jr. The syndrome of excessive thyrocalcitonin produced by medullary carcinoma of the thyroid. Proc Natl Acad Sci U S A 1968;59(4): 1216–22.
110. Elisei R, Pinchera A. Advances in the follow-up of differentiated or medullary thyroid cancer. Nat Rev Endocrinol 2012;8(8):466–75.
111. Pacini F, Castagna MG, Cipri C, et al. Medullary thyroid carcinoma. Clin Oncol (R Coll Radiol) 2010;22(6):475–85.
112. Modigliani E, Cohen R, Campos JM, et al. Prognostic factors for survival and for biochemical cure in medullary thyroid carcinoma: results in 899 patients. The GETC Study Group. Groupe d'etude des tumeurs a calcitonine. Clin Endocrinol (Oxf) 1998;48(3):265–73.
113. Stepanas AV, Samaan NA, Hill CS Jr, et al. Medullary thyroid carcinoma: importance of serial serum calcitonin measurement. Cancer 1979;43(3):825–37.
114. Ismailov SI, Piulatova NR. Postoperative calcitonin study in medullary thyroid carcinoma. Endocr Relat Cancer 2004;11(2):357–63.
115. Faggiano A, Milone F, Ramundo V, et al. A decrease of calcitonin serum concentrations less than 50 percent 30 minutes after thyroid surgery suggests incomplete C-cell tumor tissue removal. J Clin Endocrinol Metab 2010;95(9):E32–6.
116. Fugazzola L, Pinchera A, Luchetti F, et al. Disappearance rate of serum calcitonin after total thyroidectomy for medullary thyroid carcinoma. Int J Biol Markers 1994;9(1):21–4.
117. Pellegriti G, Leboulleux S, Baudin E, et al. Long-term outcome of medullary thyroid carcinoma in patients with normal postoperative medical imaging. Br J Cancer 2003;88(10):1537–42.

118. Sand M, Gelos M, Sand D, et al. Serum calcitonin negative medullary thyroid carcinoma. World J Surg Oncol 2006;4:97.
119. Borchhardt KA, Horl WH, Sunder-Plassmann G. Reversibility of 'secondary hypercalcitoninemia' after kidney transplantation. Am J Transplant 2005;5(7): 1757–63.
120. Schuetz M, Duan H, Wahl K, et al. T lymphocyte cytokine production patterns in Hashimoto patients with elevated calcitonin levels and their relationship to tumor initiation. Anticancer Res 2006;26(6B):4591–6.
121. Pratz KW, Ma C, Aubry MC, et al. Large cell carcinoma with calcitonin and vasoactive intestinal polypeptide-associated Verner-Morrison syndrome. Mayo Clin Proc 2005;80(1):116–20.
122. Machens A, Haedecke J, Holzhausen HJ, et al. Differential diagnosis of calcitonin-secreting neuroendocrine carcinoma of the foregut by pentagastrin stimulation. Langenbecks Arch Surg 2000;385(6):398–401.
123. Yocum MW, Butterfield JH, Gharib H. Increased plasma calcitonin levels in systemic mast cell disease. Mayo Clin Proc 1994;69(10):987–90.
124. Cohen R, Campos JM, Salaun C, et al. Preoperative calcitonin levels are predictive of tumor size and postoperative calcitonin normalization in medullary thyroid carcinoma. Groupe d'Etudes des Tumeurs a Calcitonine (GETC). J Clin Endocrinol Metab 2000;85(2):919–22.
125. Machens A, Schneyer U, Holzhausen HJ, et al. Prospects of remission in medullary thyroid carcinoma according to basal calcitonin level. J Clin Endocrinol Metab 2005;90(4):2029–34.
126. Maia AL, Siqueira DR, Kulcsar MA, et al. Diagnosis, treatment, and follow-up of medullary thyroid carcinoma: recommendations by the thyroid department of the Brazilian Society of Endocrinology and Metabolism. Arq Bras Endocrinol Metabol 2014;58(7):667–700.
127. Mendelsohn G, Wells SA Jr, Baylin SB. Relationship of tissue carcinoembryonic antigen and calcitonin to tumor virulence in medullary thyroid carcinoma. An immunohistochemical study in early, localized, and virulent disseminated stages of disease. Cancer 1984;54(4):657–62.
128. Barbet J, Campion L, Kraeber-Bodere F, et al. Prognostic impact of serum calcitonin and carcinoembryonic antigen doubling-times in patients with medullary thyroid carcinoma. J Clin Endocrinol Metab 2005;90(11):6077–84.
129. Laure Giraudet A, Al Ghulzan A, Auperin A, et al. Progression of medullary thyroid carcinoma: assessment with calcitonin and carcinoembryonic antigen doubling times. Eur J Endocrinol 2008;158(2):239–46.
130. van Heerden JA, Grant CS, Gharib H, et al. Long-term course of patients with persistent hypercalcitoninemia after apparent curative primary surgery for medullary thyroid carcinoma. Ann Surg 1990;212(4):395–400 [discussion: 400–1].
131. American Thyroid Association professional physician calculators. Available at: http://www.thyroid.org/thyroid-physicians-professionals/calculators/thyroid-cancer-carcinoma/. Accessed September 1, 2016.

# Biochemical Testing Relevant to Bone

Chee Kian Chew, MD, Bart L. Clarke, MD*

## KEYWORDS

- Metabolic bone disease • Calcium • Phosphorus • Vitamin D • Parathyroid hormone
- Parathyroid hormone-related protein • Biochemical markers

## KEY POINTS

- Laboratory biochemical testing is critical in the evaluation, diagnosis, and management of bone disorders.
- Assessment of mineral metabolism, including serum calcium and phosphorus, gives insight into the pathophysiology of bone diseases.
- The pathophysiology of vitamin D, parathyroid hormone, and parathyroid hormone-related protein directly impact skeletal disorders.
- Markers of bone turnover give direct insight into bone formation and resorption.

## INTRODUCTION

Laboratory biochemical testing is critical to understanding bone disorders. The most common bone disorder, osteoporosis, is characterized by low bone mass and abnormal skeletal architecture caused by genetic or acquired biochemical abnormalities that result in impaired bone strength and increased risk of fragility fracture.[1] More than 20 million Americans are affected by this common disorder, with at least 1.5 million osteoporotic fractures occurring in the United States each year.[2] Less common metabolic bone diseases, such as primary hyperparathyroidism, hypoparathyroidism, osteomalacia or rickets, Paget disease of the bone, and rare bone diseases are also clinically important, and develop owing to unique changes in skeletal physiology. This review summarizes recent data on biochemical testing relevant to bone, focusing on minerals, vitamin D, parathyroid hormone (PTH), PTH-related protein (PTHrP), and bone turnover markers (BTMs).

## MINERALS: CALCIUM AND PHOSPHORUS
### Serum Total Calcium

The adult human is estimated to contain total body calcium of about 1 kg, representing about 2% of body weight. Of this, 99% is present as calcium hydroxyapatite in the

The authors have nothing to disclose.
Division of Endocrinology, Diabetes, Metabolism, and Nutrition, Mayo Clinic, E-18A, 200 1st Street Southwest, Rochester, MN 55905, USA
* Corresponding author.
E-mail address: clarke.bart@mayo.edu

skeleton, and less than 1% is present in nonosseous intracellular or extracellular fluid. Calcium in extracellular fluid is in dynamic equilibrium with the rapidly exchangeable fraction of bone calcium. About 45% of serum total calcium is bound to proteins, mostly albumin, with about 10% found in inorganic complexes, and 45% free or ionized calcium.[3] Calcium ions are crucial for mineralization of newly formed osteoid matrix that leads to new bone. Serum total calcium is typically measured using a photometric method.

Hypocalcemia most often results from absence or impaired function of the parathyroid glands or a low vitamin D level.[4] Chronic kidney disease (CKD) may be associated with hypocalcemia owing to decreased renal 1,25-dihydroxyvitamin D (1,25-diOHD) synthesis, as well as hyperphosphatemia and skeletal resistance to the action of PTH. Hypocalcemia may cause tetany or osteomalacia.

Hypercalcemia results from either increased calcium mobilization from the skeleton or intestinal increased absorption.[5] The majority of hypercalcemia is owing to primary hyperparathyroidism or breast, prostate, thyroid, or lung carcinomas metastatic to the skeleton. Patients with primary hyperparathyroidism associated with osteoporosis or osteitis fibrosa cystica, kidney stones, nephrocalcinosis, or symptoms of hypercalcemia are candidates for parathyroidectomy.[6] Increased serum total calcium may be owing to increased albumin levels, and decreased serum calcium owing to decreased albumin levels, so albumin-corrected serum calcium should be assessed. Ideally, calcium should be measured fasting to minimize the influence of dietary or supplemental intake on the serum level.

Treatment of chronic hypocalcemia involves long-term oral therapy tailored to the specific disease causing the hypocalcemia. The therapeutic target for serum calcium level is usually 8.0 to 8.5 mg/dL, because this prevents tetany and minimizes other symptoms. For acutely symptomatic hypocalcemia, calcium is administered intravenously.[7]

Hypercalcemic symptoms develop at variable levels in different patients. Symptoms are common when serum calcium is greater than 11.5 mg/dL, although patients may still be asymptomatic at this level. Levels greater than 12.0 mg/dL are considered critical and possibly life threatening. Severe hypercalcemia greater than 15.0 mg/dL is usually considered a medical emergency.[8]

### Ionized Calcium

Ionized calcium, which accounts for about 45% of serum total calcium, is the biologically active form of calcium. Low serum ionized calcium values may be seen in CKD, severely ill patients, or patients rapidly transfused with citrated whole blood or blood products. Increased serum ionized calcium may be seen in primary hyperparathyroidism, ectopic PTH-producing tumors, excess intake of vitamin D or vitamin A, or malignancies involving the skeleton.[9] Nomograms are used to calculate serum ionized calcium from total calcium, albumin, and blood pH. Because calculated ionized calcium results may be unreliable, ion-selective electrodes are used to directly measure this in body fluids. Serum ionized calcium is used to assess calcium levels in critically ill patients with fluid shifts, acid–base imbalances, or multiple comorbidities. It is generally considered a second-order test in the evaluation of abnormal calcium values. Serum ionized calcium concentrations 50% below the lower limit of normal may result in severely reduced cardiac function. Ionized calcium is higher in children and young adults. Ionized calcium values vary inversely with pH by approximately 0.2 mg/dL per 0.1 pH unit change.

### Twenty-Four–Hour Urine Calcium

Ordinarily, about 25% to 30% of dietary calcium is absorbed, and 98% of filtered serum calcium is reabsorbed by the kidney. Trafficking of calcium between the gastrointestinal tract, bone, and kidney is tightly controlled by a complex regulatory system including vitamin D and PTH.[10]

Excessive excretion of urinary calcium is a risk factor for nephrolithiasis. Measurement of 24-hour urine calcium is useful in evaluation of calcium oxalate and calcium phosphate kidney stone risk, calculation of urinary supersaturation, and evaluation of osteoporosis and osteomalacia.

Idiopathic hypercalciuria is due to genetic deficiency or dysfunction of sodium-phosphate co-transporters 2a and 2c.[11] Patients with idiopathic hypercalciuria were previously divided into fasting and absorptive hypercalciuria, but this approach is no longer widely used. Risk of stone disease increases when 24-hour urine calcium is greater than 300 mg in men or women. Thiazide-type diuretics may be used to reduce urinary calcium excretion, with periodic 24-hour urine collections performed to monitor therapy.

Known secondary causes of hypercalciuria include hyperparathyroidism, Paget disease of the bone, prolonged immobilization, vitamin D intoxication, and destructive lesions in bone, such as metastatic cancer or multiple myeloma.

The 24-hour urine calcium excretion may be used to gauge the adequacy of calcium supplementation. In states of gastrointestinal malabsorption associated with decreased bone mineralization, such as osteomalacia, urine calcium is typically very low. Low 24-hour urine calcium is often interpreted as an indication of low calcium intake or absorption, or rapid bone mineralization, assuming the 24-hour urine sodium is not also markedly decreased, and that patients are not taking thiazide-type diuretics or lithium.[12] Decreased 24-hour urine calcium is also expected in patients with familial hypocalciuric hypercalcemia, and this level, or a calcium/creatinine clearance ratio of less than 0.01, is often used to differentiate familial hypocalciuric hypercalcemia from primary hyperparathyroidism.

### Phosphorus

Roughly 88% of total body phosphorus is localized in bone in the form of hydroxyapatite, with the remainder involved in intermediary carbohydrate metabolism or sequestered in phospholipids, nucleic acids, or ATP. Phosphorus occurs in blood as inorganic phosphate and organically bound phosphoric acid. The small amount of extracellular organic phosphorus is found exclusively in phospholipids. Serum inorganic phosphate measures approximately 2.5 to 4.5 mg/dL in photometric biochemical assays. Serum phosphate concentrations depend on meal intake and variation in the secretion of PTH. Serum phosphorus has a strong biphasic circadian rhythm, with values lowest in the morning and highest in the late afternoon and evening.

Hypophosphatemia is caused by a shift of inorganic phosphate from the extracellular to the intracellular compartment, renal tubular phosphate wasting, loss from the gastrointestinal tract, and loss from intracellular stores.[13] Hyperphosphatemia is usually secondary to an inability of the kidneys to excrete phosphate. Other causes may be owing to increased intake, or shift of phosphate from tissues into extracellular fluid.

Measuring serum phosphate is useful for diagnosis and management of a variety of disorders, including bone, parathyroid, and renal diseases. Hypophosphatemia is relatively common in hospitalized patients. Serum concentrations between 1.5 and 2.4 mg/dL are considered moderately decreased, and not usually associated with signs or symptoms. Levels of less than 1.5 mg/dL may result in muscle weakness, hemolysis of red blood cells, bone deformity, impaired bone growth, and coma, and may be life threatening.[14]

Rapid increases in serum phosphate may cause hypocalcemia, with resultant tetany, seizures, or hypotension. Soft tissue calcification may result from long-term increased serum phosphorus as a result of increased calcium $\times$ phosphate product, especially in CKD.

# VITAMIN D
## 25-Hydroxyvitamin D

Mild to moderate serum 25-hydroxyvitamin D (25-OHD) deficiency of less than 20 ng/mL may be associated with osteoporosis or secondary hyperparathyroidism. Severe deficiency of less than 10 ng/mL may lead to an inability to mineralize newly formed osteoid matrix in bone, resulting in rickets in children or osteomalacia in adults. The consequences of vitamin D deficiency in tissues other than bone are not fully known yet.

Mild to moderate 25-OHD deficiency of less than 20 ng/mL is present in about 30% of the US population.[15] More than 50% of institutionalized elderly are estimated to have vitamin D deficiency. Although much less common, severe deficiency is not rare.

Reasons for vitamin D deficiency include a lack of sunshine exposure, especially in northern latitudes during the winter; inadequate dietary or supplemental intake; malabsorption owing to celiac disease; decreased hepatic 25-hydroxylase activity owing to advanced liver disease; and liver cytochrome P450-inducing antiepileptic drugs, including phenytoin, phenobarbital, and carbamazepine, that accelerate vitamin D metabolism.[16]

In contrast with the high prevalence of 25-OHD deficiency, hypervitaminosis D is rare, and seen only after prolonged exposure to very high doses of vitamin D. With hypervitaminosis D, severe hypercalcemia and hyperphosphatemia may occur, sometimes resulting in acute renal failure.

Measurement of serum 25-OHD is useful for diagnosing vitamin D deficiency, evaluating the differential diagnosis of rickets and osteomalacia, monitoring vitamin D replacement therapy, and diagnosis of hypervitaminosis D.

Large human epidemiologic studies have shown that serum 25-OHD less than 25 ng/mL is associated with hyperparathyroidism, reduced bone mineral density, falls, and fractures, particularly in the elderly.[17] Intervention studies show fracture risk reduction with vitamin D replacement. Serum 25-OHD levels of less than 10 ng/mL may be associated with more severe abnormalities, and lead to inadequate mineralization of newly formed osteoid matrix, resulting in rickets in children or osteomalacia in adults. In affected individuals, serum calcium may be marginally low, and PTH and serum alkaline phosphatase are usually increased. Definitive diagnosis rests on the typical radiographic findings of osteomalacia, or quantitative bone histomorphometry.[18] Biochemical workup of suspected rickets or osteomalacia includes measurement of serum calcium, phosphorus, PTH, and 25-OHD. In patients where serum 25-OHD levels are greater than 10 ng/mL, alternative causes for impaired mineralization should be considered. The differential diagnosis of osteomalacia includes partially treated vitamin D deficiency, very low calcium intake, vitamin D-resistant rickets, renal failure, renal tubular mineral loss with or without renal tubular acidosis, hypophosphatemic disorders (eg, X-linked or autosomal-dominant hypophosphatemic rickets), congenital hypoparathyroidism, activating calcium-sensing receptor mutations, and osteopetrosis.[13] Measurement of serum creatinine, magnesium, and 1,25-diOHD is recommended for these patients.

Vitamin D treatment is usually given in the form of vitamin $D_2$ or $D_3$ supplementation. Lack of clinical improvement, or lack of reduction in PTH or alkaline phosphatase, may be owing to patient noncompliance, malabsorption, resistance to 25-OHD, or other factors contributing to clinical disease. Serum 25-OHD is helpful, particularly when measured by liquid chromatography-tandem mass spectrometry, because this methodology allows separation of 25-OHD3 and 25-OHD2, which are derived from animal or plant sources, respectively.

### 1,25-Dihydroxyvitamin D

Serum 1,25-diOHD plays a primary role in the maintenance of calcium homeostasis as the biologically active form of vitamin D. It promotes intestinal calcium absorption and, in concert with PTH, skeletal calcium deposition.[19] Renal calcium and phosphate reabsorption are also promoted, and prepro-PTH mRNA expression in the parathyroid glands is downregulated. The net result is positive calcium balance, increasing serum calcium and phosphate levels, and decreased PTH. Patients who present with hypercalcemia, hyperphosphatemia, and low PTH may have either ectopic unregulated conversion of 25-OHD to 1,25-diOHD, as may occur in granulomatous diseases, particularly sarcoidosis, or from hypervitaminosis D.[20] Serum 1,25-diOHD levels are increased in both groups, but only patients with hypervitaminosis D have serum 25-OHD concentrations greater than 80 ng/mL, and often greater than 150 ng/mL.

In addition to its effects on calcium and bone metabolism, serum 1,25-diOHD regulates the expression of a multitude of genes in other tissues, including immune cells, muscle, vasculature, and reproductive organs.

## PARATHYROID HORMONE AND PARATHYROID HORMONE-RELATED PROTEIN
### Parathyroid Hormone

PTH is a single-chain 84-amino-acid peptide hormone synthesized by chief cells of the parathyroid gland in response to decreased extracellular ionized calcium. It has a very short circulation half-life 3 to 8 minutes.[21] It is mostly degraded in the liver to a mixture of N-terminal, mid-region and C-terminal fragments, with most fragments cleared by the kidneys. PTH maintains bone and mineral homeostasis by increasing serum calcium owing to increased osteoclastic bone resorption, enhanced renal tubular reabsorption, stimulation of renal 1-α-hydroxylase to synthesize 1,25-diOHD (which leads to increased intestinal calcium absorption), and promotion of phosphaturia via inhibition of renal tubular transepithelial phosphate reabsorption.[22]

First-generation PTH assays are radioimmunoassays using polyclonal antibodies directed toward synthetic C-terminal (such as PTH 53-84) or a midregion (such as PTH 44-68) PTH fragments (**Fig. 1**). Other than PTH 1-84, these assays also measure fragments produced by liver catabolism in Kupffer cells. These fragments have a longer half-life than PTH 1-84, and are eliminated by the kidney.[23] Consequently, patients with CKD typically have increased PTH levels. These assays have difficulty discriminating between low and normal levels because they have low analytical sensitivity at decreased PTH concentrations.[24]

Second-generation PTH assays are 2-site assays using 2 different antibodies. The capture antibody is directed against PTH 39-84, whereas the detection antibody recognizes the proximal PTH 13-24 in the Allegro assay, or distal PTH 26-32 in the Roche Elecsys assay (Roche Diagnostics, Indianapolis, IN).[25] These assays are unable to detect C-terminal or midregion fragments, and were initially thought to measure only full-length PTH 1-84,[26] and were therefore called intact PTH assays. Although they are more accurate than first-generation assays, they overestimate severity of secondary hyperparathyroidism in CKD patients,[27] which may cause clinicians to oversuppress PTH with treatment, resulting in low turnover or adynamic bone disease. One study[28] suggested that this might be owing to an ability of the assays to recognize "non–PTH 1-84" molecules with cross-reactivity ranging from 50% to 100%, which coeluted with synthetic PTH 7-84 during high-performance liquid chromatography.

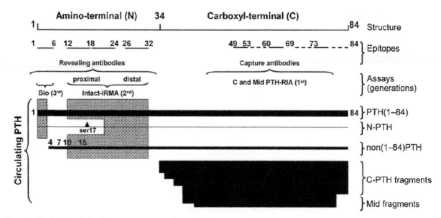

**Fig. 1.** Relationship between parathyroid hormone (PTH) structure, PTH assay generations, known PTH assay epitopes, and known circulating PTH molecular forms. With each generation, PTH assays have become more selective toward full-length PTH(1-84). (*From* Bilezikian JP, Khan A, Potts JT Jr, et al. Hypoparathyroidism in the adult: epidemiology, diagnosis, pathophysiology, target-organ involvement, treatment, and challenges for future research. J Bone Miner Res 2011;26:2325; with permission.)

Third-generation "whole" PTH assays are immunoradiometric assays using an anti–C-terminal antibody similar to "intact" PTH assays, and an N-terminal antibody directed against PTH 1-4.[29] This assay does not capture the PTH 7-84 fragment measured with second-generation assays. PTH levels measured with this assay are lower than with second-generation assays. The difference between measured values with the 2 types of assay corresponds with the concentration of PTH 7-84. In addition to PTH 1-84, the assay also measures N-terminal PTH, a molecule separate from the peak coeluting with PTH 1-84 during high-performance liquid chromatography. N-terminal PTH can be measured with second-generation assays using a distal antibody (anti–26-32), but not a proximal antibody (anti–13-24).[30] N-terminal PTH is produced excessively in patients with parathyroid carcinoma[31] or severe primary hyperparathyroidism.[30] In these patients, PTH levels measured with third-generation assays are higher than with second-generation assays using a proximal antibody.

PTH should be measured on fasting morning samples. The level detected is not affected by freeze–thaw cycles.[29] Serum PTH remains stable at room temperature for up to 6 hours before being frozen.[29] For longer delays before measurement, EDTA plasma samples are preferred,[29] but values are usually 10% to 20% higher than serum values.[32] First-generation assays are no longer used in clinical practice. Both second- and third-generation assays have good analytical quality, with within-run and interday coefficients of variation (CV) of 1% to 10%.[24] Automated assays have lower CV and detection limits than manual assays. There is no standardization among various assay methods. The UK National External Quality Assessment Service quality control study has reported significant method biases of greater than 50% between the highest and lowest reporting methods based on recovery of added synthetic human PTH 1-84.[33] The presence of different PTH fragments and their cross-reactivity by different methods are the major sources of discordance among PTH assays.

Serum PTH is used primarily as a diagnostic test to evaluate abnormal serum calcium or metabolic bone disease. A PTH result within the reference interval does not necessarily rule out a parathyroid gland abnormality.[34] A normal PTH value in a patient with hypocalcemia may suggest a lack of parathyroid gland reserve, or might be an early indicator of hypoparathyroidism. Similarly, normal serum PTH in primary hyperparathyroidism may be owing to various inhibitory fragments released by abnormal gland(s).[35] PTH results should not be interpreted in isolation, but rather in conjunction with simultaneously measured serum calcium, phosphate, vitamin D, and, if indicated, urinary calcium excretion.

Serum PTH is widely used in the management of renal osteodystrophy. Monier-Faugere and colleagues[36] reported that the ratio of PTH 1-84 to PTH 7-84 discriminated between high- and low-turnover bone disease, confirmed by iliac crest bone biopsy, significantly better than PTH measured by either a second- or third-generation assay alone. However, other studies were unable to confirm this finding.[37–39] The Kidney Disease Outcomes Quality Initiative guidelines recommend measuring PTH in CKD patients with a second-generation assay, and maintaining PTH levels within target ranges defined according to the CKD stage (ie, 150–300 pg/mL in patients with CKD stage 5).[40]

In patients undergoing thyroid or parathyroid surgery, intraoperative PTH may be used to confirm the removal of overactive parathyroid glands. Postoperative PTH may be used to assess the risk of postoperative hypocalcemia. Decreased serum PTH during surgery is an important consideration in deciding whether to stop exploration for abnormal parathyroid glands.[41] A survey by the College of American Pathologists reported that many laboratories prefer to transfer intraoperative PTH samples to a central laboratory rather than offering point-of-care testing with automated rapid assays owing to high cost and relatively poor analytical performance, with CV of around 14%.[42]

In a prospective study of 40 total thyroidectomies, serum PTH of less than 0.7 pmol/L (8 ng/L) measured 1 hour postoperatively was a strong predictor of clinically significant hypocalcemia 18 to 42 hours later.[43] Similarly, a rapid postoperative PTH value of less than 1.1 pmol/L (12 ng/L) was more sensitive and specific in predicting symptomatic hypocalcemia after thyroidectomy than an equivalent intraoperative PTH value.[44]

### Parathyroid Hormone-Related Protein

Hypercalcemia of malignancy is a common cause of hypercalcemia in hospitalized patients. Hypercalcemia of malignancy is typically associated with suppressed PTH secretion. A variety of mechanisms may lead to inappropriate hypercalcemia in hypercalcemia of malignancy. These mechanisms include impaired renal function owing to a tumor or its treatment, osteolytic activity within bony metastases, release of calcemic cytokines by nonosteolytic bony metastases, ectopic 1-alpha-hydroxylase activity in tumor tissues, secretion of humoral factors mimicking PTH action in humoral hypercalcemia of malignancy (HHM), which is usually associated with secretion of PTHrP by the primary tumor,[45] or more commonly its metastases, and other, as yet unknown factors. A single cause may not be able to be identified. Among defined causes of the condition, PTHrP oversecretion is believed to be most common.

PTHrP is a single monomeric peptide that exists in several isoforms, ranging from approximately 60 to 173 amino acids, created by differential splicing and posttranslational processing by prohormone convertases.[46] PTHrP is produced in low concentrations by virtually all tissues for autocrine or paracrine activities.

The physiologic role of PTHrP remains incompletely understood. Its functions can be broadly divided into 4 categories, not all of which are present with all PTHrP isoforms or in all tissues: (1) transepithelial calcium transport, particularly in the kidney and mammary gland, (2) smooth muscle relaxation in the uterus, bladder, gastrointestinal tract, and arterial wall, (3) regulation of cellular proliferation, cellular differentiation, and apoptosis of multiple tissues, and (4) as an indispensable component of successful pregnancy and fetal development.[47] Embryonic gene deletion of PTHrP is lethal in mammals.

The diverse functions of PTHrp are mediated by a range of different receptors, which are activated by different portions of the PTHrP molecule. Among the many receptors that respond to PTHrP is the PTH1 receptor, owing to the fact that 8 of the 13 N-terminal amino acids of PTH and the 3 common PTHrP isoforms are identical. Because most of the actions of PTHrP in normal physiology are autocrine or paracrine, with circulating levels very low, receptor cross-talk becomes relevant only when there is extreme and sustained overproduction of PTHrP. This condition is seen occasionally in pregnancy and lactation, and rarely, in a variety of nonmalignant diseases. Most commonly, it is observed when tumors secrete PTHrP ectopically. Roughly correlated to physiologic production levels of PTHrP in corresponding healthy tissues, ectopic PTHrP production is most commonly seen in carcinomas of the breast, lung (squamous), head and neck (squamous), kidney, bladder, cervix, uterus, and ovary.[45] Neuroendocrine tumors may occasionally produce PTHrP. Most other carcinomas, sarcomas, and hematologic malignancies only sporadically produce PTHrP, with the notable exceptions of T-cell lymphomas and myeloma. Patients with HHM typically have increased PTHrP before treatment, and successful treatment leads to decreased PTHrP and increased PTH levels, with decreased serum calcium.

Measurement of PTHrP is useful in patients with suspected HHM, and workup of patients with hypercalcemia of unknown origin.[3] Depending on the population, up to 80% of patients with hypercalcemia associated with malignant tumors will have HHM. Of these, 50% to 70% may have increased PTHrP. These patients also usually show typical changes of PTH receptor activation, including hypercalcemia, hypophosphatemia, hypercalciuria, hypophosphaturia, and increased serum alkaline phosphatase. PTH levels in these patients are typically less than 30 pg/mL, and occasionally are undetectable.

In patients with biochemical findings suggestive of, but not confirmatory of, primary hyperparathyroidism with hypercalcemia, normal or near-normal serum phosphate, and inappropriately normal PTH level within the reference range, but with levels greater than 30 pg/mL, HHM should be considered a possibility, particularly if the patient is elderly or has a history of malignancy or risk factors for malignancy. Increased PTHrP in this type of patient is highly suggestive of HHM.

Serum PTHrP should not be used to exclude cancer or screen tumor patients for HHM. PTHrP may be increased normally in pregnant or lactating women and newborn infants. Nonmalignant conditions that may increase plasma PTHrP levels include systemic lupus erythematosus, human immunodeficiency virus-associated lymphadenopathy, lymphedema of the pleural cavities, and benign tumors of the ovary, kidney, and neuroendocrine system.[3] Because of the complexity of PTHrP isoforms, differences between various PTHrP assays, and the lack of a common calibration standard, PTHrP measurements performed with different assays cannot be compared easily. The complex isoform mixture of PTHrP may lead to pronounced nonlinearity on serial dilution. In these situations, an accurate measurement of PTHrP may be difficult. Like all immunometric assays, PTHrP assays are susceptible to falsely low results at extremely high concentrations ("hooking"), and to rare false-positive results owing to heterophile antibody interference.

## BONE TURNOVER MARKERS

BTMs have been proposed for use in prediction of bone loss, fracture risk, monitoring treatment response with osteoporotic drugs, monitoring compliance and adherence to therapy for osteoporosis, predicting adverse effects from drug therapy, and for diagnosis and prognosis in patients with metastatic bone disease.

BTMs measured in serum or urine reflect the rate of total body bone formation or bone resorption (**Table 1**). Bone formation markers include bone-specific alkaline phosphatase (BSAP), osteocalcin (OC), procollagen type I N-terminal propeptide (PINP), and procollagen type I C-terminal propeptide (PICP). Bone resorption markers result from degradation of type I collagen, and include the intermolecular crosslinks pyridinoline and deoxypyridinoline, C-terminal telopeptide (CTX), N-terminal telopeptide (NTX), and matrix metalloprotease–generated type I collagen fragments (CTX-matrix metalloprotease). Tartrate-resistant acid phosphatase isoform 5b is secreted by and reflects the total number of osteoclasts, and is the only non–collagen-derived bone resorption marker.

BTM variability may have both preanalytical and postanalytical sources. Preanalytical sources of variability are both uncontrollable and controllable (**Table 2**).

### Preanalytical Considerations

#### Age, gender, and menopausal status
At age 25, men have BTM levels higher than women.[48] These subsequently decrease with age to a nadir between 50 and 60 years, and then increase progressively again after the age of 60.[49] In contrast, BTM levels in premenopausal women are stable and lower than in age-matched men because women finish growing and attain peak bone mineral density earlier than men.[48] Postmenopausal women have mean BTM levels that are significantly higher compared with premenopausal women.

#### Ethnicity and geography
BTMs are 5% to 15% lower in perimenopausal and postmenopausal black women than in white women.[50] Within ethnic groups, 1 study found significantly different levels of OC, BSAP, and urinary CTX in Caucasian postmenopausal women from 10 countries.[51]

**Table 1**
**Bone turnover markers**

| Marker | Biological Material | Biological Variability CVi (%) | Biological Variability CVg (%) |
|---|---|---|---|
| Bone formation markers | | | |
| BSAP | Serum | 6.6[95] | 35.6[95] |
| OC | Serum | 9.1[95] | 30.9[95] |
| PICP | Serum | 8.6[96] | 17.6[96] |
| PINP | Serum | — | — |
| Bone resorption markers | | | |
| CTX | Serum, urine | — | — |
| NTX | Urine | 14.7[96] | 26.9[96] |
| TRAP-5b | Serum | 10.8[95] | 13.3[95] |

*Abbreviations:* CVg, interindividual variation; CVi, intraindividual variability; TRAP-5b, tartrate-resistant acid phosphatase isoform 5b.

*Modified from* Banfi G, Lombardi G, Colombini A, et al. Bone metabolism markers in sports medicine. Sports Med 2010;40:697–714.

**Table 2**
**Sources of preanalytical variability in BTMs**

| Source | Importance | Nature of Effect |
|---|---|---|
| Uncontrollable sources | | |
| Age | Very important | BTM increase with age in men and women |
| Menopausal status | Very important | BTM increase within a few months after the last menstrual period |
| Gender | Very important | BTM are higher in older women than older men |
| Fractures | Important—limits evaluation of case control studies | BTM increase after a fracture (maximal at 2–12 wk, but effect has for ≤52 wk) |
| Pregnancy and lactation | Important | BTM are increased during pregnancy; highest levels during third trimester, even higher postpartum |
| Drugs | Important: corticosteroids, anticonvulsants, heparin, GnRH agonists | BTM may be decreased (glucocorticoids) or increased (anticonvulsants) |
| Disease | Important: thyroid disease, diabetes, renal impairment, liver disease | BTM often increased (thyrotoxicosis, chronic kidney disease) |
| Bed rest/ immobility | Important | Bone formation markers decrease and resorption markers increase |
| Geography | Somewhat important | Small changes among countries, usually explained by differences in lifestyle |
| Ethnicity | Not important | Small changes, such as lower OC in African Americans vs Caucasians |
| Oral contraception | Not important, except in women >35 y | Lower values for BTM |
| Controllable sources | | |
| Circadian | Extremely important | Most striking for bone resorption markers; highest values in second half of night and on waking; lowest values in afternoon and evening |
| Fasting status | Important for specific markers | Feeding results in a decrease in BTM; eg, s-CTX decreases by 20% after breakfast |
| Exercise | Important—chronic and acute effects | Changes occur but depend on type of exercise and age of subjects |
| Menstrual | Not important | Small decreases in bone resorption and increases in bone formation during luteal phase |
| Seasonal | Not important for individual, but may be for longitudinal studies | Small decreases in BTM over winter |
| Diet | Not important | Small reduction in BTM immediately after calcium supplementation |

*Abbreviations:* BTM, bone turnover markers; GnRH, gonadotropin-releasing hormone.
*From* Vasikaran S, Eastell R, Bruyère O, et al. Markers of bone turnover for the prediction of fracture risk and monitoring of osteoporosis treatment: a need for international reference standards. Osteoporosis Int 2011;22:393; with permission.

### Pregnancy and lactation
At term, urinary NTX, CTX, and pyridinoline are 2- to 3-fold higher than before pregnancy or in the first trimester, whereas PICP, PINP, and BSAP are 35% to 100% higher in the third trimester.[52] In contrast, OC decreases in the first 2 trimesters and only returns to prepregnancy levels in the third trimester and after delivery.[53] BTMs decrease gradually for 6 to 12 months postpartum, but less rapidly in lactating mothers.[53,54] After weaning, BTMs gradually decrease to the same levels as in nonlactating women.[54]

### Drugs
Glucocorticoid therapy reduces serum OC and PICP by up to 40% to 50% within a few days of initiation of therapy,[55] but has little effect on bone resorption markers.[56] Long-term anticonvulsant treatment causes a significant increase in bone turnover; this is greater in men (50%–100%) than in women (10%–30%).[57] Thiazide-type diuretics reduce OC by 25% in postmenopausal women,[58] whereas gonadotropin-releasing hormone agonist treatment in premenopausal women increases urinary NTX by 2-fold.[59] One week of high-dose heparin therapy reduces OC by 40%,[60] but warfarin has no effect. The effect of oral contraceptives on BTMs seems to be age dependent. Results of studies in young women are conflicting. However, significant decreases of 15% to 30% are seen in older women aged 35 to 49 years.[61]

### Disease
BTMs are increased in primary hyperparathyroidism[62] and thyrotoxicosis.[63] In Paget disease of the bone, there is a large increase in total and bone alkaline phosphatase, but only a small increase in OC.[64] Patients with types 1 or 2 diabetes mellitus have lower BTM levels than nondiabetics.[65] Serum OC is significantly increased in renal impairment because OC is primarily metabolized by the kidney,[66] but may be decreased in liver disease.[67] BSAP and procollagen propeptide may increase in liver disease owing to impaired clearance by the liver. The increase seen in BSAP may be owing to cross-reactivity with the liver isoform in the assay.

### Fractures
Ivaska and colleagues[68] found that BTMs were not affected shortly after fractures occurred, but significantly increased 4 months after fractures, and remained increased for up to 12 months after fractures. Increases were most pronounced after hip fracture. However, serum OC was decreased 4 hours after hip fracture, possibly owing to the trauma-related increase in serum cortisol.[69]

### Immobility
Bone resorption markers increase significantly after 2 to 4 days of bed rest, and by 30% to 50% after 1 week, whereas bone formation markers remain unchanged or only increase slightly.[70] During remobilization, bone resorption markers gradually return to normal levels, and interestingly, PICP may increase paradoxically.[70]

### Circadian rhythm
Circadian variability has a greater impact on BTMs than other sources of variability. Most BTMs peak in the early morning between 0200 and 0800 hours, and reach a nadir between 1300 and 2300 hours, with the amplitude of the rhythm greater for resorption markers than formation markers.[71] Fasting results in a decrease of about 75% in the circadian rhythm of serum and urinary CTX.[72]

### Menstrual cycle
Gass and colleagues[73] reported that serum CTX is higher in the early and midfollicular phase than during the midluteal and late luteal phases, with a difference of about 9.5%

between the follicular and luteal phases. BSAP is 7.2% lower[74] in women close to ovulation compared with those at the beginning or end of the menstrual cycle. These changes are small and may be regarded as insignificant.

### Seasonal variation

Seasonal variability of BTMs is low, and may account for up to a 20% difference between winter and summer months.[74] In winter, serum CTX and BSAP and urinary pyridinoline and deoxypyridinoline are highest, with a nadir in serum 25-OHD levels and rise in serum intact PTH, but OC and PICP seem to have no seasonal rhythm.

### Diet

Nakamura and colleagues[75] reported that a high-sodium diet has no effect on BTMs, but Park and colleagues[76] observed increases of 21.3% in serum CTX and 15.7% in serum OC in those with high urinary sodium excretion ($\geq$2 g/d). Calcium supplementation decreases urinary deoxypyridinoline and NTX and serum CTX and PINP,[75] whereas vitamin D supplementation decreases serum OC, BSAP and tartrate-resistant acid phosphatase isoform 5b.[77]

### Exercise

Eliakim and colleagues[78] found increases of 10% to 20% in formation markers (BSAP, PICP, and OC) and a decrease of 17% of urinary NTX, with no change in serum CTX after 5 weeks of aerobic exercise. After an acute bout of exercise, serum CTX but not PINP and BSAP are increased for 4 days.[79] Subjects should be asked about their exercise habits and refrain from exercise for at least 24 hours before samples are taken for BTM measurement.

### Postanalytical Considerations

The use of reference intervals with BTMs is limited owing to their large degrees of variability between and within individuals. Biological variability within the individual, measured by the coefficient of variation CVi, is the random natural variation around an individual's homeostatic set point. The CVi of the markers are the key factors in determining how much a marker's concentration must vary between 2 results before the change is considered to be clinically significant. This difference is called the least significant change (LSC). In general, serum markers show less day to day variability than markers of bone turnover measured in urine. Serum markers vary by around 10% to 15%, compared with urinary markers, which vary by around 20% to 30%.[80]

### Bone formation markers

**Bone-specific alkaline phosphatase** Alkaline phosphatase is a ubiquitous membrane-bound enzyme that plays an important role in osteoid matrix formation and mineralization. Several isoforms originate from the liver, bone, intestine, spleen, kidney, and placenta. In adults with normal liver function, approximately 50% of serum total alkaline phosphatase in serum is derived from the liver, and the remaining 50% arises from bone. In children and adolescents, BSAP predominates, with up to 90% of serum total alkaline phosphatase coming from bone because of rapid skeletal growth. Serum BSAP has a reported CVi of 4.2%, with an optimal manufacturer-reported LSC of 25%.[81] Advantages of BSAP are low circadian variation owing to its half-life of 1 to 2 days, sample stability, wide availability of assays, and lack of renal clearance.[82] However, cross-reactivity of 15% to 20% with the liver isoform immunoassays results in artificially high levels of BSAP in patients with liver disease.

**Osteocalcin** OC is a hydroxyapatite-binding protein exclusively synthesized by osteoblasts, odontoblasts, and hypertrophic chondrocytes. Serum levels of immunoreactive OC correlate well with bone formation rate assessed by histomorphometry.[83] Patients do not need to be fasting for OC measurement.[72] However, OC has a circadian rhythm, peaking at approximately 4 AM, and is affected by renal clearance. OC concentrations are decreased by freeze–thaw cycles and hemolysis. OC in the serum is rapidly degraded to fragments that are detected by antibody-based assays, along with the full-length molecule. Existing assays measuring OC have low analytical variability of less than 10%.[84] Assays recognizing both the intact molecule and the large N-terminal fragment (N-MID, amino acids 1–43) are more stable, sensitive, and reproducible compared with assays detecting only intact OC, which are particularly affected by in vitro degradation.[83]

**N-terminal and C-terminal propeptides of type I procollagen** Type I collagen is synthesized by osteoblasts in the form of pre-procollagen, and secreted as procollagen into the extracellular space, where it is cleaved at both its amino-terminal and carboxy-terminal ends to give rise to PINP and PICP. PICP and PINP are cleared by liver reticuloendothelial cells via the mannose receptor and the scavenger receptor, respectively.[85,86] As a marker, PINP is preferred to PICP because the mannose receptor is regulated by growth hormone and thyroid hormone, thus complicating interpretation in subjects with pituitary or thyroid dysfunction.[85] PINP has several advantages, including its low diurnal variability and stability at room temperature.[87] Patients do not need to be fasting, and its clearance is unaffected by renal dysfunction.[86] The intraindividual coefficient of variation is 12.4%.[88] PINP is released into the circulation in a trimeric form that is unstable at 37°C, and rapidly converted to its monomeric form. Assays measuring trimeric and monomeric forms have similar precision, intraindividual variation, and an LSC of 20%.[87] The International Osteoporosis Foundation and International Federation of Clinical Chemistry and Laboratory Medicine recommend serum PINP as the preferred marker for bone formation.[89]

### Bone resorption markers

NTX and CTX are discussed herein because they are widely used clinically compared with other bone resorption markers.

**Amino-terminal cross-linking telopeptide of type I collagen** NTX is a type I collagen breakdown product from osteoclastic bone resorption that can be measured in either serum or urine with immunoassays using a monoclonal antibody specific for an N-terminal epitope.[90] Serum NTX is less sensitive than urinary NTX in detecting changes induced by antiresorptive therapies. NTX fragments are stable in urine for days, and samples can be stored at −20°C for years without significant deterioration. Dietary influences are small, but there is significant circadian variation of up to 20%, and standardized sampling with a fasting second morning void is important.[91] Therefore, measurement of NTX in 24-hour urine has the advantage of overcoming variability owing to circadian changes, and the results are less sensitive to dietary collagen intake.[90] However, the CVi of urinary NTX is high (>20%) owing to additional variance from creatinine adjustment.[92]

**Carboxy-terminal cross-linking telopeptide of type I collagen** CTX is a C-terminal telopeptide composed of an octapeptide of the C-terminus of the $\alpha_1$ type I collagen. The CTX–$\alpha_1$ chain of type I collagen undergoes β-isomerization and racemization, which is an age-dependent process. Urine and serum CTX correlate well, but the serum assay eliminates the need for urine collection and creatinine measurement, therefore minimizing variability.[92] The CVi is also lower for serum CTX (<15%) compared with urine CTX (23%–48%).[92] Disadvantages of serum CTX include pronounced circadian variability, with a peak in the early morning and a nadir in the afternoon, with food intake leading to a decreased level.[72] Therefore, sample collection needs to be standardized and performed in the fasting state and at the same time in the morning. The development of an automated assay has greatly reduced the analytical variability to less than 5%.[93] The assay for serum β-CrossLaps (Roche Diagnostics) has a reported precision of 5% and LSC of 27%.[94] The International Osteoporosis Foundation and International Federation of Clinical Chemistry and Laboratory Medicine recommend serum CTX as the preferred marker for bone resorption.[89]

## SUMMARY

Biochemical testing is critical for the diagnosis and management of skeletal disorders. Focused evaluation of serum and urine minerals, serum vitamin D, PTH, and PTHrP, and serum and urine BTMs is necessary in evaluating bone disease of many different types. Without these assessments, elucidation of the pathophysiology of these disorders would not be possible.

Of course, other biochemical assessments are also often used in evaluation of skeletal disorders that could not be addressed here owing to space limitation. Serum gonadal sex steroids, complete blood count with differential, erythrocyte sedimentation rate, serum and urine protein electrophoresis, serum and urine cortisol, serum tryptase, serum magnesium, and urine N-methylhistamine, as well as other tests in the appropriate setting, may all be required for evaluation of different patients in the appropriate clinical circumstance. The challenge remaining for the clinician is to judiciously select the highest yield tests for the clinical situation to confirm the diagnosis and to guide therapy.

## REFERENCES

1. McClung MR. Emerging therapies for osteoporosis. Endocrinol Metab (Seoul) 2015;30:429–35.
2. Bone health and osteoporosis: a report of the Surgeon General. Rockville (MD): Office of the Surgeon General (US); 2004.
3. Horwitz MJ, Hodak SP, Stewart AF. Non-parathyroid hypercalcemia. In: Rosen CJ, editor. Primer on the metabolic bone diseases and disorders of mineral metabolism. 8th edition. Washington, DC: American Society for Bone and Mineral Research; 2008. p. 562–71.
4. Shoback DM. Hypoparathyroidism in the differential diagnosis of hypocalcemia. In: Bilezikian JP, editor. The parathyroids. 3rd edition. Amsterdam: Elsevier; 2015. p. 687–96.
5. Streeten EA, Jaimungal S. The differential diagnosis of hypercalcemia. In: Bilezikian JP, editor. The parathyroids. 3rd edition. Amsterdam: Elsevier; 2015. p. 607–16.
6. Silverberg SJ, Clarke BL, Peacock M, et al. Current issues in the presentation of asymptomatic primary hyperparathyroidism: proceedings of the Fourth International Workshop. J Clin Endocrinol Metab 2014;99:3580–94.
7. Bilezikian JP, Khan A, Potts JT Jr, et al. Hypoparathyroidism in the adult: epidemiology, diagnosis, pathophysiology, target-organ involvement, treatment, and challenges for future research. J Bone Miner Res 2011;26:2317–37.

8. Fitzpatrick LA. Acute primary hyperparathyroidism. In: Bilezikian JP, editor. The parathyroids. 3rd edition. Amsterdam: Elsevier; 2015. p. 401–7.

9. Bandeira F, Correa A. Clinical presentation of primary hyperparathyroidism: a global perspective. In: Bilezikian JP, editor. The parathyroids. 3rd edition. Amsterdam: Elsevier; 2015. p. 309–15.

10. Brown EM. Control of parathyroid hormone secretion by its key physiologic regulators. In: Bilezikian JP, editor. The parathyroids. 3rd edition. Amsterdam: Elsevier; 2015. p. 101–18.

11. Coe FL, Worcester EM, Evan AP. Idiopathic hypercalciuria and formation of calcium renal stones. Nat Rev Nephrol 2016;12:519–33.

12. Reilly RF, Huang CL. The mechanism of hypocalciuria with NaCl cotransporter inhibition. Nat Rev Nephrol 2011;7:669–74.

13. Ruppe MD, Jan de Beur S. Disorders of phosphate homeostasis. In: Rosen CJ, editor. Primer on the metabolic bone diseases and disorders of mineral metabolism. 8th edition. Washington, DC: American Society for Bone and Mineral Research; 2013. p. 601–12.

14. White KE, Econs MJ. Fibroblast growth factore-23 (FGF23). In: Rosen CJ, editor. Primer on the metabolic bone diseases and disorders of mineral metabolism. 8th edition. Washington, DC: American Society for Bone and Mineral Research; 2013. p. 188–94.

15. Schleicher RL, Sternberg MR, Lacher DA, et al. The vitamin D status of the US population from 1988 to 2010 using standardized serum concentrations of 25-hydroxyvitamin D shows recent modest increases. Am J Clin Nutr 2016;104:454–61.

16. Gallagher JC. Vitamin D insufficiency and deficiency. In: Rosen CJ, editor. Primer on the metabolic bone diseases and disorders of mineral metabolism. 8th edition. Washington, DC: American Society for Bone and Mineral Research; 2013. p. 624–31.

17. Gallagher JC. Vitamin D and falls - the dosage conundrum. Nat Rev Endocrinol 2016;12:680–4.

18. Chang CY, Rosenthal DI, Mitchell DM, et al. Imaging findings of metabolic bone disease. Radiographics 2016;36:1871–87.

19. Bickle D, Adams JS, Christakos S. Vitamin D: production, metabolism, mechanism of action, and clinical requirements. In: Rosen CJ, editor. Primer on the metabolic bone diseases and disorders of mineral metabolism. 8th edition. Washington, DC: American Society for Bone and Mineral Research; 2013. p. 235–47.

20. Tebben PJ, Singh RJ, Kumar R. Vitamin D-mediated hypercalcemia: mechanisms, diagnosis, and treatment. Endocr Rev 2016;37:521–47.

21. Bieglmayer C, Kaczirek K, Prager G, et al. Parathyroid hormone monitoring during total parathyroidectomy for renal hyperparathyroidism: pilot study of the impact of renal function and assay specificity. Clin Chem 2006;52:1112–9.

22. Murray TM, Rao LG, Divieti P, et al. Parathyroid hormone secretion and action: evidence for discrete receptors for the carboxy-terminal region and related biological actions of carboxyl-terminal ligands. Endocr Rev 2005;26:78–113.

23. D'Amour P, Brossard JH. Carboxyl-terminal parathyroid hormone fragments: role in parathyroid hormone physiopathology. Curr Opin Nephrol Hypertens 2005;14:330–6.

24. Souberbielle J-C, Friedlander G, Cormier C. Practical considerations in PTH testing. Clin Chim Acta 2006;366:81–9.

25. D'Amour P, Brossard JH, Räkel A, et al. Evidence that the amino-terminal composition of non-(1-84) parathyroid hormone fragments starts before position 19. Clin Chem 2005;51:169–76.

26. Nussbaum S, Zahradnik R, Lavigne J, et al. Highly sensitive two-site immunora-diometric assay of parathyrin, and its clinical utility in evaluating patients with hy-percalcemia. Clin Chem 1987;33:1364–7.
27. Wang M, Herez G, Sherrard D, et al. Relationship between intact PTH (1–84) parathyroid hormone and bone histomorphometry parameters in dialysis patients without aluminum toxicity. Am J Kidney Dis 1995;26:836–44.
28. Lepage R, Roy L, Brossard JH, et al. A non (1–84) circulating parathyroid hor-mone fragment interferes significantly with intact PTH commercial assay mea-surements in uremic samples. Clin Chem 1998;44:805–9.
29. Gao P, Scheibel S, D'Amour P, et al. Development of a novel immunoradiometric assay exclusively for biologically active whole parathyroid hormone 1–84: impli-cation for improvement of accurate assessment of parathyroid function. J Bone Miner Res 2001;16:605–14.
30. Räkel A, Brossard JH, Patenaude JV, et al. Overproduction of an amino-terminal form of PTH distinct from human PTH (1–84) in a case of severe primary hyper-parathyroidism: influence of medical treatment and surgery. Clin Endocrinol 2005;62:721–7.
31. Rubin M, D'Amour P, Cantor T, et al. A molecular form of PTH distinct from PTH (1–84) is produced in parathyroid carcinoma. J Bone Miner Res 2004;19(Suppl 1):S327.
32. Omar H, Chamberlin A, Walker V, et al. Immulite 2000 parathyroid hormone assay: stability of parathyroid hormone in EDTA blood kept at room temperature for 48 h. Ann Clin Biochem 2001;38:561–3.
33. Sturgeon CM, Ellis AR, Al-Sadie R. UK NEQAS annual review 2005. Edinburgh (United Kingdom): NEQAS; 2005.
34. Lafferty FW, Hamlin CR, Corrado KR, et al. Primary hyperparathyroidism with a low–normal, atypical serum parathyroid hormone as shown by discordant immu-noassay curves. J Clin Endocrinol Metab 2006;91:3826–9.
35. Boudou P, Ibrahim F, Cormier C, et al. Unexpected serum parathyroid hormone profiles in some patients with primary hyperparathyroidism. Clin Chem 2006; 52:757–60.
36. Monier-Faugere MC, Geng Z, Mawad H, et al. Improved assessment of bone turnover by the PTH-(1–84)/large C-PTH fragments ratio in ESRD patients. Kidney Int 2001;60:1460–8.
37. Coen G, Bonucci E, Ballanti P, et al. PTH 1–84 and PTH '7–84' in the noninvasive diagnosis of renal bone disease. Am J Kidney Dis 2002;40:348–54.
38. Salusky IB, Goodman WG, Kuizon BD, et al. Similar predictive value of bone turn-over using first- and second-generation immunometric PTH assays in pediatric patients treated with peritoneal dialysis. Kid Int 2003;63:1801–8.
39. Lehmann G, Stein G, Huller M, et al. Specific measurement of PTH (1–84) in various forms of renal osteodystrophy (ROD) as assessed by bone histomorph-ometry. Kid Int 2005;68:1206–14.
40. National Kidney Foundation. K/DOQI clinical practice guidelines for bone meta-bolism and disease in chronic kidney disease. Am J Kidney Dis 2003;42:S1–201.
41. Carneiro-Pla DM, Solorzano CC, Irvin GL III. Consequences of targeted parathy-roidectomy guided by localization studies without intraoperative parathyroid hor-mone monitoring. J Am Coll Surg 2006;202:715–22.
42. Hortin GL, Carter AB. Intraoperative parathyroid hormone testing: survey of testing program characteristics. Arch Pathol Lab Med 2002;126:1045.
43. Lam A, Kerr PD. Parathyroid hormone: an early predictor of post-thyroidectomy hypocalcemia. Laryngoscope 2003;113:2196.

44. McLeod IK, Arciero C, Noordzij JP, et al. The use of rapid parathyroid hormone assay in predicting postoperative hypocalcemia after total or completion thyroidectomy. Thyroid 2006;16:259–65.
45. Wysolmerski JJ. Parathyroid hormone-related protein. In: Rosen CJ, editor. Primer on the metabolic bone diseases and disorders of mineral metabolism. 8th edition. Washington, DC: American Society for Bone and Mineral Research; 2013. p. 215–23.
46. Strewler GJ. The physiology of parathyroid hormone-related protein. N Engl J Med 2000;342:177–85.
47. Philbrick WM, Wysolmerski JJ, Galbraith S, et al. Defining the roles of parathyroid hormone-related protein in normal physiology. Physiol Rev 1996;76:127–73.
48. Gundberg CM, Looker AC, Nieman SD, et al. Patterns of osteocalcin and bone alkaline phosphatase by age, gender, and race or ethnicity. Bone 2002;31:703–8.
49. Fatayerji D, Eastell R. Age-related changes in bone turnover in men. J Bone Miner Res 1999;14:1203–10.
50. Perry HM III, Horowitz M, Morley JE, et al. Aging and bone metabolism in African American and Caucasian women. J Clin Endocrinol Metab 1996;81:1108–17.
51. Cohen FJ, Eckert S, Mitlak BH. Geographic differences in bone turnover: data from a multinational study in healthy postmenopausal women. Calcif Tissue Int 1998;63:277–82.
52. Naylor KE, Iqbal P, Fledelius C, et al. The effect of pregnancy on bone density and bone turnover. J Bone Miner Res 2000;15:129–37.
53. Cole DE, Gundberg CM, Stirk LJ, et al. Changing osteocalcin concentrations during pregnancy and lactation: implications for maternal mineral metabolism. J Clin Endocrinol Metab 1987;65:290–4.
54. Kalkwarf HJ, Specker BL, Ho M. Effects of calcium supplementation on calcium homeostasis and bone turnover in lactating women. J Clin Endocrinol Metab 1999;84:464–70.
55. Oikarinen A, Autio P, Vuori J, et al. Systemic glucocorticoid treatment decreases serum concentrations of carboxyterminal propeptide of type I procollagen and aminoterminal propeptide of type III procollagen. Br J Dermatol 1992;126:172–8.
56. Gram J, Junker P, Nielsen HK, et al. Effects of short-term treatment with prednisolone and calcitriol on bone and mineral metabolism in normal men. Bone 1998; 23:297–302.
57. Valimaki MJ, Tiihonen M, Laitinen K, et al. Bone mineral density measured by dual-energy x-ray absorptiometry and novel markers of bone formation and resorption in patients on antiepileptic drugs. J Bone Miner Res 1994;9:631–7.
58. Dawson-Hughes B, Harris S. Thiazides and seasonal bone change in healthy postmenopausal women. Bone Miner 1993;21:41–51.
59. Marshall LA, Cain DF, Dmowski WP, et al. Urinary N-telopeptides to monitor bone resorption while on GnRH agonist therapy. Obstet Gynecol 1996;87:350–4.
60. Cantini F, Niccoli L, Bellandi F, et al. Effects of short-term, high dose, heparin therapy on biochemical markers of bone metabolism. Clin Rheumatol 1995;14:663–6.
61. Garnero P, Sornay-Rendu E, Delmas PD. Decreased bone turnover in oral contraceptive users. Bone 1995;16:499–503.
62. Cortet B, Cortet C, Blanckaert F, et al. Bone ultrasonometry and turnover markers in primary hyperparathyroidism. Calcif Tissue Int 2000;66:11–5.
63. Pantazi H, Papapetrou PD. Changes in parameters of bone and mineral metabolism during therapy for hyperthyroidism. J Clin Endocrinol Metab 2000;85: 1099–106.

64. Duda RJ, O'Brien JF, Katzman JA, et al. Concurrent assay of circulating bone Gla-protein and bone alkaline phosphatase: effect of sex, age, and metabolic bone disease. J Clin Endocrinol Metab 1998;66:951–7.
65. Farr JN, Khosla S. Determinants of bone strength and quality in diabetes mellitus in humans. Bone 2016;82:28–34.
66. Delmas PD, Wilson DM, Mann KG, et al. Effect of renal function on plasma levels of bone Gla-protein. J Clin Endocrinol Metab 1983;57:1028–30.
67. Steinberg KK, Bonkovsky HL, Caudill SP, et al. Osteocalcin and bone alkaline phosphatase in the serum of women with liver disease. Ann Clin Lab Sci 1991; 21:305–14.
68. Ivaska KK, Gerdhem P, Akesson K, et al. Effect of fracture on bone turnover markers: a longitudinal study comparing marker levels before and after injury in 113 elderly women. J Bone Miner Res 2007;22:1155–64.
69. Barton RN, Weijers JW, Horan MA. Increase rates of cortisol production and urinary free cortisol excretion in elderly women 2 weeks after proximal femur fracture. Eur J Clin Invest 1993;23:171–6.
70. Zerwekh JE, Ruml LA, Gottschalk F, et al. The effects of twelve weeks of bed rest on bone histology, biochemical markers of bone turnover, and calcium homeostasis in eleven normal subjects. J Bone Miner Res 1998;13:159–61.
71. Delmas PD, Eastell R, Garnero P, et al. The use of biochemical markers of bone turnover in osteoporosis. Committee of Scientific Advisors of the International Osteoporosis Foundation. Osteoporos Int 2000;11(Suppl):S2–17.
72. Schlemmer A, Hassager C. Acute fasting diminishes the circadian rhythm of biochemical markers of bone resorption. Eur J Endocrinol 1999;140:332–7.
73. Gass ML, Kagan R, Kohles JD, et al. Bone turnover marker profile in relation to the menstrual cycle of premenopausal healthy women. Menopause 2008;15: 667–75.
74. Woitge HW, Scheidt-Nave C, Kissling C, et al. Seasonal variation of biochemical indexes of bone turnover: results of a population-based study. J Clin Endocrinol Metab 1998;83:68–75.
75. Nakamura K, Hori Y, Nashimoto M, et al. Dietary calcium, sodium, phosphate, and protein and bone metabolism in elderly Japanese women: a pilot study using the duplicate portion sampling method. Nutrition 2004;20:340–5.
76. Park SM, Joung JY, Cho YY, et al. Effect of high dietary sodium on bone turnover markers and urinary calcium excretion in Korean postmenopausal women with low bone mass. Eur J Clin Nutr 2015;69:361–6.
77. Herrmann W, Kirsch SH, Kruse V, et al. One year B and D vitamins supplementation improves metabolic bone markers. Clin Chem Lab Med 2013;51:639–47.
78. Eliakim A, Raisz LG, Brasel JA, et al. Evidence for increased bone formation following a brief endurance-type training intervention in adolescent males. J Bone Miner Res 1997;12:1708–13.
79. Scott JP, Sale C, Greeves JP, et al. The effect of training status on the metabolic response of bone to an acute bout of exhaustive treadmill running. J Clin Endocrinol Metab 2010;95:3918–25.
80. Garnero P, Mullerman D, Munoz F, et al. Long-term variability of markers of bone turnover in postmenopausal women and implication for their clinical use: the OFELY study. J Bone Miner Res 2003;18:1789–94.
81. Ostase product information. ullerton (CA): Beckman Coulter Inc.; 1998.
82. Brown JP, Albert C, Nassar BA, et al. Bone turnover markers in the management of postmenopausal osteoporosis. Clin Chem 2009;42:929–42.

83. Delmas PD, Malaval L, Arlot ME, et al. Serum bone Gla-protein compared to bone histomorphometry in endocrine diseases. Bone 1985;6:339–41.
84. Schmidt-Gayk H, Spanuth E, Kotting J, et al. Performance evaluation of auto-mated assays for beta-CrossLaps, N-MID-Osteocalcin and intact parathyroid hor-mone (BIOROSE Multicenter Study). Clin Chem Lab Med 2004;42:90–5.
85. Smedsrod B, Melkko J, Risteli L, et al. Circulating C-terminal propeptide of type I procollagen is cleared mainly via the mannose receptor in liver endothelial cells. Biochem J 1990;271:345–50.
86. Melkko J, Hellevik T, Risteli L, et al. Clearance of NH2-terminal propeptides of type I and III procollagen is a physiological function of the scavenger receptor in liver endothelial cells. J Exp Med 1994;179:405–12.
87. Garnero P, Vergnaud P, Hoyle N. Evaluation of a fully automated serum assay for total N-terminal propeptide of type I collagen in postmenopausal osteoporosis. Clin Chem 2008;54:188–96.
88. Scariono JK, Garry PJ, Montoya GD, et al. Critical differences in the serial mea-surement of three biochemical markers of bone turnover in the sera of pre- and postmenopausal women. Clin Biochem 2001;34:639–44.
89. Vasikaran S, Cooper C, Eastell R, et al. International Osteoporosis Foundation and International Federation of Clinical Chemistry and Laboratory Medicine posi-tion on bone marker standards in osteoporosis. Clin Chem 2011;49:1271–4.
90. Clemens JD, Herrick MV, Singer FR, et al. Evidence that serum NTX (collagen-type I N-telopeptides) can act as an immune chemical marker of bone resorption. Clin Chem 1997;43:2058–63.
91. Gertz BJ, Clemens JD, Holland SD, et al. Application of a new serum assay for type I collagen cross-linked N-telopeptide: assessment of diurnal changes in bone turnover with and without alendronate treatment. Calcif Tissue Int 1998; 63:102–6.
92. Herrmann M, Siebel M. The amino- and carboxyterminal cross-linked telopepti-des of collagen type I, NTX and CTX-I: a comparative review. Clin Chim Acta 2008;393:57–75.
93. Garnero P, Borel O, Delmas PD. Evaluation of a fully automated serum assay for C-terminal cross-linking telopeptide of type I collagen in osteoporosis. Clin Chem 2001;47:694–702.
94. Okabe R, Nakatsuka K, Inaba M, et al. Clinical evaluation of the Elecsys beta-CrossLaps serum assay, a new assay for degradation products of type I collagen C-telopeptides. Clin Chem 2001;47:1410–4.
95. Panteghini M, Pagani F. Biological variation in bone-derived biochemical markers in serum. Scand J Clin Lab Invest 1995;55:609–16.
96. Panteghini M. Variabilità analitica e biologica degli indicadori biochimica di rimo-dellamento osseo. Ligand Assay 1998;3:176–8.

# Biochemical Testing in Neuroendocrine Tumors

Vidya Aluri, MD, MS, Joseph S. Dillon, MB, BCh*

## KEYWORDS

- Neuroendocrine tumor • Carcinoid • Tumor marker • Diagnostic test
- Prognostic indicator • Disease monitoring

## KEY POINTS

- Neuroendocrine tumors secrete chemicals that can be used as circulating biomarkers.
- Tumors originating from different sites may differ in the tumor markers secreted.
- All tumor markers have potential for false-positive and false-negative results.

Neuroendocrine cells are widely distributed throughout the body. They are characterized by the ability to produce, store, and secrete peptides and biogenic amines, in response to neural, chemical, and other stimuli. Most tumors arising from these cells are found in the intestine (particularly the jejunoileum), pancreas, and lung. As with tumors arising in other endocrine organs, the neuroendocrine tumors (NET) may be functional (secreting 1 or more products associated with a clinical syndrome) or nonfunctional. Nonfunctional tumors either fail to secrete any known product, or may secrete a product with no known associated clinical outcome. Diagnosis of NET involves analysis of the patients' clinical features, imaging (including somatostatin receptor-based imaging), biomarkers, and biopsy. Blood or urine concentrations of amines and peptides secreted by NET have proved to be useful biomarkers for the diagnosis and monitoring of these tumors. Although biomarkers may include cellular, biochemical, or molecular alterations that are measurable in biological media such as human tissues, cells, or fluid, we focus herein on currently available biochemical testing of blood or urine for gastroenteropancreatic (GEP) and lung NET.

Timely diagnosis of NET can be challenging for multiple reasons:

1. The incidence of these tumors is low, although it does seem to be increasing. Incidence of NET from all sites was 5 in 100,000 in 2004, increased from 1 in 100,000 in 1973.[1]

The authors have nothing to disclose.
Division of Endocrinology, University of Iowa, 200 Hawkins Drive, Iowa City, Iowa 52242, USA
* Corresponding author.
*E-mail address:* joseph-dillon@uiowa.edu

2. The primary tumor may be very small and is often metastatic at the time of diagnosis. Data from US and European cancer registries suggest that 30% to 75% of patients have distant metastases at the time of diagnosis.[1–3]

3. Clinical presentation may vary depending on the site of origin of the primary tumor. Traditionally, NET are described as arising from the foregut (bronchopulmonary, thymus, gastric, proximal duodenum, pancreas), midgut (distal duodenum, jejunum, ileum, ascending colon), or hindgut (distal colon, rectum). Primary tumors arising from these different anatomic zones differ in their tumor secretions (**Table 1**). For example, tumors originating in the midgut secrete serotonin and are more likely than tumors of other origins to present with carcinoid syndrome. Carcinoid syndrome, when present, may include the following symptoms: flushing (94%), diarrhea (78%), abdominal cramping (50%), valvular heart disease (50%), telangiectasia (25%), wheezing (15%), or edema (19%).[4–6] Pulmonary tumors are less likely to secrete serotonin (although they may secrete the serotonin precursor, 5-hydroxytryptophan) and more likely to secrete histamine. Although foregut tumors can present with flushing and wheezing, the full carcinoid syndrome with diarrhea is unusual. Hindgut tumors rarely secrete serotonin or cause carcinoid syndrome.

4. The clinical presentation may vary between tumors of the same originating site, based on the tumor grade and stage. Some biochemical tests have been suggested as markers of tumor grade or differentiation, for example, neuron-specific enolase. Although only about 10% of NET present with features of carcinoid syndrome, this number increases with greater tumor bulk (later stage), especially when liver metastatic disease increases.

Because of the low incidence, early diagnosis requires highly sensitive and specific biomarkers. It should be noted, however, that although the incidence of NET is low, the prevalence is relatively high because of slow tumor progression. The estimated prevalence is 3-fold that of pancreatic cancer and is greater than that of esophageal and gastric cancers combined.[1] Because of relatively slower progression and prolonged follow-up period, markers of tumor growth, response to therapy, prognosis, and differentiation state are important.

**Table 1**
**Neuroendocrine tumor sites of origin, potential associated symptoms, and specific biomarker tests**

| Primary Tumor Location | Symptom | Test |
| --- | --- | --- |
| Bronchopulmonary and thymic | Local symptoms<br>Flushing, wheezing<br>Cushing syndrome | CgA, serotonin,<br>5-HIAA, 5 hydroxytryptophan<br>ACTH, cortisol |
| Jejunoileal | Local symptoms<br>Carcinoid syndrome | Serotonin<br>CgA<br>Pancreastatin<br>NKA |
| Colorectal | Local symptoms<br>Incidental findings | CgA |
| Pancreaticoduodenal | | |
| Nonfunctional | Local symptoms/incidental | CgA, (serotonin), PP |
| Functional (see **Table 2**) | Specific syndrome | See **Table 2** |

*Abbreviations:* 5-HIAA, 5-hydroxyindoleacetic acid; ACTH, adrenocorticotrophic hormone; CgA, chromogranin A; NKA, neurokinin A; PP, pancreatic polypeptide.

More than 20 different secretory products of NET have been described (**Tables 2 and 3**).[7] Many of these are not assayed in commercial laboratories. Thus, although certain tumor secretions, for example, chromogranin A (CgA), are widely expressed by NET of different tissues, there are cases of clearly functional tumors with negative biochemical testing for the common tumoral secretions. Thus, owing to the heterogeneity of the originating cells and their secretory capacities for amines and peptides, a single biomarker may not allow accurate diagnosis or follow-up.

Most of the available biochemical tests do not predict behavior of the tumor or prognosticate survival well. Furthermore, all of the specific biochemical testing used for NET diagnosis and monitoring have specific causes of inaccuracy (see **Table 3**). For different assays, these issues include the effect of diet, fasting state, technique of phlebotomy, and handling of sample. Standardization of the assays in different laboratories is frequently a concern. This is particularly the case with CgA in the United States, where there are multiple assays in commercial use. In Europe, this assay has been standardized across countries and is more clinically useful in follow-up.

## BIOMARKERS IN NEUROENDOCRINE TUMORS

Some patients present with well-defined symptoms associated with overproduction of circulating biologically active hormones, peptides, and amines (see **Table 2**). This situation is similar to other functional endocrine tumors, for example, prolactinoma, where specific symptoms are associated with specific hormonal secretion. In these patients with functional NET, the specific clinical presentation should guide the initial choice of biochemical testing. Besides NET associated with carcinoid syndrome (most frequently midgut in origin), most of the functional NET are pancreatic endocrine tumors, and assessment of the specific hormone or related fragments allows diagnosis. Other NET may not have an identifiable clinical syndrome and may be asymptomatic or cause local symptoms like obstruction or bleeding. For these tumors, screening tests might include CgA, urine or plasma 5-hydroxyindoleacetic acid, or blood or serum serotonin.

Because of the difficulties of choosing an optimal biomarker, along with the interpretation issues of each test, professional societies have not provided strong recommendations related to minimal biochemical testing. In general, guidelines from expert committees (European and American NET societies and the National Comprehensive Cancer Network) suggest consideration of CgA for small intestinal, nonfunctional pancreatic, pulmonary, high-grade GEP-NET, and metastases of unknown origin. A 24-hour urine 5-hydroxyindoleacetic acid test could be considered for small intestinal and pulmonary NET and for all tumors with carcinoid syndrome. Pancreatic polypeptide is recommended for nonfunctional pancreatic NET, and neuron-specific enolase can be considered for high-grade tumors. Specific markers to assess functionality in patients with syndromes should be guided by the specific symptoms (eg, urine or plasma 5-hydroxyindoleacetic acid for carcinoid syndrome, insulin for hypoglycemia, etc). Our own practice is to test a broad range of markers initially and then follow markers that are positive.

### Novel Neuroendocrine Tumor Biomarkers

Despite the development of multiple biomarkers and imaging studies, the diagnosis of NET is often delayed by years and the disease is frequently metastasized at the time of diagnosis. This observation suggests that the existing markers are not sufficiently sensitive for diagnosis. There is also an unmet need for markers that offer greater diagnostic and prognostic value, as well as information about response to therapy. An

**Table 2**
Specific syndromes associated with pancreaticoduodenal NET tumor sites and suggested biochemical testing

| Syndromes | Site of Tumor | Symptoms | Diagnosis | Marker |
|---|---|---|---|---|
| Insulinoma | Pancreas | Hyperinsulinemic hypoglycemic syndrome | Hypoglycemia with nonsuppressed insulin in a 72-h fast | Insulin<br>Proinsulin<br>C-peptide |
| Gastrinoma/ZES | Duodenum<br>Pancreas | Recurrent peptic ulcers<br>Diarrhea | Fasting plasma gastrin >1000 pg/mL; gastric pH <2.5 | Gastrin |
| Glucagonoma | Pancreas | Glucose intolerance<br>Weight loss Erythematous rash<br>Venous thrombosis | Plasma glucagon levels 500–1000 pg/mL | Glucagon |
| VIPoma | Pancreas<br>Pheochromocytoma | Secretory diarrhea<br>Hypokalemia<br>Dehydration | Plasma VIP >200 pg/mL | VIP |
| Somatostatinoma | Pancreas<br>Duodenum | Diabetes mellitus<br>Gallstones<br>Diarrhea<br>Weight loss<br>Steatorrhea | Increased plasma somatostatin with histologically confirmed NET | Somatostatin |
| Cushing | Pancreas<br>Lung/thymus | Easy bruising<br>Facial plethora<br>Myopathy<br>Purple striae<br>Hypertension<br>Osteoporosis | Urine 24-h cortisol, late night salivary cortisol, or 1 mg overnight dexamethasone suppression test | Cortisol<br>ACTH<br>CRH |
| Acromegaly | Pancreas<br>Lung | Acral enlargement<br>Prognathism | Nonsuppressible GH after glucose ingestion | GHRH<br>IGF-1 |

*Abbreviations:* ACTH, adrenocorticotropic hormone; CRH, corticotrophin releasing hormone; GH, growth hormone; GHRH, growth hormone-releasing hormone; IGF-1, insulin-like growth factor-1; NET, neuroendocrine tumor; VIP, vasoactive intestinal polypeptide; ZES, Zollinger-Ellison syndrome.

**Table 3**
Specific blood and urine markers for NET

| Marker | Sensitivity (%) | Specificity (%) | Advantages | Disadvantages | Comments | Reference |
|---|---|---|---|---|---|---|
| CgA | 43–100 | 10–96 | Most widely accepted test as it is secreted by almost all NET particularly metastatic midgut carcinoids and pancreatic tumors<br>Levels independent of functional status<br>Correlates with tumor load and tends to be highest in metastatic cancer | Expressed in healthy tissue<br>Elevated in other neoplasia like pancreatic, small bowel, prostate cancer<br>Elevated in inflammatory conditions, cardiac disorders, renal failure, PPI use<br>Not increased in 15%–40% patients<br>Not standardized between laboratories | Granin family of peptides are water soluble acidic glycoproteins expressed in excretory vessels in neurons and endocrine cells<br>Often used to confirm diagnosis, establish baseline, and provide insight into tumor burden | 13–17 |
| PP | 50–80 | No data | May be useful for early detection of NET of pancreatic origin in context of MEN1 | Increased PP release after meals, exercise and hypoglycemia; decreased by IV glucose and somatostatin<br>Falsely elevated levels with laxative abuse, age, inflammatory processes of gut, chronic renal disease | Produced by NET of pancreas and colon and thought to play a role in autoregulation of pancreatic and gastrointestinal secretion and hepatic glycogen levels | 18,19 |
| Pancreastatin | 64 | 58–100 | Not affected by PPI use<br>More stable measurement of tumor activity<br>Possibly greater sensitivity and specificity compared with CgA | Levels elevated in diabetics and hyperparathyroidism | Derivative of CgA | 20–23 |
| NSE | 33 | Up to 100 | Used in diagnosis of small cell lung cancer or neuroblastoma<br>Increased in poorly differentiated NET where CgA might be normal<br>Possible use as early response marker with mTOR inhibitor therapy | Cannot differentiate between different subtypes of NET<br>No particular benefit over CgA<br>Poor sensitivity (33%)<br>Erythrocytes have large amount of NSE and can cause falsely elevated levels | NSE is an enolase present in neurons and neuroendocrine cells and can indicate tumors derived from these cell types<br>Located in cell cytoplasm and enters circulation after tumor lysis | 17 |

(continued on next page)

**Table 3**
*(continued)*

| Marker | Sensitivity (%) | Specificity (%) | Advantages | Disadvantages | Comments | Reference |
|---|---|---|---|---|---|---|
| NKA | 88 | No data | Predominantly secreted by midgut NET<br>Correlates with poor outcomes in midgut tumors<br>Signals response to somatostatin analogues | | | 24 |
| 24-h urine 5-HIAA | 35 | Up to 100 | Specific marker for carcinoid syndrome and midgut NET | Many substances affect urinary 5-HIAA levels including:<br>• Foods rich in tryptophan (avocado, pineapples, banana etc)<br>• Drugs (acetaminophen, guaifenesin, caffeine, mesalamine)<br>Falsely low values can occur with concomitant use of ethanol, levodopa, MAO inhibitors, heparin, methyldopa | | 25,26 |
| Whole blood or serum serotonin | 75–80 | Up to 100 | Specific marker for carcinoid syndrome and midgut NET<br>Less cumbersome to obtain than a 24-h urine 5-HIAA | Levels are somewhat affected by diet and stress (see 5-HIAA)<br>Not all NET secrete serotonin<br>Single level can vary during the day compared with 24-h urine 5-HIAA | Most circulating serotonin is stored in the platelets<br>The preferred specimens for serotonin analysis are either whole blood (containing all of the platelets) or serum from clotted specimens (because the clotting process releases almost all platelet serotonin) | 25,27–29 |
| Plasma 5-HIAA | 89–95 | 75–85 | Specific marker for carcinoid syndrome and midgut NET<br>Less cumbersome to obtain than a 24-h urine 5-HIAA | Assay not standardized across laboratories<br>Does not offer a significant advantage over blood serotonin levels | | 25,27 |

*Abbreviations:* 5-HIAA, 5-hydroxyindoleacetic acid; CgA, chromogranin A; IV, intravenous; MAO, monoamine oxidase; mTOR, mammalian target of rapamycin; NET, neuroendocrine tumor; NSE, neuron-specific enolase; NKA, neurokinin A; PPI, proton pump inhibitors; PP, pancreatic polypeptide.

ideal biomarker would have low false-positive and false-negative rates, measure the aggressiveness of the tumor, identify treatment response to medical or surgical treatment, measure the aggressiveness of remnant disease, detect relapse, and serve as a prognostic indicator.

Although new individual biomarkers continue to be assessed, for example, connective tissue growth factor for carcinoid heart disease or paraneoplastic Ma antigen 2 for small intestinal NET,[8] there is an increasing interest in multianalyte assays that address the deficiencies of the current mono-analyte or single marker assays. These tests use multiple simultaneous measurements of different parameters related to the disease, along with algorithms, which improve sensitivity and specificity. This concept is already used for other conditions, for example, FibroSure test for hepatitis C[9] or MammaPrint for metastatic breast cancer.[10] There have been recent developments in nucleic acid–based technologies, like microRNA profiling, and strategies to collect circulating tumor cells, which may become helpful in future for NET diagnosis and management. At this time, however, the only commercially available multianalyte NET test, which may be clinically helpful, is the NETest.

The NETest, developed by Wren Laboratories (Branford, CT), is a multianalyte quantitative reverse-transcriptase polymerase chain reaction assay, based on 51 marker genes with an algorithmic analysis, claims a high sensitivity (>95%) and specificity (>95%) in the detection of all GEP-NET tumors. The test offers an assessment of disease status and treatment effectiveness.[11,12] Early data suggest that the NETest may be more accurate than single biomarker or monoanalyte tests and it is not known to be affected by age, gender, fasting status, or use of proton pump inhibitors. The test requires a single laboratory, Wren Laboratories, to offer the specialized analysis. More information is needed on whether the test is positive in non–GEP-NET or cancers with mixed epithelial and NET phenotype, for example, prostate cancer. Additionally, more prospective verification studies by investigators independent of the manufacturing company are needed. At this time, there is no specific recommendation from any professional organization supporting the NETest.

## REFERENCES

1. Yao JC, Hassan M, Phan A, et al. One hundred years after "carcinoid": epidemiology of and prognostic factors for neuroendocrine tumors in 35,825 cases in the United States. J Clin Oncol 2008;26(18):3063–72.

2. Lawrence B, Gustafsson BI, Chan A, et al. The epidemiology of gastroenteropancreatic neuroendocrine tumors. Endocrinol Metab Clin North Am 2011; 40(1):1–18, vii.

3. Lombard-Bohas C, Mitry E, O'Toole D, et al. Thirteen-month registration of patients with gastroenteropancreatic endocrine tumours in France. Neuroendocrinology 2009;89(2):217–22.

4. Caplin ME, Buscombe JR, Hilson AJ, et al. Carcinoid tumour. Lancet 1998; 352(9130):799–805.

5. Modlin IM, Kidd M, Latich I, et al. Current status of gastrointestinal carcinoids. Gastroenterology 2005;128(6):1717–51.

6. Vinik A, Moattari AR. Use of somatostatin analog in management of carcinoid syndrome. Dig Dis Sci 1989;34(3 Suppl):14S–27S.

7. Vinik AI, Silva MP, Woltering EA, et al. Biochemical testing for neuroendocrine tumors. Pancreas 2009;38(8):876–89.

8. Cui T, Hurtig M, Elgue G, et al. Paraneoplastic antigen Ma2 autoantibodies as specific blood biomarkers for detection of early recurrence of small intestine neuroendocrine tumors. PLoS One 2010;5(12):e16010.

9. Poynard T, Imbert-Bismut F, Munteanu M, et al. Overview of the diagnostic value of biochemical markers of liver fibrosis (FibroTest, HCV FibroSure) and necrosis (ActiTest) in patients with chronic hepatitis C. Comp Hepatol 2004;3(1):8.

10. Kittaneh M, Montero AJ, Gluck S. Molecular profiling for breast cancer: a comprehensive review. Biomark Cancer 2013;5:61–70.

11. Modlin IM, Aslanian H, Bodei L, et al. A PCR blood test outperforms chromogranin A in carcinoid detection and is unaffected by proton pump inhibitors. Endocr Connect 2014;3(4):215–23.

12. Modlin IM, Drozdov I, Kidd M. The identification of gut neuroendocrine tumor disease by multiple synchronous transcript analysis in blood. PLoS One 2013;8(5): e63364.

13. Campana D, Nori F, Piscitelli L, et al. Chromogranin A: is it a useful marker of neuroendocrine tumors? J Clin Oncol 2007;25(15):1967–73.

14. Hsiao RJ, Mezger MS, O'Connor DT. Chromogranin A in uremia: progressive retention of immunoreactive fragments. Kidney Int 1990;37(3):955–64.

15. Lawrence B, Gustafsson BI, Kidd M, et al. The clinical relevance of chromogranin A as a biomarker for gastroenteropancreatic neuroendocrine tumors. Endocrinol Metab Clin North Am 2011;40(1):111–34, viii.

16. Marotta V, Nuzzo V, Ferrara T, et al. Limitations of chromogranin A in clinical practice. Biomarkers 2012;17(2):186–91.

17. Modlin IM, Gustafsson BI, Moss SF, et al. Chromogranin A–biological function and clinical utility in neuro endocrine tumor disease. Ann Surg Oncol 2010; 17(9):2427–43.

18. Langstein HN, Norton JA, Chiang V, et al. The utility of circulating levels of human pancreatic polypeptide as a marker for islet cell tumors. Surgery 1990;108(6): 1109–15 [discussion: 1115–6].

19. Metz DC, Jensen RT. Gastrointestinal neuroendocrine tumors: pancreatic endocrine tumors. Gastroenterology 2008;135(5):1469–92.

20. Calhoun K, Toth-Fejel S, Cheek J, et al. Serum peptide profiles in patients with carcinoid tumors. Am J Surg 2003;186(1):28–31.

21. Ito T, Igarashi H, Jensen RT. Serum pancreastatin: the long sought universal, sensitive, specific tumor marker for neuroendocrine tumors? Pancreas 2012;41(4): 505–7.

22. Raines D, Chester M, Diebold AE, et al. A prospective evaluation of the effect of chronic proton pump inhibitor use on plasma biomarker levels in humans. Pancreas 2012;41(4):508–11.

23. Stridsberg M, Oberg K, Li Q, et al. Measurements of chromogranin A, chromogranin B (secretogranin I), chromogranin C (secretogranin II) and pancreastatin in plasma and urine from patients with carcinoid tumours and endocrine pancreatic tumours. J Endocrinol 1995;144(1):49–59.

24. Turner GB, Johnston BT, McCance DR, et al. Circulating markers of prognosis and response to treatment in patients with midgut carcinoid tumours. Gut 2006;55(11):1586–91.

25. Tellez MR, Mamikunian G, O'Dorisio TM, et al. A single fasting plasma 5-HIAA value correlates with 24-hour urinary 5-HIAA values and other biomarkers in midgut neuroendocrine tumors (NETs). Pancreas 2013;42(3):405–10.

26. Vinik AI, Woltering EA, Warner RR, et al. NANETS consensus guidelines for the diagnosis of neuroendocrine tumor. Pancreas 2010;39(6):713–34.

27. Carling RS, Degg TJ, Allen KR, et al. Evaluation of whole blood serotonin and plasma and urine 5-hydroxyindole acetic acid in diagnosis of carcinoid disease. Ann Clin Biochem 2002;39(Pt 6):577–82.
28. Beck O, Wallén NH, Bröijersén A, et al. On the accurate determination of serotonin in human plasma. Biochem Biophys Res Commun 1993;196(1):260–6.
29. Meijer WG, Kema IP, Volmer M, et al. Discriminating capacity of indole markers in the diagnosis of carcinoid tumors. Clin Chem 2000;46(10):1588–96.

# Biochemical and Imaging Diagnostics in Endocrinology: Predictors of Fertility

Erica B. Mahany, MD*, John F. Randolph Jr, MD

## KEYWORDS

- Ovarian reserve • Ovulatory status • Gamete transport • Male factor • Infertility

## KEY POINTS

- An appropriate diagnostic evaluation of the infertile couple includes ovarian reserve testing, determination of ovulatory status, evaluation of anatomy as it relates to gamete transport, and evaluation of the male, if applicable.
- In a couple who fulfills the criteria for the diagnosis of infertility, biochemical modalities are particularly useful for evaluating the ovaries and ovulatory status, and imaging is the appropriate way to evaluate transport.
- Although much has been elucidated about the diagnostic evaluation of the infertile couple, current testing has limited predictability for the ultimate achievement of a live birth.

## INTRODUCTION

Infertility has traditionally been defined as the inability to achieve a successful pregnancy after 12 months or more of regular unprotected intercourse. This definition applies to heterosexual couples, because approximately 85% achieve a pregnancy within that time frame without medical assistance. Conversely, this means that 15% of heterosexual couples warrant an evaluation for causes of infertility. In women older than the age of 35, earlier evaluation is recommended (following 6 months of subfertility) because of the increased prevalence of ovarian reserve concerns in this group. Furthermore, an evaluation before 12 months may also be indicated for patients with clinical situations, such as oligomenorrhea or amenorrhea, known or suspected peritoneal disease, severe endometriosis, or male factor infertility.[1] In addition, same sex couples and single women may also benefit from a baseline evaluation to try and screen for potential fertility issues beyond lack of exposure to gametes.

One of the limiting factors of fertility testing is the relative inefficiency of human reproduction, because a couple without infertility has a fecundability rate of only

The authors have nothing to disclose.

Division of Reproductive Endocrinology and Infertility, Department of Obstetrics and Gynecology, Michigan Medicine, 1500 East Medical Center Drive, L4000 University Hospital South, Ann Arbor, MI 48109, USA

* Corresponding author.

*E-mail address:* emahany@med.umich.edu

15% to 20% per month.[2] A careful history and physical examination must be performed on each patient to inform the particular diagnostic tests that are chosen, and to create a meaningful treatment plan. The testing parameters, such as sensitivity, specificity, positive predictive value (PPV), and negative predictive value, can help to interpret test results, although there is no perfect screening test for the various causes of infertility. This article describes the four major categories of testing for infertility: (1) ovarian reserve, (2) ovulatory status, (3) gamete transport, and (4) male factor (if applicable) (**Box 1**).

## OVARIAN RESERVE
### Review of Reproductive Physiology

Under normal circumstances, each month, a woman of reproductive age has a cohort of ovarian follicles. These follicles are destined for atresia, although one follicle is "rescued" from the group and is selected as the dominant follicle based on a variety of factors, such as the ability to express follicle-stimulating hormone (FSH) receptors, and to produce aromatase and estradiol. Inhibin B and estradiol from the follicle exert negative feedback on the hypothalamus and pituitary, until estradiol levels surpass a threshold, prompting a shift to positive feedback, inducing a luteinizing hormone (LH) surge and ovulation. The follicle remodels and becomes the corpus luteum, making progesterone, estradiol, and inhibin A. These hormones exhibit negative feedback with resultant suppression of gonadotropins. If a woman is not pregnant in a given cycle, the hormones from the corpus luteum rapidly decline to basal levels, which decreases the negative feedback, and FSH rises to start the process again.[3]

Ovarian follicle number and oocyte quality decrease continually from a midfetal peak until the loss of any ovulatory follicles around menopause. With ovarian aging, the corpus luteum function declines, with decrease in negative feedback. This results in an earlier rise in FSH, earlier recruitment of new follicles, and a shorter follicular phase. Antimüllerian hormone (AMH), produced by the total cohort of primary, secondary, and early antral follicles, decreases as the size of the cohort steadily decays. Although the exact role of AMH remains to be clarified, AMH is the least variable direct measure of follicular secretory activity and is constant throughout the menstrual cycle[2,4] (**Table 1**).

### Diminished Ovarian Reserve

Diminished ovarian reserve (DOR) is the most pressing concern in women of advanced maternal age. Unlike men, who produce new sperm on a daily basis, women reach peak oocyte number between 16 and 24 weeks of gestation with steady decline in numbers and quality until after menopause.[3] Biochemical measures of ovarian reserve include AMH, a direct estimate of the total number of the primordial follicles, and early follicular FSH and estradiol, estimating the pituitary response to diminished negative feedback from a decreasing follicular pool. As of yet, there are no age-specific reference ranges for AMH, and lack of calibration among assays limits generalizability of

---

**Box 1**
**Categories of testing for infertility**

Ovarian reserve

Ovulatory status

Gamete transport

Male factor (if applicable)

| Table 1 | |
|---|---|
| **Diagnostic evaluation of ovarian reserve** | |
| **Ovarian Reserve Testing** | **Test** |
| Biochemical | Antimüllerian hormone |
| | Day 3 follicle-stimulating hormone, estradiol |
| Imaging | Antral follicle count |

existing data.[5] In general, a low AMH level (<1 ng/mL) correlates with decreased in vitro fertilization (IVF) pregnancy rates.[6] Higher AMH levels (>4.9 ng/mL) have been associated with polycystic ovarian syndrome (PCOS),[7] although most data about AMH and ovarian reserve are from infertility patients.[8] Furthermore, because of the inhibitory role of AMH on follicular development, a high AMH level (>7.4 ng/mL) may portend poor response to ovulation induction regimens.[9] A direct morphologic assessment of the antral follicle pool with a transvaginal ultrasound, the antral follicle count (AFC), correlates well with AMH levels (see **Table 1**). Ovarian reserve markers should aid in the diagnosis of infertility, keeping in mind that the PPV of ovarian reserve testing for older women (where the prevalence of DOR is high) is higher than for younger women (where the prevalence of DOR is lower).[2]

Cycle-dependent biochemical testing was the original modality for ovarian reserve assessment. Measurement of FSH and estradiol on Cycle Days 2 to 5 of the menstrual cycle provides information about the hypothalamic-pituitary-gonadal axis. If FSH is elevated (typically defined as >10 IU/L) in the context of a normal estradiol level (<60 pg/mL), this suggests a compensatory response to declining negative feedback. High FSH levels have also been shown to correlate with poor response in IVF cycles[10]; however, significant intercycle and intracycle variability limit the reliability. An early rise in serum estradiol suggests earlier recruitment of follicles because of decreased negative feedback in the preceding luteal phase, and may mask an abnormal FSH level that is being suppressed into the normal range. The clomiphene citrate challenge test is a dynamic test that measures serum FSH before (Cycle Day 3) and after (Cycle Day 10) administration of clomiphene citrate, although it is rarely performed today because of limited sensitivity and specificity.[2]

Importantly, the available tests are quantitative, and as of yet, there are no good tests for egg quality or embryo competence. Patients undergoing assisted reproductive technology have the option of having a trophectoderm biopsy performed on embryos on Day 5 or 6 following oocyte retrieval for preimplantation genetic screening for aneuploidy of individual embryos. Because meiotic errors tend to increase with ovarian aging, the ability to generate euploid embryos correlates with oocyte quality. However, this is invasive and expensive, and cannot be used for screening.

### Primary Ovarian Insufficiency

Primary ovarian insufficiency is the depletion or dysfunction of ovarian follicles with cessation of menses before age 40 years. It may be caused by genetic factors (*FMR1* gene mutations or Turner karyotype), exposure to chemotherapy or radiation, autoimmune causes (presumed antiovarian antibodies, for which a reliable assay has yet to be developed), or an idiopathic cause. The diagnosis must exclude other causes of oligomenorrhea or amenorrhea, and the hallmark biochemical findings are low estradiol, high gonadotropins, and undetectable AMH. Although 5% to 10% of patients with primary ovarian insufficiency conceive spontaneously, ovulation cannot be stimulated with fertility treatments. Primary ovarian insufficiency also can increase the risk of bone loss and cardiovascular disease, and can be associated with other autoimmune endocrine disorders; hormone therapy is usually recommended to replace sex steroids to which the patient would otherwise be exposed. Emotional support should be provided to patients and families because of the emotional import of this diagnosis.[11]

### Postchemotherapy

Besides age, other factors can cause DOR. Many chemotherapy regimens destroy primordial follicles.[12] With the increase in survivorship from cancer treatments, women of reproductive age are returning posttherapy and wanting to conceive. Although some women have had the opportunity to freeze oocytes or embryos before fertility-threatening treatments, most women have not. The American Society of Clinical Oncology guidelines recommend that oncologists address the possibility for infertility with all patients of child-bearing potential who may desire future fertility.[13]

With any chemotherapy regimen, it is difficult to counsel an individual patient on her personal risk for developing permanent chemotherapy-related amenorrhea (CRA). Risk stratification tools have been created based on the specific regimen and age, although these often give a wide range of risk. A standard cyclophosphamide-containing regimen has a 30% to 70% chance of causing CRA in a 30-year-old woman.[14] Furthermore, most of the published studies have evaluated return of menses, the most common time point being 12 months following chemotherapy,[15] as the primary end point, and not live birth. A recent systematic review and meta-analysis evaluated factors associated with return of ovarian function after breast cancer chemotherapy. The authors found that age less than 40 years and exposure to a gonadotropin-releasing hormone agonist were positively associated with menses recovery (odds ratio, 6.07 and 2.03, respectively), but exposure to taxanes adversely affected recovery (odds ratio, 0.49).[16]

AMH levels are beginning to show some promise in terms of prognosis for recovery of ovarian activity. Three studies in women with breast cancer have shown that higher pretreatment AMH level was associated with postchemotherapy ovarian activity.[15,17,18] In addition, pretreatment AMH levels have been shown to be associated with posttreatment levels.[12] It has been proposed that intrinsic patient factors (baseline AMH) could potentially be combined with extrinsic factors (the proposed treatment)[19] to better counsel patients on their prognosis for developing CRA. The end points of live birth, menopause, and ovarian endocrine function require more studies.

## OVULATORY STATUS

Historically, regular menses have been a hallmark of inferring if a patient is ovulatory.[3] Currently, over-the-counter urinary assessments of a midcycle LH surge are effective for estimating the occurrence and timing of ovulation, although they are neither sensitive nor specific. These enzyme-linked immunosorbent assay–based tests are confounded by urinary volume and dilution, patient difficulty in interpretation, and persistently positive tests in patients with PCOS with tonically high LH levels. An estimate of peak corpus luteum function at the time of implantation with a serum progesterone level (drawn days 7–9 following an LH surge) can verify ovulation and assess corpus luteum adequacy. Before current practice, basal body temperature measurements and endometrial biopsies have been performed, although these are imprecise and are no longer used.[3] Serial ultrasonography can document follicular growth and collapse. The presence of a dominant follicle at midcycle is highly suggestive of a functioning hypothalamic-pituitary-gonadal axis (**Fig. 1**). Progressive growth and

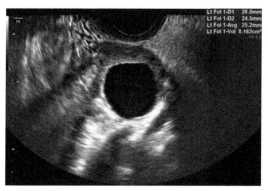

**Fig. 1.** A mature follicle at midcycle.

echotexture of the endometrium supports the assessment of ovulatory status (**Table 2**).

## Considerations of Anovulation

### Polycystic ovarian syndrome

PCOS is a disease of metabolic and ovulatory dysfunction that affects 5% to 10% of reproductive-age women.[7] Clinical criteria for the diagnosis of PCOS include two of the three following: oligomenorrhea or amenorrhea, clinical or biochemical evidence of hyperandrogenism, and polycystic-appearing ovaries on ultrasound ($\geq$12 antral follicles 2–9 mm in each ovary or ovarian volume >10 mL), with exclusion of other causes (the Rotterdam criteria).[20] Hyperandrogenism can also be caused by androgen-secreting tumors from the ovary or adrenal glands, screened for with a serum total testosterone and dehydroepiandrosterone-sulfate, or adrenal hypersecretion from congenital adrenal hyperplasia, screened for with 17-hydroxyprogesterone. Cushing syndrome should also be ruled out based on clinical suspicion. Other causes of ovulatory dysfunction should be ruled out with a thyroid-stimulating hormone and prolactin. The AFC is a useful test, because higher AFC values have a high likelihood of a diagnosis of PCOS.[21] Imaging of the adrenals should be performed if suspicion is high for adrenal hypersecretion.

PCOS is characterized by an increased number of growing follicles at all stages of development. In particular, there are an increased number of preantral and small antral follicles, each of which produces AMH.[7] With the increase in use of AMH as an ovarian reserve marker, it has been established that patients with PCOS have a two to four

| Table 2 | |
|---|---|
| **Diagnostic evaluation of ovulatory status** | |
| **Ovulatory Status** | **Test** |
| Biochemical | Urinary LH testing (qualitative) |
| | Luteal progesterone (Day 7, 8, or 9 following LH surge) |
| Imaging | Serial ultrasounds (especially midcycle) |
| | Mature-sized follicle |
| | Endometrium |
| Other | Basal body temperature |
| | Endometrial biopsy |

times increased AMH compared with age-matched control subjects without PCOS.[22] In addition, elevated AMH has been associated with decreased chances of response to ovulation induction,[9,23] because of an inhibitory effect on the development of antral follicles, and decreased sensitivity of the follicles to FSH.[7] Higher levels also correlate with overresponse in the setting of assisted reproductive technology.[5,24] However, there are persistent limitations to the use of AMH as a marker of ovarian function.[25,26]

### Hypothalamic amenorrhea

Some women are anovulatory because of insufficient release of gonadotropin-releasing hormone from the hypothalamus, with resultant decreased release of LH and FSH from the pituitary. These women often have low body weight, high physical stress, or high emotional stress. On serum testing, these patients may have low or normal estradiol levels, and low or normal LH and FSH levels. These women often can become ovulatory and conceive with behavior modification, such as decreased exercise and increased caloric intake or with ovulation induction.

### Advanced maternal age

As women approach perimenopause, they begin to have cycle variability with decreasing probability of ovulatory cycles each month.[27] Because ovarian reserve biomarker and menstrual changes portend menopause,[28,29] cycle variability is a useful indicator of decreased fecundability.

## GAMETE TRANSPORT

Under normal circumstances, after the oocyte is released from the follicle, it is captured by the fimbriae of the fallopian tubes, with subsequent transport for fertilization in the ampulla. If sperm are present and fertilize the oocyte, the resulting embryo is transported to the uterus. Thus, transport of the gametes and early embryo requires normal tubal anatomy.[3] Fallopian tube disease should be suspected in a patient with a prior history of sexually transmitted infections, documented pelvic inflammatory disease, known endometriosis, or extensive abdominal surgery. The presence of anti-chlamydial antibodies is associated with tubal pathology, although this test has limited clinical use because of low sensitivity and low PPV.[1] Hysterosalpingography (HSG) is the primary imaging procedure to confirm tubal patency, although false-positives occur in 39%, in which further evaluation with laparoscopy is required to evaluate for true occlusion versus tubal spasm.[1] Saline infusion sonography (SIS) is an alternate way to assess tubal patency, and may be a more comprehensive way to evaluate the pelvis. It has a lower PPV than HSG,[30] but better sensitivity and specificity (>90%) for detecting intrauterine pathology, such as myomas and endometrial polyps.[1,30] Hysteroscopy is the gold standard for diagnosis and treatment of intrauterine pathology, although tubal patency cannot be determined from hysteroscopy alone. Hysteroscopy can be reserved for further evaluation and treatment of intrauterine pathology after HSG or SIS has been performed.[1] MRI may be considered in cases where a uterine anomaly is suspected or significant fibroids are present (**Table 3**).

## MALE FACTOR

In a heterosexual couple, male factor is primarily responsible for the infertility approximately 20% of the time, and may contribute to an additional 30% to 40% of cases.[31,32] Most men with infertility are asymptomatic. At minimum, the initial screening evaluation should include a thorough reproductive history and analysis of at least one semen sample. If the evaluation is abnormal, a physical examination

**Table 3**
**Diagnostic evaluation of gamete transport**

| Gamete Transport | Test | Test attributes |
|---|---|---|
| Biochemical | None | |
| Imaging | Hysterosalpingogram | Best noninvasive test for tubal patency, limited assessment of uterus |
| | Saline infusion sonogram | Most comprehensive noninvasive test for uterus/ovaries, but less specific for tubal occlusion |
| | Hysteroscopy | Gold standard for uterine cavity evaluation, but no information on tubal patency |
| | Laparoscopy | Invasive, although best test for tubal patency and evaluation for adhesive disease |
| | MRI | Best test for uterine anomalies and myomas, but does not assess tubal status |

should be performed, and referral to a provider with experience in male reproduction is recommended.[31]

The semen analysis is the initial screening test for all infertile men. It is an efficient test, because it evaluates sperm production and transport. Semen is collected by masturbation into a specimen cup, or by intercourse with the use of semen collection condoms. The standard conditions for semen testing include a 2- to 5-day interval since the last ejaculation, collection at the testing site, and evaluation within an hour after production. It should be processed in a laboratory that adheres to Clinical Laboratory Improvement Amendments standards.[31]

The parameters tested include semen volume, sperm concentration, percent motility, total sperm count, and percent normal morphology. The standard reference is the World Health Organization's guideline, which evaluated more than 4500 men from four continents that had achieved a pregnancy in the preceding 12 months. The lower limit of normal total sperm count is 39 million, motility of at least 40%, and morphology of at least 4% normal forms.[33] A normal semen analysis is highly suggestive of normal male reproductive capacity, but occult fertilization failure can occur. If any of the parameters are abnormal, referral for further evaluation is warranted and may include physical examination, biochemical and genetic testing, transscrotal ultrasound, and testicular biopsy/aspiration (**Table 4**).

**Table 4**
**Diagnostic evaluation of male factor**

| Male Factor | Test |
|---|---|
| Initial evaluation | Semen analysis<br>If abnormal, see secondary evaluation below |
| Secondary evaluation | |
| Physical examination | Evaluate for vas deferens bilaterally, varicocele |
| Biochemical | Total testosterone, LH, FSH, estradiol, prolactin |
| Imaging | +/− Scrotal ultrasound |
| Genetic evaluation | If azoospermia or severe oligospermia (karyotype, Y chromosome microdeletion) |
| Testicular biopsy/aspiration | If azoospermia, aspiration of testes to evaluate for sperm |

## UNEXPLAINED INFERTILITY

In a small percentage of couples seeking infertility, no cause is found, after evaluating for DOR, ovulatory dysfunction, uterine/tubal pathology, and abnormal semen parameters.[34] These patients have comparable IVF success rates compared with age-matched control subjects with other infertility diagnoses,[35] and some studies have shown that 6% to 27% of patients conceive spontaneously if expectant management is offered.[34] In these patients, treatment should be individualized and may include empiric therapy with ovulation-induction agents, intrauterine insemination, and IVF. If no source for infertility is identified, referral to an infertility specialist is warranted.

## FUTURE CONSIDERATIONS/SUMMARY

An appropriate diagnostic evaluation of the infertile couple includes ovarian reserve testing, determination of ovulatory status, evaluation of anatomy as it relates to gamete transport, and evaluation of the male, if applicable. In a couple who fulfills the criteria for the diagnosis of infertility, biochemical modalities are particularly useful for evaluating the ovaries and ovulatory status, and imaging is the appropriate way to evaluate transport. Semen analysis is the primary way to evaluate the male, if applicable. Although much has been elucidated about the diagnostic evaluation of the infertile couple, current testing has limited predictability for the ultimate achievement of a live birth. As technology pushes the boundaries of current knowledge, a better understanding of ovarian aging and oocyte competence, and the benefits and limitations of preimplantation genetic screening of embryos, will be developed. This information is needed to better interpret the quantitative ovarian reserve markers in a meaningful way, especially as regards chances of, and treatment to enable, live birth.

---

**VIGNETTES**

1. Ovarian reserve: A 34-year-old woman with breast cancer completed her chemotherapy regimen, which included taxanes, 3 months ago. She is amenorrheic, and she is interested in learning about her fertility potential. You measure biochemical tests of ovarian reserve, which are the following:
   a. AMH <0.3 ng/mL
   b. FSH 20 IU/L
   c. Estradiol 15 pg/mL

   How long should she wait before repeat testing?
   • Repeat testing at 12 months following chemotherapy

   In addition, you counsel her that return of menses and ovarian reserve values are inadequate predictors of fertility in young women postchemotherapy. A good prognostic factor is that she was younger than the age of 40 during her treatment.

2. Ovulatory status: A 28-year-old woman presents with irregular menses every 30 to 55 days, and acne and bothersome hair along her chin line. Her body mass index is 32 kg/m². She is interested in conceiving and has not become pregnant despite 18 months of unprotected intercourse. You measure biochemical tests, which are the following:
   a. AMH 11 ng/mL, FSH 8.0 IU/L, estradiol 40 pg/mL
   b. Testosterone, 17-OH P, dehydroepiandrosterone-sulfate within normal limits
   c. Thyroid-stimulating hormone and prolactin are within normal limits
   d. Semen analysis is normal
   e. Saline infusion sonography confirms patent fallopian tubes, and polycystic-appearing ovaries with an AFC of 55 (Fig. 2)

   You counsel her about next steps, primarily weight loss through lifestyle modifications. She conceives 7 months later.

3. Gamete transport: A 24-year-old woman with 2 years of primary infertility presents for evaluation. On review of her records, you notice that she had asymptomatic chlamydia identified on cervical screening at her annual gynecology appointment. The patient and her partner were treated. You order the following:
   a. HSG: shows bilateral tubal occlusion and hydrosalpinx (**Fig. 3**)

You refer to her a fertility specialist, because she needs IVF to conceive.

4. Male factor: A 30-year-old woman presents with 5 years of primary infertility. You order an initial evaluation, and her husband is found to be azoospermic. Her testing is normal. His history is unremarkable. You do an examination, which shows the presence of bilateral vas deferentia and normal-sized testes. You order biochemical tests (FSH, LH, estradiol, testosterone, and prolactin), all of which are normal. You refer him to a reproductive urologist for testicular aspiration, and sperm are seen. They undergo IVF and conceive.

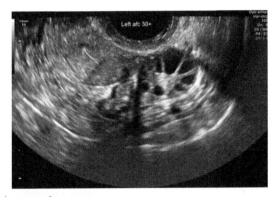

**Fig. 2.** A polycystic-appearing ovary.

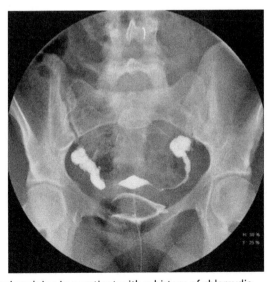

**Fig. 3.** Bilateral hydrosalpinx in a patient with a history of chlamydia.

## REFERENCES

1. Practice Committee of the American Society for Reproductive Medicine. Diagnostic evaluation of the infertile female: a committee opinion. Fertil Steril 2015; 103(6):e44–50.
2. Practice Committee of the American Society for Reproductive Medicine. Testing and interpreting measures of ovarian reserve: a committee opinion. Fertil Steril 2015;103(3):e9–17.
3. Fritz MA, Speroff L. Clinical gynecologic endocrinology and infertility. 8th edition. Philadelphia: Lippincott Williams & Wilkins; 2011.
4. La Marca A, Pati M, Orvieto R, et al. Serum anti-müllerian hormone levels in women with secondary amenorrhea. Fertil Steril 2006;85(5):1547–9.
5. Anderson RA. Towards improving analysis and interpretation of antimüllerian hormone in women. Fertil Steril 2016;106(5):1051–2.
6. Reijnders IF, Nelen WL, IntHout J, et al. The value of anti-mullerian hormone in low and extremely low ovarian reserve in relation to live birth after in vitro fertilization. Eur J Obstet Gynecol Reprod Biol 2016;200:45–50.
7. Dumont A, Robin G, Catteau-Jonard S, et al. Role of anti-müllerian hormone in pathophysiology, diagnosis and treatment of polycystic ovary syndrome: a review. Reprod Biol Endocrinol 2015;13:137.
8. Grossman LC, Safier LZ, Kline MD, et al. Utility of ovarian reserve screening with anti-mullerian hormone for reproductive age women deferring pregnancy. J Womens Health 2016;26:345–51.
9. Mumford SL, Legro RS, Diamond MP, et al. Baseline AMH level associated with ovulation following ovulation induction in women with polycystic ovary syndrome. J Clin Endocrinol Metab 2016;101(9):3288–96.
10. La Marca A, Ferraretti AP, Palermo R, et al. The use of ovarian reserve markers in IVF clinical practice: a national consensus. Gynecol Endocrinol 2015;32(1):1–5.
11. American College of Obstetricians and Gynecologists Committee on Adolescent Health Care. Committee Opinion No. 605: primary ovarian insufficiency in adolescents and young women. Obstet Gynecol 2014;124(1):193–7.
12. Dillon KE, Sammel MD, Prewitt M, et al. Pretreatment anti-müllerian hormone levels determine rate of posttherapy ovarian reserve recovery: acute changes in ovarian reserve during and after chemotherapy. Fertil Steril 2013;99(2):477–83.
13. Lee SJ, Schover LR, Partridge AH, et al. American Society of Clinical Oncology recommendations on fertility preservation in cancer patients. J Clin Oncol 2006;24(18):2917–31.
14. SaveMyFertility. 2011. Available at: http://www.savemyfertility.org. Accessed October 23, 2016.
15. Anders C, Kelly Marcom P, Peterson B, et al. A pilot study of predictive markers of chemotherapy-related amenorrhea among premenopausal women with early stage breast cancer. Cancer Invest 2008;26(3):286–95.
16. Silva C, Caramelo O, Almeida-Santos T, et al. Factors associated with ovarian function recovery after chemotherapy for breast cancer: a systematic review and meta-analysis. Hum Reprod 2016;31(12):2737–49.
17. Anderson RA, Cameron DA. Pretreatment serum anti-müllerian hormone predicts long-term ovarian function and bone mass after chemotherapy for early breast cancer. J Clin Endocrinol Metab 2011;96(5):1336–43.
18. Henry NL, Xia R, Schott AF, et al. Prediction of postchemotherapy ovarian function using markers of ovarian reserve. Oncologist 2014;19(1):68–74.

19. Anderson RA, Wallace WH. Anti-müllerian hormone, the assessment of ovarian reserve, and the reproductive outcome of the young patient with cancer. Fertil Steril 2013;99(6):1469–75.
20. Rotterdam ESHRE/ASRM-Sponsored PCOS Consensus Workshop Group. Revised 2003 consensus on diagnostic criteria and long-term health risks related to polycystic ovary syndrome (PCOS). Fertil Steril 2004;81(1):19–25.
21. Dewailly D, Lujan ME, Carmina E, et al. Definition and significance of polycystic ovarian morphology: a task force report from the Androgen Excess and Polycystic Ovary Syndrome Society. Hum Reprod Update 2014;20(3):334–52.
22. Pellatt L, Rice S, Dilaver N, et al. Anti-müllerian hormone reduces follicle sensitivity to follicle-stimulating hormone in human granulosa cells. Fertil Steril 2011; 96(5):1246–51.
23. Wiweko B, Maidarti M, Priangga MD, et al. Anti-müllerian hormone as a diagnostic and prognostic tool for PCOS patients. J Assist Reprod Genet 2014; 31(10):1311–6.
24. Knez J, Kovacic B, Medved M, et al. What is the value of anti-müllerian hormone in predicting the response to ovarian stimulation with GnRH agonist and antagonist protocols? Reprod Biol Endocrinol 2015;13:58.
25. Pankhurst MW, Harnh Chong Y. Variation in circulating antimüllerian hormone precursor during the periovulatory and acute postovulatory phases of the human ovarian cycle. Fertil Steril 2016;106(5):1238–43.
26. Hadlow N, Brown S, Habib A, et al. Quantifying the intraindividual variation of antimüllerian hormone in the ovarian cycle. Fertil Steril 2016;106(5):1230–7.
27. O'Connor KA, Ferrell R, Brindle E, et al. Progesterone and ovulation across stages of the transition to menopause. Menopause 2009;16(6):1178–87.
28. Sowers MR, Eyvazzadeh AD, McConnell D, et al. Anti-müllerian hormone and inhibin B in the definition of ovarian aging and the menopause transition. J Clin Endocrinol Metab 2008;93(9):3478–83.
29. Hall JE. Endocrinology of the menopause. Endocrinol Metab Clin North Am 2015; 44(3):485–96.
30. Luciano DE, Exacoustos C, Luciano AA. Contrast ultrasonography for tubal patency. J Minim Invasive Gynecol 2014;21(6):994–8.
31. Practice Committee of the American Society for Reproductive Medicine. Diagnostic evaluation of the infertile male: a committee opinion. Fertil Steril 2015; 103(3):e18–25.
32. Thonneau P, Marchand S, Tallec A, et al. Incidence and main causes of infertility in a resident population of three French regions. Hum Reprod 1991;6(6):811–6.
33. Cooper TG, Noonan E, von Eckardstein S, et al. World Health Organization reference values for human semen characteristics. Hum Reprod Update 2010;16(3): 231–45.
34. Gunn D, Wright Bates G. Evidence-based approach to unexplained infertility: a systematic review. Fertil Steril 2016;105(6):1457–8.
35. Society for Assisted Reproductive Technology. SART National Summary Report. 2014. Available at: https://www.sartcorsonline.com/rptCSR_PublicMultYear.aspx? ClinicPKID=0. Accessed October 24, 2016.

# Thyroid Cancer
## Ultrasound Imaging and Fine-Needle Aspiration Biopsy

Michelle Melany, MD[a],*, Sardius Chen, MD[b]

### KEYWORDS

- Thyroid ultrasound • Nodule • Papillary cancer • FNA

### KEY POINTS

- Ultrasound is critical in diagnosis and management of thyroid nodules. Nodules detected by imaging or palpation should undergo further characterization with diagnostic ultrasound to determine whether sonographic features suggest malignancy and the need for fine-needle aspiration.
- Preoperative and postoperative diagnostic ultrasound evaluation of cervical lymph nodes and ultrasound-guided intervention are also critical to management of thyroid cancer.
- Future developments in thyroid ultrasound, including elastography and refinements in thyroid ultrasound reporting lexicon, may impact future management and may obviate the need for follow-up in certain low-risk or frankly benign lesions.
- Advances in molecular testing may result in a test with strong predictive capability that could potentially prevent unnecessary thyroid surgery in significant numbers of patients.

### INTRODUCTION

Ultrasound is a widely available, highly sensitive imaging modality for detection and characterization of thyroid nodules. Updated consensus guidelines from the American Thyroid Association (ATA) and other medical societies continue to highlight advantages of ultrasound and maintain that thyroid ultrasound with attention to cervical lymph nodes should be performed in all patients with suspected or known thyroid nodules.[1]

When thyroid cancer is diagnosed, if not previously performed, focused ultrasound evaluation of lateral compartment cervical lymph nodes is performed before surgery.

Disclosure Statement: The authors have nothing to disclose.
[a] Department of Imaging, Cedars Sinai Imaging, Greater Los Angeles VA Medical Center, David Geffen School of Medicine at University of California, Los Angeles, 8700 Beverly Boulevard, Suite M335, Los Angeles, CA 90048, USA; [b] Department of Imaging, Cedars Sinai Imaging, Cedars Sinai Medical Center, 8700 Beverly Boulevard, Suite M335, Los Angeles, CA 90048, USA
* Corresponding author.
E-mail address: Michelle.melany@cshs.org

Endocrinol Metab Clin N Am 46 (2017) 691–711
http://dx.doi.org/10.1016/j.ecl.2017.04.011
0889-8529/17/Published by Elsevier Inc.

endo.theclinics.com

"Lymph node mapping" refers to a detailed ultrasound examination by an experienced sonographer or sonologist as preoperative evaluation for potential nodal metastatic disease. Although often described as operator dependent, ultrasound in experienced hands is more accurate than other imaging modalities, including magnetic resonance (MR), computed tomography (CT), PET/CT, and whole body iodine scan (WBS) in detecting cervical metastases from thyroid cancer.[2] All patients undergoing thyroidectomy for malignancy should undergo preoperative neck ultrasound to evaluate central, right, and left lateral compartment nodes.[1] Should abnormal lateral compartment nodes be detected preoperatively, the patient may undergo FNA of suspicious nodes and, if appropriate, will be offered thyroidectomy with neck dissection to surgically remove involved or suspicious nodal groups. Ultrasound of the thyroid bed (central compartment) and lateral compartments is used in routine thyroid cancer follow-up after treatment. Ultrasound is more sensitive than WBS and serum thyroglobulin (Tg) in detecting local recurrence, residual disease, and lateral compartment metastases, and is the initial test in follow-up of patients with thyroid cancer.[3]

Diagnosis of malignant thyroid nodules, nodal metastases, and central compartment recurrence with fine-needle aspiration biopsy (FNAB) is often performed with ultrasound guidance. Other ultrasound-guided interventional procedures include preoperative localization with charcoal/dye, percutaneous ethanol, and radiofrequency ablation of metastatic lesions in the central and lateral compartments.[4,5]

Neck CT and MRI are not used in the *initial* evaluation of thyroid nodules. Routine use of neck CT, MR, PET and PET/CT imaging is not supported in patients with differentiated thyroid malignancy. However, in patients with invasive thyroid cancer who have extension outside the gland, these modalities may be preferable to investigate involvement of adjacent structures, including the carotid artery, jugular vein, larynx, and trachea. Regional or distant metastases may be detected with the previously described imaging modalities.[1,6]

## THYROID NODULES

Thyroid nodules are discrete lesions within the gland that are radiographically distinct from adjacent thyroid parenchyma. Increased use of neck and chest PET/CT, CT, MRI, and neck ultrasound for imaging has dramatically increased diagnostic ultrasound and ultrasound-guided fine-needle aspiration (FNA) of nonpalpable thyroid nodules. Major clinical societies involved in thyroid cancer diagnosis disagree about guidelines for FNA of these "incidentalomas."[7] Maximizing detection of clinically relevant thyroid cancer while decreasing FNA of benign nodules is critical to managing health care dollars spent on thyroid evaluation. This article includes discussion of ultrasound features of thyroid cancer, including pattern recognition of benign nodules and features that suggest papillary thyroid cancer (PTC).

## ULTRASOUND FEATURES OF THYROID CANCER

Ultrasound features that suggest thyroid nodule malignancy include solid composition, hypoechoic/markedly hypoechoic, intranodular blood flow, calcification, lack of a well-defined halo, ill-defined or spiculated margins, and "taller-than-wide" configuration. Review of the literature reveals these features to have highly variable sensitivities, specificities, and positive and negative predictive values (PPV and NPV). No single ultrasound feature is adequately sensitive or specific to confirm or rule out malignancy.

Multiple studies report ultrasound features *in combination* may better stratify malignancy risk. For example, nodules with no suspicious features carry less than 2% risk, whereas lesions with at least 2 features listed previously carry significantly higher risk.[8] When multiple malignant features are present in a nodule, specificity for detecting cancer increases, but a requirement that multiple features be present to detect a cancerous nodule will decrease sensitivity.[9–11]

Pattern recognition may be more accurate for predicting a thyroid nodule is benign. Rather than rely on individual sonographic features, this method groups nodules into reproducible morphologic patterns. Bonavita and colleagues[12] described the following 4 patterns to have 100% specificity in predicting benignity: "spongiform" or "honeycomb" lesions composed of greater than 50% adjacent linear cysts, avascular or iso-vascular compared with thyroid parenchyma (**Fig. 1**), cysts with avascular internal echoes, "giraffe pattern" nodules (globular areas of hyperechoic thyroid tissue surrounded by thin linear hypoechoic tissue), and diffusely hyperechoic nodules.

Similar to Breast Imaging-Reporting and Data System (BI-RADS) created by the American College of Radiology (ACR), Thyroid Imaging-Reporting and Data Systems (TI-RADS) have been proposed by various investigators and medical societies.[7,13–16] Ideally, a single reporting system will emerge to create a cost-effective strategy to reduce unnecessary thyroid biopsies and follow-up scans, aid in diagnosis of clinically relevant cancers, and improve management of patients with thyroid nodules.[15–17]

### Calcifications

Calcifications occur in benign and malignant thyroid conditions and are reported to be one of the most reproducible sonographic features with high interobserver reliability.[18] Thyroid calcifications are classified as microcalcifications, macrocalcifications, or peripheral calcifications. Any calcification in a nodule increases the chance of malignancy.[19,20]

Microcalcifications are punctate echogenic foci (**Fig. 2A**) that do not, as single entities, shadow. A cluster of microcalcifications may cast an acoustic shadow. Histologically, microcalcifications represent infarcted, calcified papillae called psammoma bodies, characteristic of papillary cancer.[20] Microcalcifications in a solid nodule lead to a threefold increase in cancer risk. Among sonographic features of malignancy, microcalcifications have the highest PPV, but have low sensitivity and are present in only 26% to 59% of cancers.[8]

Colloid crystals can be difficult to distinguish from microcalcifications. Colloid crystals often reverberate on contact with the ultrasound beam, causing characteristic triangular-shaped "posterior ring-down" or "comet-tail artifacts" (**Fig. 3**). FNA of thyroid lesions with comet-tail artifacts typically reveals significant colloid at cytology in 85% of cases. If punctate echogenic foci in a solid nodule or solid component of a nodule *do not* have convincing comet-tail artifact, it can be difficult

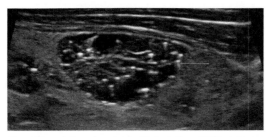

**Fig. 1.** Spongiform thyroid nodule composed of more than 50% cysts, many of which have a linear configuration. Echogenic foci with posterior ring-down artifact (*arrow*) are colloid crystals in this benign nodule.

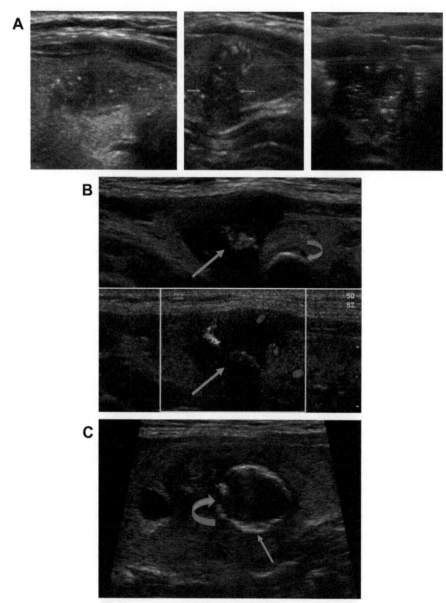

**Fig. 2.** Thyroid nodule calcifications. (*A*) Microcalcifications in 3 different hypoechoic nodules are characteristic of PTC. Arrows denote a cluster of microcacifications that together cast an acoustic shadow. (*B*) Macrocalcifications (*straight arrows*) in a markedly hypoechoic papillary thyroid malignancy with intranodular blood flow. An adjacent nodule has peripheral rim calcification (*curved arrow*). (*C*) Peripheral rim calcification is thick (*straight arrow*) and interrupted (*curved arrow*) in this hypoechoic papillary thyroid cancer.

to differentiate colloid from microcalcification. In this scenario, when using ultrasound to evaluate the risk of cancer, one should assume echogenic foci are microcalcifications rather than colloid crystals and err on the side of performing FNA of the nodule.[8]

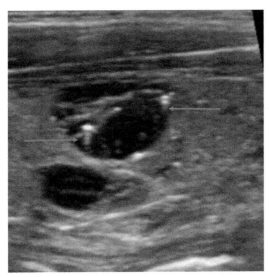

**Fig. 3.** Colloid crystals characterized by punctate or short linear echogenic foci with triangular-shaped "comet-tail" artifacts marked by arrows.

Macrocalcifications (**Fig. 2**B) are coarse calcifications that may cast an acoustic shadow and likely represent fibrosis/degeneration of thyroid tissue.[20] Macrocalcifications are seen in chronic thyroid nodules and Hashimoto thyroiditis.[21] Despite being associated with benign thyroid processes, coarse macrocalcifications also occur in malignant thyroid nodules and, when present *in a nodule*, increase risk of malignancy twofold.[8] If present in combination with additional suspicious features, such as marked hypoechogenicity, ill-defined margins and taller-than-wide shape, macrocalcifications in a nodule further increase cancer risk.[22]

Peripheral rim or "eggshell" calcifications in a nodule (**Fig. 2**C) are features that previously suggested benignity; however, in the past decade, these calcifications are reported to carry an approximately 20% malignancy risk.[23] Some investigators further stratify rim calcification as being lower risk if continuous and smooth, and higher risk if interrupted and thick (>5 mm).[24–26]

### Margins

Similar to neoplasms in other parts of the body, thyroid nodules that are benign typically have sharp, well-defined margins, whereas malignant lesions often have ill-defined margins. Additional descriptions of thyroid nodule margins include smooth, lobulated, and spiculated (**Fig. 4**).[8,20] The terms spiculated and ill-defined imply malignant infiltration into adjacent parenchyma. The definition of an ill-defined thyroid nodule is one in which more than 50% of its margin is not discernible. The reported sensitivity and specificity of ill-defined margins in thyroid nodules is variable. One study found well-defined margins in 47% of PTC. Many of these nodules were encapsulated at histology.[27] Benign nodules with ill-defined margins have been reported in 15% to 59% of cases.[10,18] Due to variable specificity and sensitivity, the single feature of nodular margin is not reliable in diagnosing malignancy except when obvious invasion through the thyroid capsule is noted.[28]

### Halo

A halo or hypoechoic periphery encircling a nodule may be created by surrounding blood vessels, a fibrous connective tissue pseudocapsule, chronic inflammatory

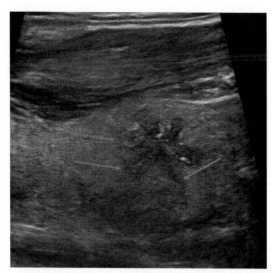

**Fig. 4.** Spiculated margins (*single arrow*) and ill-defined margins (*double arrows*) in a hypo-echoic papillary cancer with microcalcifications.

infiltrates, or compressed thyroid tissue (**Fig. 5**A).[28–30] The feature of a completely uniform halo is closely correlated with benignity (specificity = 95%). However, sensitivity is poor in that more than 50% of benign nodules lack a halo and, conversely, a complete or incomplete halo is present in 10% to 24% of PTC.[27,28] Aggressive thyroid cancers may demonstrate thick, irregular, hypovascular halos, likely due to adjacent compressed thyroid tissue (**Fig. 5**B).[29]

### Shape

Thyroid nodule shape is useful for predicting malignancy risk. Shape "taller than wide" or greater in anterior-posterior dimension compared with transverse dimension is associated with higher malignancy risk (**Fig. 6**).[20,31,32] Malignant nodules are thought to disrespect normal tissue planes and invade through them, resulting in "taller-than-wide" appearance, whereas benign nodules expand parallel to normal tissue planes.[20]

### Composition: Solid Versus Cystic

Malignant thyroid nodules are mostly solid.[33] Solid composition sensitivity rates range from 69% to 86%, making it the most sensitive feature for malignancy. The PPV is, however, low with only 15% to 27% chance that a given solid nodule is malignant.

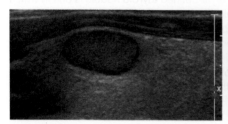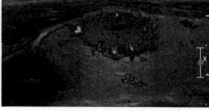

**Fig. 5.** A partially uniform halo composed of blood vessels and compressed thyroid tissue in a benign follicular adenoma.

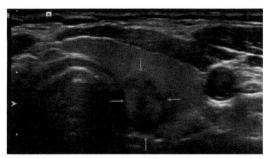

**Fig. 6.** Thyroid nodule shape taller than wide (*blue arrows*) in a papillary thyroid cancer with hypoechoic and markedly hypoechoic tissue and a thick irregular halo.

An inverse relationship between cystic or partially cystic nodules and risk of malignancy has been reported. Although a simple cyst is highly specific for benignity, it represents fewer than 1% to 2% of thyroid lesions.[1,9] A mixed solid and cystic lesion with more than 50% solid component has a greater risk of malignancy. Eccentric location of the solid component with microcalcifications further increases the malignancy risk[34] (**Fig. 7**). Studies describing "spongiform" nodules demonstrated greater than 99% specificity for benignity. Avascular or isovascular spongiform nodules were always benign. A single case of a malignant hypervascular spongiform lesion is reported in the literature.[20,34,35]

Cystic thyroid nodules are defined as containing more than 50% fluid. Cystic PTC represents approximately 5% to 7% of PTC. These lesions contain a vascularized solid component and/or microcalcifications, and this component needs to be sampled during FNA to achieve accurate diagnosis (**Fig. 8**).[27]

### Echotexture

Malignant thyroid nodules are usually solid and hypoechoic relative to adjacent thyroid parenchyma. These 2 sonographic features, in combination, reportedly have sensitivity of 87% for thyroid malignancy.[10] In the same series, benign nodules were also

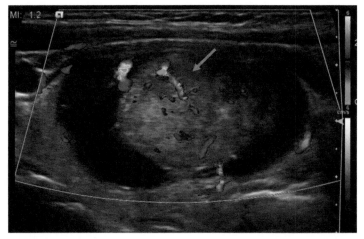

**Fig. 7.** Mixed solid and cystic papillary thyroid carcinoma with a >50% solid component that has intranodular flow (*blue arrow*) and scattered microcalcifications.

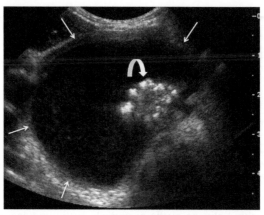

**Fig. 8.** Cystic papillary thyroid carcinoma (*straight arrows*) is more than 50% fluid. FNAB was directed at the solid component with microcalcifications (*curved arrow*).

solid and hypoechoic in 55%, yielding low specificity (15%–27%) and PPV for this combination of features.[8,28] Increased specificity up to 94% is obtained when the solid component of a nodule is *markedly hypoechoic*, defined as more hypoechoic than adjacent neck strap muscles; however, sensitivity is reduced to 12% (**Fig. 9**).

### Multinodularity

The risk of multiple nodules harboring cancer is approximately 14%, similar to the risk for a solitary nodule.[9,21] When multiple discrete nodules are present, the lesion(s) with suspicious morphology should be aspirated rather than the dominant lesion (**Fig. 10**). In the absence of suspicious features, some recommend biopsy of the dominant nodule. When multiple similar nodules are present in a diffusely enlarged gland without adjacent normal thyroid tissue, FNA is likely not needed.[1,8]

### Color Doppler Imaging

Color and power Doppler are used to distinguish thyroid nodule vascular patterns or combinations of patterns, including absent flow, perinodular flow, and intranodular flow (**Fig. 11**). Nodular vascular pattern is an additional feature used to stratify risk of malignancy; however, broad interobserver variability yields significant differences in sensitivity and specificity of this feature.

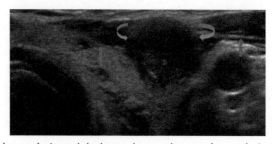

**Fig. 9.** Markedly hypoechoic nodule (*curved arrows*), more hypoechoic than the adjacent strap muscles (*straight arrows*), has high specificity for papillary thyroid malignancy.

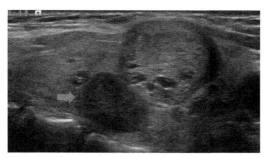

**Fig. 10.** Multinodular gland: the dominant nodule contains linear cysts, a small focus of colloid (*thin arrow*) and is a benign adenomatous nodule. The smaller, adjacent markedly hypoechoic nodule (*thick arrow*) is a medullary carcinoma.

Intranodular hypervascularity, flow in the center of a nodule, more than the surrounding tissue, is present in in 69% to 74% of thyroid malignancies and is the most common vascular pattern reported.[10,27] This finding is, however, not specific and more than 50% of solid hypervascular nodules are benign.[36]

Perinodular flow pattern, vessels surrounding at least 25% of the circumference of a nodule, is more common in benign nodules but has been described in 22% of carcinomas.[6,27,28] Complete lack of blood flow is seen in hyperplastic lesions and is unlikely to be seen in thyroid malignancy.[6,27]

## Size

As with other isolated ultrasound features, size of a nodule does not predict or exclude thyroid malignancy. The different societies that publish consensus guidelines recommending thyroid nodule FNA disagree about which features, including size criteria, should prompt a biopsy. Recent ATA guidelines recommend FNA for highly suspicious nodules once they reach 1 cm. Nodules smaller than 1 cm with suspicious ultrasound features are acknowledged as targets for FNA if patients are considered high risk or have suspicious cervical nodes.[1,21] The ATA defines a high-risk history as follows: personal history of radiation therapy in childhood, family history of thyroid cancer, prior partial thyroidectomy with cancer in the surgical specimen, and presence of PET-positivity in a thyroid nodule.

The sensitivity, specificity, PPV, and NPV of malignant ultrasound features when applied to nodules smaller than 1 cm are similar to nodules larger than 1 cm.[37] In

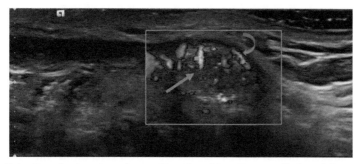

**Fig. 11.** Color Doppler imaging of a papillary thyroid malignancy that contains peripheral (*curved arrow*) and intranodular (*straight arrow*) blood flow.

features applied to nodules smaller than 5 mm demonstrated
es and inadequate cytologic accuracy was also reported. This
to advise against routine FNA of subcentimeter thyroid nodules
us ultrasound features were thought to be present.[38] Recent
agreement between biopsy results and ultrasound features sug-
y and have shown adequate diagnostic sampling in subcentimeter
everal of which were smaller than 5 mm.[39]

SIONS

licular lesion" includes follicular thyroid adenoma and follicular thyroid
TC) and the latter can be distinguished only by the presence of vascular
ar invasion in the surgical specimen. Differentiating benign from malignant
sions with cytology or even core biopsy is often not possible; however, mo-
sting of FNA specimens may improve diagnostic accuracy in the future. FTC
its 5% to 15% of all thyroid malignancy, is more prevalent in iodine-deficient
,[6] and is thought to evolve from preexisting adenoma. FTC metastasizes pri-
hematogenously to lung, liver, bone, and brain. Local cervical nodal metastases
less commonly.

ecause FTC usually lacks characteristic ultrasound features of PTC outlined thus
in this article, sonographic differentiation of benign from malignant follicular lesions
challenging. Seventy percent of FTC is solid and homogeneous.[40] FTC is more often
oechoic to hyperechoic, may have a thick, irregular halo, and often lacks microcalcification (**Fig. 12**).[41] In large solid lesions with otherwise benign ultrasound features,
lack of cystic degeneration supports but is not completely diagnostic of a follicular
neoplasm.[16,42] Features that suggest malignancy in follicular lesions include intranodular, chaotic blood flow, with or without perinodular flow. Benign follicular lesions tend
to have perinodular flow.[6,29] Reportedly, follicular cancers smaller than 2 cm do not
present with metastatic disease.[43]

## MEDULLARY THYROID CANCER

Medullary thyroid carcinoma (MTC) accounts for approximately 5% of thyroid cancer
and arises from parafollicular C-cells that secrete calcitonin. Calcitonin can be a useful
tumor marker for disease recurrence/progression, which often initially occurs in the

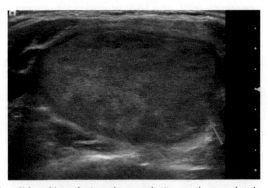

**Fig. 12.** FTC that is solid and isoechoic to hyperechoic, nearly completely replaces the gland
and has an irregular halo of adjacent compressed thyroid parenchyma. The halo appears
thick posteriorly and a focal indistinct portion of the halo (*blue arrow*) histologically repre-
sented an area of frank invasion.

neck and mediastinum. At presentation, 50% have regional nodal metastases and 15% to 25% distant metastases. Familial MTC occurs in 20% of cases. When associated with multiple endocrine neoplasia II syndrome, MTC is more aggressive and has a worse prognosis, with approximately 55% 5-year survival.[6,29]

Sonographically, MTC typically is solid, hypoechoic with intranodular flow, and mimics PTC, except that MTC tends to have rounded or ovoid, rather than irregular shape.[44] Punctate echogenic foci seen in 80% to 90% of MTC are the result of calcification from amyloid deposition, rather than psammomatous calcification seen in PTC (**Fig. 13**). These calcifications are also found in 50% to 60% of MTC nodal metastases.

## THYROID LYMPHOMA

Thyroid lymphoma (TL) comprises only 1% to 4% of all thyroid cancers, frequently is non-Hodgkin, and, in 70% to 80% of cases, arises in the setting of Hashimoto thyroiditis. Presenting symptoms include dyspnea, dysphagia, and history of a rapidly growing mass.[45] The stage of disease at presentation predicts prognosis with 90% 5-year survival in early-stage presentation versus 5% in advanced disease.

Sonographic features of TL when a focal lesion is present include hypoechogenicity, hypovascularity, and lobulated shape. When TL involves a lobe or the entire gland, the thyroid parenchyma is typically heterogeneous or diffusely enlarged and hypoechoic (**Fig. 14**). Similar to lymphoma in other organs, a pseudocystic appearance with posterior acoustic enhancement is possible. Late presentation of TL is characterized by encasement of vessels and adjacent head and neck structures. Any adjacent thyroid parenchyma not involved with tumor may demonstrate features of underlying chronic Hashimoto thyroiditis with fine echogenic linear fibrous strands.[6,29,46] Enlarged, hypoechoic, rounded lateral and central compartment cervical nodes, seen in chronic thyroiditis, are commonly seen in TL. When TL is considered, multiple FNA specimens or, if possible, core biopsy may be obtained for flow cytometry, which is required for cytologic diagnosis.

## ANAPLASTIC THYROID CANCER

Anaplastic thyroid carcinoma is among the most aggressive head and neck malignancies and represents fewer than 5% of all thyroid cancer. It occurs in advanced age, presents as a rapidly growing mass that invades adjacent structures, and has the worst prognosis of all thyroid malignancies with greater than 95% mortality at 5 years. These cancers may represent dedifferentiation of an existing neoplasm and

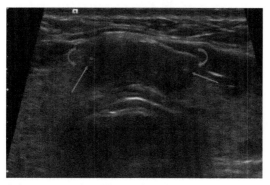

**Fig. 13.** MTC in the isthmus is ovoid and hypoechoic (*curved arrows*) with microcalcifications from amyloid deposition (*straight arrows*) and mimics PTC.

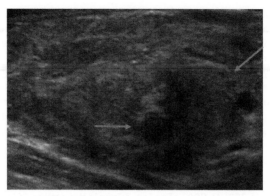

**Fig. 14.** TL is a hypoechoic mass (*arrows*) and the background heterogeneous thyroid paren-chyma demonstrates features of Hashimoto thyroiditis with echogenic linear fibrous strands.

are often associated with PTC or FTC at pathology. Patients are typically inoperable at time of diagnosis and may present with airway compression or vascular thrombosis due to local invasion.

Sonographically, anaplastic thyroid cancer is characterized by an ill-defined, infiltra-tive, hypoechoic mass with intranodular flow and areas of necrosis. The mass typically involves at least an entire lobe and demonstrates extracapsular extension, invasion of adjacent neck muscles, and encasement and/or invasion of adjacent vascular struc-tures. Local nodal involvement, often with necrosis, and/or distant metastases, is often present at diagnosis (**Fig. 15**). The extensive nature of anaplastic malignancies limits the usefulness of ultrasound, and contrast-enhanced neck CT and MRI more accurately illustrate extent of disease.[6,29,47]

## RECURRENT THYROID CANCER

Thyroid cancer, when it recurs locally, is often detected initially in the postoperative bed and may also locally metastasize to central compartment and/or lateral compart-ment nodes. Recurrent PTC is typically circumscribed and hypoechoic but may be irregular in shape. If intranodular flow, cystic change, or microcalcifications are

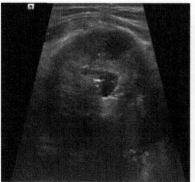
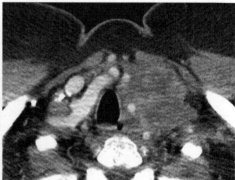

**Fig. 15.** Anaplastic thyroid carcinoma is a large ill-defined, hypoechoic mass with a cystic area of necrosis on the ultrasound. The CT scan demonstrates invasion of neck muscles and encasement/invasion of adjacent vessels.

present, recurrent or central compartment metastatic disease is favored over postoperative change (**Fig. 16**). Postoperative suture granuloma may present as an avascular, circumscribed, hypoechoic thyroid bed nodule. These may contain suture material characterized by larger than 1-mm central or paracentral, paired, parallel, irregular-shaped, echogenic foci that mimic calcification.[48]

## LYMPH NODE METASTASES

Ultrasound is indicated in preoperative evaluation of lateral compartment (level 2–5) lymph node metastases for operative planning. Ultrasound also can detect central compartment nodal metastases and extrathyroidal tumor extension. CT has been reported to have greater sensitivity than ultrasound in detection of central compartment (level 6) nodal metastases, but evaluation and management of the central compartment is typically performed intraoperatively by the surgeon.[2]

Macroscopic lateral compartment nodal metastases impact recurrence rates and may influence survival. For this reason, preoperative ultrasound mapping of lateral compartment nodes before surgery is routine in management of newly diagnosed thyroid cancer.[49] Identification of pathologic nodes in the central and/or lateral compartments allows for excision at the time of initial thyroidectomy.[50]

Ultrasound criteria that suggest malignant nodal morphology include cystic change, calcification, rounded rather than elongated shape, abnormal blood flow, and focal or diffuse hyperechoic changes (**Fig. 17**). Absent fatty hilum was once considered a potential feature of malignant adenopathy, but has been reported in subsequent studies to be much less accurate than the features listed in the preceding sentence. Negative cytology in nodes with suspicious features does not exclude metastatic involvement.[51] The above-described ultrasound criteria are used in predicting malignancy in the *lateral* compartment; however, only 2 of the features, calcification and abnormal blood flow, are reported to accurately predict metastases in the *central*

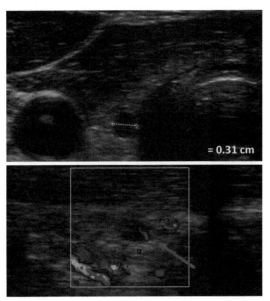

**Fig. 16.** Recurrent papillary thyroid carcinoma characterized by a 3-mm circumscribed nodule with intranodular blood flow (*blue arrow*).

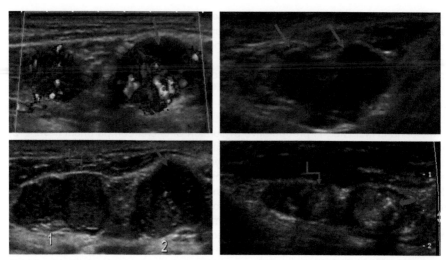

**Fig. 17.** Metastatic papillary thyroid carcinoma in multiple cervical nodes in the same patient. Several of the nodes are rounded in shape with abnormal "disorganized" blood flow. Straight arrows denote cystic change; curved arrow depicts microcalcifications; and arrows with 90° angles point to echogenic foci in these nodes, all of which are metastatic.

compartment.[52] Preoperative ultrasound of cervical lymph nodes plays a major role in preoperative planning in patients with thyroid cancer, specifically in evaluating the need for and extent of lateral neck dissection.[53]

Patients with Hashimoto thyroiditis may present with thyroid nodules and cervical lymphadenopathy. Numerous enlarged and/or hypoechoic lymph nodes with rounded shape can be seen in these patients. In patients with Hashimoto thyroiditis and thyroid malignancy, cystic change and calcification in the lateral compartment nodes are features that suggest metastatic disease.[54]

## ULTRASOUND-GUIDED FINE-NEEDLE ASPIRATION

Although ultrasound features may provide risk stratification or signal high suspicion for cancer, FNAB is the gold standard for diagnosis of malignancy in thyroid nodules and lymph nodes.[1] Ultrasound-guided FNA has lower rates of nondiagnostic cytology than palpation-guided FNA. Ultrasound both identifies and enables sampling of nonpalpable nodules and improves cytologic adequacy through targeted aspiration of solid, vascularized components in partially cystic nodules.[55] The false-negative rate is lower in ultrasound-guided FNA compared with palpation-guided FNA (1.0% vs 2.3%).[56]

Diagnosis of recurrent or metastatic cancer can be aided by Tg assay of material aspirated from abnormal neck masses in the central and lateral compartments should cytology in these lesions be nondiagnostic or negative.[57] Tg assay of lesions in the central compartment is of limited usefulness in patients who have *not* undergone radioactive iodine ablation, as lesions in this compartment may represent benign regenerated or residual thyroid tissue that normally produces Tg. FNAB is usually performed with the initial aspirate placed on a slide for cytology. The needle can then be rinsed in 1 to 2 mL sterile saline and saved for Tg analysis if the cytology is inconclusive or negative. Accuracy and sensitivity in diagnosis of metastases are improved when FNAB-Tg is combined with FNAB-cytology compared with FNAB-cytology alone. Investigators report improved accuracy in detection of metastases in small lymph nodes with FNAB-Tg.[58]

## FUTURE CONSIDERATION
### Thyroid Imaging-Reporting and Data Systems

Lexicons for standardizing ultrasound reporting assign risk levels to thyroid nodules. In the spirit of the BI-RADS system used in breast imaging, Horvath and colleagues[15] built a pattern-based model, stratifying thyroid nodules into 10 different patterns and assigned a TI-RADS risk category to each pattern. The distinction between TI-RADS 3 and 4 marked a significant increase in risk of malignancy. Kwak and colleagues[59] used similar risk categories, but rather than patterns, described suspicious features that suggest significant association with malignancy and assigned a TI-RADS category according to the absolute number of suspicious findings in a particular nodule. Currently, the ATA uses a system of pattern-based ultrasound findings with varying size criteria for FNAB, depending on the presence or absence of specific ultrasound findings.[1] One soon-to-be-published study by Chung and colleagues retrospectively characterized 1059 previously biopsied thyroid nodules using the following 3 methods: TI-RADS as defined by Kwak and colleagues[59] and the most recent ATA[1] and Society of Radiologists in Ultrasound (SRU) guidelines.[7] TI-RADS outperformed ATA and SRU guidelines in PPV, NPV, and accuracy; however, sensitivity was highest using ATA guidelines.[60]

In 2015, the ACR released its own TI-RADS classification system and described 6 categories of findings: nodule composition, echogenicity, shape, size, margin, and presence/absence of echogenic foci.[14] Definitions of each subcategory were released in 2015 and risk stratification into specific TI-RADS categories was published in May 2017.[61]

### Papillary Thyroid Microcarcinomas

Papillary thyroid microcarcinomas (PTMCs) are defined as cancers that are 1 cm or smaller. Controversy exists about whether patients with low-risk PTMCs can safely avoid surgery and undergo surveillance ultrasound. Ito and colleagues[62] followed low-risk Japanese patients with PTMCs for periods ranging from 18 to 187 months (average 74 months). Patients were monitored with serial sonograms and serum Tg. Tumor enlargement by at least 3 mm occurred in 16.0% at 10 years and development of lymph node metastasis in 3.4% at 10 years. PTMC progression was significantly more common in patients younger than 40 years compared with older subjects. Currently, no other clinical features or molecular abnormalities have been proven to predict progression of PTMC. So far, the only ultrasound feature of PTMC reported to suggest risk of future growth is hypervascularity.[63] The ATA currently recommends surgery for any biopsy-proven thyroid malignancy, but the group acknowledges surveillance in PTMC may be appropriate for low-risk or poor surgical candidates.[1] Should long-term clinical follow-up become acceptable management of PTMC, development of consistent ultrasound lexicon for these lesions will be critical (**Fig. 18**).

### Molecular Testing

Several molecular tests exist that further characterize FNAB specimens designated "atypia of undetermined significance" (AUS) or "follicular lesion of undetermined significance" (FLUS). AUS/FLUS lesions are classified as Bethesda III nodules in the Bethesda cytology classification system.

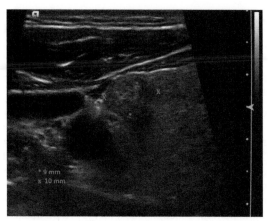

**Fig. 18.** Papillary thyroid micro carcinoma is hypoechoic with microcalcifications and measures 10 mm in this patient who elected to undergo surveillance rather than surgical management.

Afirma is a molecular test that compares the expression of 167 gene transcripts in AUS/FLUS samples to known benign profiles. Afirma had a high NPV (94%) in a large but sponsored clinical validation study and is considered a "rule-out" test that may reduce unnecessary surgical intervention.[64] Asuragen miRInform is a "rule-in" mutational analysis test for common point mutations of BRAF and RAS and 2 additional rearrangement mutations. Validation studies have supported a high PPV of 87% to 95%, suggesting a role for this test for "ruling in" malignancy.[65] Most recently, Thyroseq is a test that amplifies mRNA and DNA content of thyroid FNA samples for comparison to libraries of mutations and expressed proteins. Thyroseq, in some studies, has both high PPVs and NPVs that may allow it to serve as both a "rule-in" and "rule-out" test.[66] Other molecular tests available include serum measurement of thyroid stimulating hormone receptor levels as an indicator of malignancy and assessment of galecin-3 expression.

Currently there is no consensus regarding using molecular testing to guide surgical decision making. Some researchers argue that diagnosis of a Bethesda III nodule with a mutation such as BRAF might justify consideration of total rather than hemithyroidectomy. Currently, molecular testing may help direct treatment or provide prognostic information in some proven malignancy cases, but these tests provide only supplemental data in the setting of AUS/FLUS lesions and overall clinical utility in affecting long-term outcomes has yet to be established.[67]

### Elastography

Firm or stiff nodule consistency is associated with increased malignancy risk. Strain and shear wave elastography have emerged as tools to acquire stiffness measurements. In the context of other grayscale ultrasound findings, these are used to increase specificity and diagnostic confidence for thyroid malignancy.

Application of *strain* elastography requires application of uniform compression over a nodule either manually or with commercially available elastography systems, but is reliable only in evaluation of solid nodules. It is unreliable in heterogeneous tissue, including thyroid isthmus, exophytic masses, and lesions adjacent to the carotid artery and cannot be reliably used with deep lesions or cystic, rim-calcified, or coalescent nodules.[68,69] Larger single-center studies[70] and meta-analyses[71] found elastography had better overall diagnostic performance compared with *single* ultrasound features; however, its utility compared with multiple ultrasound findings or patterns is undetermined. *Shear wave* elastography uses ultrasound push pulses (similar to Doppler) but it has yet to be robustly studied. Some elastography research has demonstrated high sensitivity and specificity for PTC[72–74]; however, investigators have also reported interobserver unreliability for diagnosis of malignancy.[75] At this time, elastography provides supplemental information and cannot replace grayscale ultrasound examination for nodule characterization.

## SUMMARY

Ultrasound is critical in diagnosis and management of thyroid nodules. Nodules detected by imaging or palpation should undergo further characterization with diagnostic ultrasound to determine whether sonographic features suggest malignancy and the need for FNA. Recall that the classic ultrasound features of PTC and FTC differ. PTC tends to be solid and hypoechoic with intranodular flow and irregular margins and, therefore, conforms to current sonographic criteria for malignancy. Microcalcification is specific for PTC but can be difficult to distinguish from colloid. If decision for FNA is guided by these classic malignancy criteria, FTC which often lacks microcalcification and is isoechoic to hyperechoic with a thick irregular halo, will be missed.[41]

Preoperative and postoperative diagnostic ultrasound evaluation of cervical lymph nodes and ultrasound-guided intervention are also critical to management of thyroid cancer. Future developments in thyroid ultrasound, including elastography and, perhaps more importantly, refinements in thyroid ultrasound reporting lexicon may impact future management and may obviate the need for follow-up in certain low-risk or frankly benign lesions. Longitudinal studies with large numbers of patients will likely lead to established criteria for future management of PTMC. And finally, advances in molecular testing may result in a test with strong predictive capability that could potentially prevent unnecessary thyroid surgery in significant numbers of patients.

## REFERENCES

1. Haugen BRM, Alexander EK, Bible KC, et al. 2015 American Thyroid Association management guidelines for adult patients with thyroid nodules and differentiated thyroid cancer. Thyroid 2015;26:1–133.
2. Choi JS, Kim J, Kwak JY, et al. Preoperative staging of papillary thyroid carcinoma: comparison of ultrasound imaging and CT. Am J Roentgenol 2009; 193(3):871–8.
3. Frasoldati A, Presenti M, Gallo M, et al. Diagnosis of neck recurrences in patients with differentiated thyroid carcinoma. Cancer 2003;97(1):90–6.
4. Monchik JM, Donatini G, Iannuccilli J, et al. Radiofrequency ablation and percutaneous ethanol injection treatment for recurrent local and distant well-differentiated thyroid carcinoma. Ann Surg 2006;244(2):296–304.
5. Sippel RS, Elaraj DM, Poder L, et al. Localization of recurrent thyroid cancer using intraoperative ultrasound-guided dye injection. World Surg 2009;33:434–9.
6. Wong KT, Ahuja AT. Ultrasound of thyroid cancer. Cancer Imaging 2005;5(1): 157–66.
7. Frates MC, Benson CB, Charboneau JW, et al. Management of thyroid nodules detected at US: Society of Radiologists in Ultrasound consensus conference statement. Ultrasound Q 2006;22:231–40.

8. Bastin S, Bolland MJ, Croxson MS. Role of ultrasound in the assessment of nodular thyroid disease. J Med Imaging Radiat Oncol 2009;53(2):177–87.

9. Frates MC, Benson CB, Doubilet PM, et al. Prevalence and distribution of carcinoma in patients with solitary and multiple thyroid nodules on sonography. J Clin Endocrinol Metab 2006;91:3411–7.

10. Papini E, Guglielmi R, Bianchini A, et al. Risk of malignancy in non-palpable thyroid nodules: predictive value of ultrasound and color Doppler features. J Clin Endocrinol Metab 2002;87:1941–6.

11. Capelli C, Castellano M, Pirola I, et al. Thyroid shape suggests malignancy. Eur J Endocrinol 2006;155:27–31.

12. Bonavita JA, Mayo J, Babb J, et al. Pattern recognition of benign thyroid nodules at ultrasound: which nodules can be left alone? Am J Roentgenol 2009;193(1): 207–13.

13. Park JY, Lee HJ, Jang HW, et al. A proposal for a thyroid imaging reporting and data system for ultrasound features of thyroid nodules. Thyroid 2009;19(11): 1257–64.

14. Grant E, Tessler F, Hoang J, et al. Thyroid Ultrasound Reporting Lexicon: White Paper of the ACR Thyroid Imaging, Reporting and Data System (TIRADS) Committee. J Am Coll Radiol 2015;12:1272–9.

15. Horvath E, Majlis S, Rossi R, et al. An ultrasonogram reporting system for thyroid nodules stratifying cancer risk for clinical management. J Clin Endocrinol Metab 2009;94(5):1748–51.

16. ACR practice Guidelines for the Performance of Thyroid and Parathyroid Ultrasound Examinations, revised 2007. Available at: http://www.acr.org/SecondaryMainMenuCategories/quality_safety/guidelines/us/us_thyroid_parathyroid.aspx. Accessed June 10, 2010.

17. Liu YI, Kamaya A, Desser TS, et al. A Bayesian classifier for differentiating benign versus malignant thyroid nodules using sonographic features. AMIA Annu Proc 2008;6:419–23.

18. Wienke JR, Chong WK, Fielding JR, et al. Sonographic features of benign thyroid nodules: interobserver reliability and overlap with malignancy. J Ultrasound Med 2003;22:1027–31.

19. Moon WJ, Jung SL, Lee JH, et al. Benign and malignant thyroid nodules: US differentiation—multicenter retrospective study. Radiology 2008;247(3):602–4.

20. Wang N, Xu Y, Ge C, et al. Association of sonographically detected calcification with thyroid carcinoma. Head Neck 2006;28:1077–83.

21. Sipos JA. Advances in ultrasound for the diagnosis and management of thyroid cancer. Thyroid 2009;19(12):1363–72.

22. Kim MJ, Kim EK, Kwak JY, et al. Differentiation of thyroid nodules with macrocalcifications: role of suspicious sonographic findings. J Ultrasound Med 2008; 27(8):1179–84.

23. Yoon DY, Lee JW, Chang SK, et al. Peripheral calcification in thyroid nodules: ultrasonographic features and prediction of malignancy. J Ultrasound Med 2007; 26:1349–55.

24. Lee SK, Rho BH. Follicular thyroid carcinoma with an eggshell calcification: report of 3 cases. J Ultrasound Med 2009;28(6):801–6.

25. Park M, Shin JH, Han BK, et al. Sonography of thyroid nodules with peripheral calcifications. J Clin Ultrasound 2009;37(6):324–8.

26. Kim BM, Kim MJ, Kim EK, et al. Sonographic differentiation of thyroid nodules with eggshell calcifications. J Ultrasound Med 2008;27(10):1425–30.

27. Chan BK, Desser TS, McDougall IR, et al. Common and uncommon sonographic features of papillary thyroid carcinoma. J Ultrasound Med 2003;22(10):1083–90.
28. Hoang JK, Lee WK, Lee M, et al. Ultrasound features of thyroid malignancy: pearls and pitfalls. Radiographics 2007;27:847–65.
29. Solbiati L, Charnoneau JW, James EM, et al. The thyroid gland. In: Rumack CM, Wilson SR, Charboneau JW, editors. Diagnostic ultrasound. St Louis (MO): Mosby-Yearbook, Inc; 1998. p. 713–4.
30. Propper RA, Skolnick ML, Weinstein BJ, et al. The nonspecificity of the thyroid halo sign. J Clin Ultrasound 1980;8(2):129–32.
31. Kim EK, Park CS, Chung WY, et al. New sonographic criteria for recommending fine-needle aspiration biopsy of nonpalpable solid nodules of the thyroid. Am J Roentgenol 2002;178:687–91.
32. Alexander EK, Marqusee E, Orcutt J, et al. Thyroid nodule shape and prediction of malignancy. Thyroid 2004;14:953–8.
33. Baier ND, Hahn PF, Gervais DA, et al. Fine-needle aspiration biopsy of thyroid nodules: experience in a cohort of 944 patients. Am J Roentgenol 2009;193(4): 1175–9.
34. Lee MJ, Kim EK, Kwak JY, et al. Partially cystic thyroid nodules on ultrasound: probability of malignancy and sonographic differentiation. Thyroid 2009;19(4): 341–6.
35. Reading CC, Charboneau JW, Hay ID, et al. Sonography of thyroid nodules: a "classic pattern" diagnostic approach. Ultrasound Q 2005;21:157–65.
36. Frates MC, Benson CB, Doubilet PM, et al. Can color Doppler sonography aid in the prediction of malignancy of thyroid nodules? J Ultrasound Med 2003;22(2): 127–31.
37. Kwak JY, Kim EK, Kim MJ, et al. Significance of sonographic characterization for managing subcentimeter thyroid nodules. Acta Radiol 2009;50(8):917–23.
38. Mazzeferri EL, Sipos J. Should all patients with subcentimeter thyroid nodules undergo fine-needle aspiration biopsy and preoperative neck ultrasonography to define the extent of tumor invasion? Thyroid 2008;18(6):597–602.
39. Sharma A, Gabriel H, Nemcek A, et al. Subcentimeter thyroid nodules: utility of sonographic characterization and ultrasound-guided needle biopsy. AJR Am J Roentgenol 2011;197:6.
40. Lin JD, Hsueh C, Chao TC, et al. Thyroid follicular neoplasms diagnosed by high-resolution ultrasonography with fine needle aspiration cytology. Acta Cytol 1997; 41:687–91.
41. Jeh SK, Jung SL, Kim BS, et al. 2007 Evaluating the degree of conformity of papillary carcinoma and follicular carcinoma to the reported ultrasonographic findings of malignant thyroid tumor. Korean J Radiol 2007;8:192–7.
42. Murakami T. Ultrasonography. In: Clark OH, Noguchi S, editors. Thyroid cancer diagnosis and treatment. St Louis (MO): Quality Medical Publishing, Inc; 2000. p. 209–25.
43. Machens A, Holzhausen HJ, Dralle H. The prognostic value of primary tumor size in papillary and follicular thyroid carcinoma. Cancer 2005;103:2269–73.
44. Kim SH, Kim BS, Jung SL, et al. Ultrasonographic findings of medullary thyroid carcinoma: a comparison with papillary thyroid carcinoma. Korean J Radiol 2009;10(2):101–5.
45. Ruggiero FP, Frauenhoffer E, Stack BC Jr. Thyroid lymphoma: a single institution's experience. Otolaryngol Head Neck Surg 2005;133:888–96.
46. Kasagi K, Hatabu H, Tokuda Y, et al. Lymphoproliferative disorders of the thyroid gland: radiological appearances. Br J Radiol 1991;64:569–75.

47. Nel CJC, Van Heerden JA, James EM, et al. Anaplastic carcinoma of the thyroid: a clinicopathologic study of 82 cases. Mayo Clin Proc 1985;60:51–8.
48. Kim JH, Lee JH, Shong YK, et al. Ultrasound features of suture granulomas in the thyroid bed after thyroidectomy for papillary thyroid carcinoma with an emphasis on their differentiation from locally recurrent thyroid carcinoma. Ultrasound Med Biol 2009;35(9):1452–7.
49. Marshall CL, Lee JE, Xing Y, et al. Routine pre-operative ultrasonography for papillary thyroid cancer: effects on cervical recurrence. Surgery 2009;146(6): 1063–72.
50. Sippel RS, Chen H. Controversies in the surgical management of newly diagnosed and recurrent/residual thyroid cancer. Thyroid 2009;19(12):1373–80.
51. Sohn YM, Kwak JY, Kim EK, et al. Diagnostic approach for evaluation of lymph node metastasis from thyroid cancer using ultrasound and fine-needle aspiration. Am J Roentgenol 2010;194(1):38–43.
52. Park J, Son KR, Na DG, et al. Performance of preoperative sonographic staging of papillary thyroid carcinoma based on sixth edition AJCC/UICC TNM classification system. Am J Roentgenol 2009;192(3):66–72.
53. Roh JL, Park JY, Kim JM, et al. Use of preoperative ultrasonography as guidance for neck dissection in patients with papillary thyroid carcinoma. J Surg Oncol 2009;99(1):28–31.
54. Paksoy N, Yazal K. Cervical lymphadenopathy associated with Hashimoto's thyroiditis: an analysis if 22 cases by fine needle aspiration cytology. Acta Cytol 2009;53(5):491–6.
55. Cesur M, Corapcioglu D, Bulut S, et al. Comparison of palpation-guided fine needle aspiration biopsy to ultrasound-guided fine needle aspiration biopsy in the evaluation of thyroid nodules. Thyroid 2006;16(6):555–61.
56. Danese D, Sciacchitano S, Farsetti A, et al. Diagnostic accuracy of conventional versus sonography guided fine needle aspiration biopsy of thyroid nodules. Thyroid 1998;8:15–21.
57. Bruno R, Giannasio P, Chiarella R, et al. Identification of a neck lump as a lymph node metastasis from an occult contralateral papillary microcarcinoma. Thyroid 2009;19(5):531–3.
58. Jeon SJ, Kim E, Park JS. Diagnostic benefit of thyroglobulin measurement in fine needle aspiration for diagnosing metastatic cervical lymph nodes from papillary thyroid cancer: correlations with US features. Korean J Radiol 2009;10(2):106–11.
59. Kwak JY, Han KH, Yoon JH, et al. Thyroid Imaging Reporting and Data System for US features of nodules: a step in establishing better stratification of cancer risk. Radiology 2011;260:892–9.
60. Chung H, Tan N, Ragavendra N et al. Performance of Societal Guidelines for Thyroid Cancer Detection after FNA. American Roentgen Ray Society Meeting. Los Angeles (CA), April 18, 2016.
61. Tessler FN, Middleton WD, Grant EG, et al. ACR thyroid imaging, reporting and data system (TI-RADS): white paper of the ACR TI-RADS committee. J Am Coll Radiol 2017;14(5):587–95.
62. Ito Y, Miyauchi A, Inoue H, et al. An observational trial for papillary thyroid microcarcinoma in Japanese patients. World J Surg 2010;34:28–35.
63. Sugitani I, Toda K, Yamada K, et al. Three distinctly different kinds of papillary thyroid microcarcinoma should be recognized: our treatment strategies and outcomes. World J Surg 2010;34:1222–31.
64. Alexander EK, Kennedy GC, Baloch ZW, et al. Preoperative diagnosis of benign thyroid nodules with indeterminate cytology. N Engl J Med 2012;367:705–15.

65. Nikiforov YE, Ohori NP, Hodak SP, et al. Impact of mutational testing on the diagnosis and management of patients with cytologically indeterminate thyroid nodules: a prospective analysis of 1056 FNA samples. J Clin Endocrinol Metab 2011;96:3390–7.

66. Nikiforov Y, Carty S, Chiosea S, et al. Impact of the multi-gene ThyroSeq next-generation sequencing assay on cancer diagnosis in thyroid nodules with atypia of undetermined significance/follicular lesion of undetermined significance cytology. Thyroid 2015;25(11):1217–23.

67. Bernet V, Hupart KH, Parangi S, et al. Molecular diagnostic testing of thyroid nodules with indeterminate cytopathology. Writing Group for the AACE Thyroid Scientific Committee. 2014.

68. Wang Y, Dan HJ, Dan HY, et al. Differential diagnosis of small single solid thyroid nodules using real-time ultrasound elastography. J Int Med Res 2010;38:466–72.

69. Cosgrove D, Barr R, Bojunga J, et al. World Federation for Ultrasound in Medicine & Biology Guidelines and recommendations on the clinical use of ultrasound elastography: Part 4. Thyroid. Ultrasound Med Biol 2016;1–23.

70. Azizi G, Keller J, Lewis M, et al. Performance of elastography for the evaluation of thyroid nodules: a prospective study. Thyroid 2013;23:734–40.

71. Razavi S, Hadduck T, Sadigh G, et al. Comparative effectiveness of elastographic and B-Mode ultrasound criteria for diagnostic discrimination of thyroid nodules: a meta-analysis. Am J Radiol 2013;200:1317–26.

72. Rago T, Vitti P. Potential value of elastography in the diagnosis of malignancy in thyroid nodules. Q J Nucl Med Mol Imaging 2009;53(5):455–63.

73. Friedrich-Rust M, Sperber A, Holzer K, et al. Real-time elastography and contrast-enhanced ultrasound for the assessment of thyroid nodules. Exp Clin Endocrinol Diabetes 2009;118(9):602–9.

74. Hong Y, Liu X, Li Z, et al. Real-time ultrasound elastography in the differential diagnosis of benign and malignant thyroid nodules. J Ultrasound Med 2009;28:861–7.

75. Park SH, Kim SJ, Ek Kim, et al. Interobserver agreement in assessing the sonographic and elastographic features of malignant thyroid nodules. Am J Roentgenol 2009;193(5):W416–23.

# Pituitary Imaging

Barry D. Pressman, MD

## KEYWORDS

- Pituitary imaging • MRI • CT

## KEY POINTS

- In the past, a number of indirect techniques including plain radiography, pnenmoencephalography, and angiography were used to diagnose pituitary masses.
- The advent of CT allowed for diagnosis of pituitary lesions by direct visualization of the gland. However, contrast sensitivity to lesions with CT is limited, although CT does offer advantages in that it is particularly excellent for detecting calcification bone detail such as erosion of the sella turcica.
- MRI offers superb contrast resolution and very good special resolution. Therefore, it can be used to detect, characterize pituitary and parasellar regions with great accuracy. MRI permits follow up of lesions and their response to treatment, without subjecting the patient to ionizing radiation.

## INTRODUCTION

Modern pituitary imaging *is* MRI, as explored in this article. However, computed tomography (CT) still has limited usefulness, such as the occasional CT angiogram when magnetic resonance angiography proves insufficient, and in those cases when MRI is contraindicated. In addition, because CT offers much better bone detail and calcium detection, there are some cases where such additional information is necessary.

Before the advent of CT, plain radiography, pneumoencephalography, and angiography were used to diagnose pituitary masses. Plain radiography allowed for evaluation of the size, shape, and bony erosion of the sella turcica. Pneumoencephalography offered indirect evaluation of the superior shape and size of the pituitary gland as it extended into the suprasellar space. Angiography demonstrated lateral displacement of the carotid arteries by macroadenomas that impressed on or extended into the cavernous sinus. More recently CT, and then especially MRI, made it possible to primarily delineate lesions within and around the pituitary gland rather than depending on secondary information that could only suggest their presence.

The author has nothing to disclose.
Department of Imaging, S. Mark Taper Foundation Imaging Center, Cedars-Sinai, 8700 Beverly Boulevard, Los Angeles, CA 90048, USA
*E-mail address:* Barry.Pressman@cshs.org

## IMAGING TECHNIQUE

The pituitary gland is a small structure, usually no more than 8 mm in height. Microadenomas, especially adrenicotropic producing, may be 1 mm in size. It is therefore crucial that imaging be of the highest possible quality including excellent spatial resolution and high signal to noise ratio. If the signal to noise ratio is inadequate, graininess of the image may obscure small lesions. Higher signal to noise is achieved with higher magnetic field strength (measured in units of Tesla) and/or longer acquisition time. There is a direct linear relationship between the signal to noise ratio and these two parameters. Therefore, 3-T MRI is preferable to 1.5-T because it offers twice the signal to noise ratio in the same acquisition time or, alternatively, allows for reduction in acquisition time. Furthermore, the higher the signal to noise ratio, the thinner the slices that may be obtained without excessive graininess. Longer acquisition times with a 1.5-T MRI can achieve signal to noise ratios comparable with that of 3-T, but at the risk of patient motion and image degradation.

MRI sections should be no thicker than 2 mm, without an intervening gap. Even a 1-mm gap can result in missing a 1-to-2-mm lesion. There are multiple two-dimensional and three-dimensional protocols available to accomplish high-resolution 2-mm images without a gap (**Box 1**). Each manufacturer has a different variation on this same theme. Radiologists should be strongly encouraged to use a sequence that achieves thin slices, high spatial resolution, and excellent signal to noise ratios.

Generally, coronal and sagittal T1-weighted precontrast and postcontrast images suffice to evaluate the pituitary gland as to size, shape, signal homogeneity, the presence of a mass within or contiguous to the gland, the infundibulum, the optic chiasm, and the cavernous sinuses and their contents. T1-weighted images of the pituitary offer superb anatomic detail and allow for recognition and characterization of most lesions when precontrast and postcontrast studies are performed. On occasion, T2-weighted images may be useful, particularly if there is a contraindication to the administration of contrast (gadolinium-based contrast), and for the definition of large masses that may be invading or displacing brain parenchyma.

Timing of image acquisition after contrast administration is important. Normal pituitary tissue generally enhances more quickly than do tumors and it is this temporal contrast differential that allows for differentiation of tumor from normal tissue. Therefore, contrast should be administered in a bolus and imaging started immediately thereafter.

Dynamic imaging further capitalizes on this temporal enhancement differential. Imaging is obtained using fast scanning technique with repetitive 10-minute acquisitions just before and after contrast bolus administration, over approximately 1 minute. Lesions that otherwise may not be detected on routine imaging because the lesion has enhanced equally to the normal gland by the time the imaging is completed (routine high-resolution images take several minutes to acquire) may be detected by these lower-resolution images because of the contrast differential. Dynamic imaging is generally reserved for those cases in which routine scans fail to detect a lesion, especially in hypercortisolemia (**Box 2, Fig. 1**).[1–4]

CT still has a limited role in pituitary/sella imaging. Since the advent of helical imaging, it is possible to obtain isotropic voxels (ie, same geometry in all dimensions) in the sagittal and coronal planes after axial acquisition. It is no longer necessary to angle the patients head and/or the CT imaging gantry to obtain true coronal imaging.

CT imaging is also best performed with noncontrast, and immediate postcontrast imaging. Sections in the axial planes should be 0.625 mm to 1.3 mm in thickness with the sagittal and coronal reformations of equal size.

---

**Box 1**
**Sample MRI pituitary imaging parameters**

*Sagittal T1 tse*

Field of view = 20 cm

Slice thickness = 2 mm (no gap)

Usually used 15 slices

TR = 650 ms

TE = 9.7 ms

ETL = 3

Resolution = 320 × 240

Band width = 274 Hx/px

Averages = 4

*Coronal T1 tse*

Field of view = 20 cm

Slice thickness = 2 mm (no gap)

Usually used 15 slices

TR = 650 ms

TE = 9.5 ms

ETL = 3

Resolution = 384 × 307

Band width = 271 Hx/px

Averages = 4

*Coronal T2 tse*

Field of view = 18 cm

Slice thickness = 2 mm (no gap)

Usually used 16 slices

TR = 3700 ms

TE = 108 ms

ETL = 25

Resolution = 384 × 384

Band width = 362 Hx/px

Averages = 3

---

## NORMAL ANATOMY/MRI APPEARANCE

The normal pituitary is isointense to brain on noncontrast T1-weighted images. It enhances moderately and homogeneously with contrast. In neonates up to approximately 3 months and in pregnant women, the pituitary is most often hyperintense on T1-weighted images (**Figs. 2** and **3**).

A small gland of less than 4 mm is not necessarily abnormal, especially in the elderly, but is common in primary hypopituitarism.[5–7] A small pituitary gland may be

---

**Box 2**
**Sample parameters for dynamic contrast-enhanced pituitary MRI**

Field of view = 18 cm

Slice thickness = 2 mm (no gap)

Usually used 12 slices

TR = 150 ms

TE = 4.0 ms

Flip angles = 70°

Resolution = 250 × 192

Band width = 250 Hx/px

Averages = 1

Number of measurements = 7 (one precontrast and six postcontrast)

Contrast given as a bolus and imaging begins immediately

---

associated with a small sella turcica, especially when developmental in origin (**Fig. 4**). The gland is usually 7 mm to 8 mm maximum in height and is superiorly flat, although mild superior convexity is frequent.

The pituitary is not uncommonly larger in menstruating women, 9 mm or even greater in height, with superior convexity, and it may impress on the undersurface of the chiasm (**Fig. 5**). Differentiating such normal hyperplasia from pathology may be difficult and requires close correlation with hormonal and clinical status. Unless a distinct lesion is visualized, caution is prudent.[8,9]

Another condition that has been increasingly recognized is intracranial hypotension, often associated with spontaneous spinal cerebrospinal fluid (CSF) leak. In such patients the pituitary gland may enlarge, and regress in size after successful treatment of the leak (**Fig. 6**).

The infundibulum extends from the tuber cinereum at the floor of the hypothalamus, to the superior pituitary gland, passing through the hiatus of the diaphragma sella. It is usually midline in position and no more than 2 mm to 3 mm in width. It is isointense to

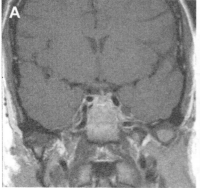
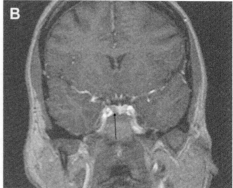

**Fig. 1.** (*A*) T1-weighted postcontrast image of a normal-appearing pituitary. (*B*) Dynamic series image of same patient with low signal microadenoma (*arrow*).

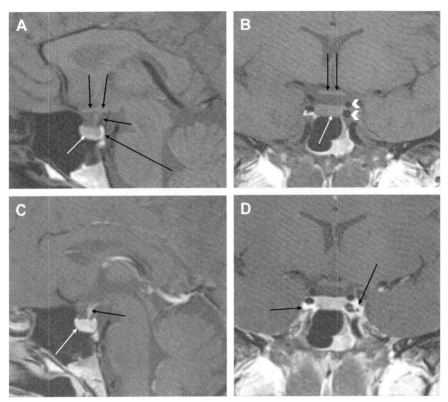

**Fig. 2.** (*A, B*) T1-weighted noncontrast sagittal and coronal images, respectively. Optic chiasm (*double arrows*), infundibulum (*single short black arrow*), pituitary (*white arrow*), and hyperintense posterior pituitary (*long black arrow*) all have normal appearance. The upper and lower loops of the cavernous carotid artery are visible on the coronal image (*arrowheads*). (*C, D*) T1-weighted postcontrast sagittal and coronal images, respectively. Contrast-enhanced infundibulum (*C, black arrow*), contrast-enhanced pituitary (*C, white arrow*), and contrast-enhanced cavernous sinus (*D, arrows*).

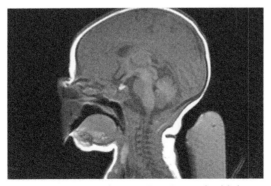

**Fig. 3.** T1-weighted noncontrast sagittal image in a 2 month old demonstrates high signal of the pituitary (*arrow*).

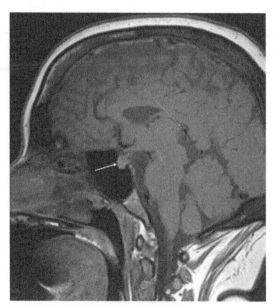

**Fig. 4.** T1-weighted noncontrast sagittal image demonstrates small sella turcica and pituitary gland (*arrow*). The long arrow points to the normal appearing pineal gland.

brain on T1-weighted images and because it does not have a blood-brain barrier, it normally enhances avidly with contrast (see **Fig. 2**).

The optic chiasm is isointense to brain on T1-weighted noncontrast images. It has a blood-brain barrier similar to brain parenchyma, and therefore does not enhance with

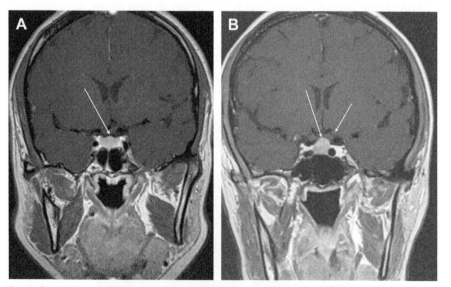

**Fig. 5.** (*A, B*) T1-weighted postcontrast coronal images of two different menstruating females. Both demonstrate superiorly convex pituitary glands (*long arrows*). In addition, in image (*B*), the gland is markedly impinging on the undersurface of the chiasm (*short arrow*).

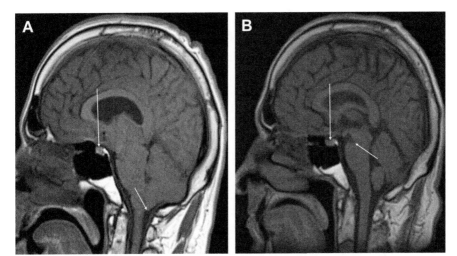

**Fig. 6.** T1-weighted noncontrast sagittal images. (*A*) The pituitary gland is mildly superiorly convex (*long arrow*), with low-lying cerebellar tonsils (*short arrow*) and a sagging mid-brain, with no visualization of the interpeduncular cistern. (*B*) After the CSF leak was repaired the superior margin of the pituitary gland (*long arrow*) is superiorly concave, the cerebellar tonsils are no longer caudally displaced, and the interpeduncular cistern is visualized (*short arrow*).

contrast. Typically it is horizontal in course and flat unless impressed on by an extrinsic mass (most often a pituitary macroadenoma from below) or herniated downward in the instance of an empty sella (see **Fig. 2**).

The normal pituitary typically fills the sella turcica but there may be a small amount intrasellar CSF present. If there is an abundance of fluid superior to the gland, that is termed a primary or secondary "empty sella." Primary empty sella is a result of long-term CSF pulsation through an incompetent diaphragm sella (**Fig. 7**). In marked cases the sella is enlarged and the superior gland may be concave. This is rarely a significant process. Secondary empty sella suggests that there was a previous intrasellar lesion, most often a pituitary mass, that had been surgically removed or medically treated. Such cases often evidence downward displacement and/or angulation of the optic chiasm (**Fig. 8**).

The cavernous sinuses on either side of the sella turcica are anatomically complex and medically exceptionally important. Because they are primarily blood-containing they are primarily hypointense on noncontrast T1-weighted images and strongly enhance. The third, fourth, and sixth cranial nerves, the first and second divisions of the fifth cranial nerve, and the carotid arteries, all pass through the cavernous sinus. Cranial nerves 3, 4, and the first and second division of cranial nerve 5, are lateral within the sinus, whereas the sixth nerve is inferomedial. The nerves are seen as moderately hypointense filling defects and the arteries are very hypointense because flowing blood results in a signal void (no signal). The cavernous carotid artery loops 180° within the cavernous sinus. Therefore, on coronal sections the upper and lower loops are seen, appearing as two separate vessels (see **Fig. 2**; **Fig. 9**).

Importantly, the inferior petrosal sinuses (IPS) drain into the cavernous sinuses and the cavernous sinuses drain the pituitary gland (discussed later in the section on cavernous sinus venous sampling).

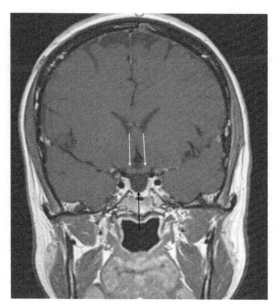

**Fig. 7.** T1-weighted postcontrast coronal image with a primary empty sella turcica filled with CSF (*black arrow*). Note the optic chiasm (*white arrows*) is in normal position and has a normal appearance.

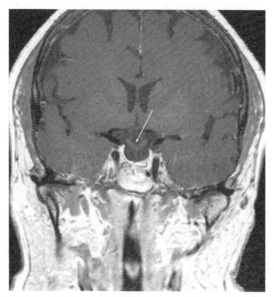

**Fig. 8.** T1-weighted noncontrast coronal image in a patient with a secondary empty sella turcica after medical treatment of a pituitary adenoma. Note that the sella turcica is enlarged and fluid filled and that the optic chiasm is downwardly displaced and angulated (*arrow*).

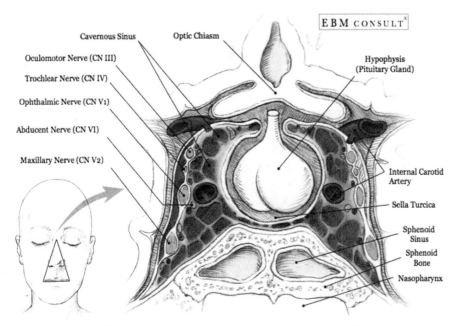

**Fig. 9.** Diagram of the cavernous sinuses. A, abducens nerve; C, carotid artery; M, Meckel cave; T, trochlear nerve; O, oculomotor nerve branches (upper B1 and lower B3). (*From* EBM Consult. Available at: http://www.ebmconsult.com/articles/anatomy-cavernous-sinus.)

The posterior pituitary lies within the posterior aspect of the sella turcica nestled anterior to the dorsum sellae (see **Figs. 2** and **22**). It is normally hyperintense on T1-weighted images secondary to the phospholipid membranes of the vesicles which envelop the posterior pituitary hormones.[10] These hormones, oxytocin and vasopressin, are formed in the hypothalamus and pass through the infundibulum to the posterior pituitary. The posterior pituitary is not always visible even in patients with normal posterior pituitary function. However, it is usually absent in diabetes insipidus. It may be ectopic in position, that is anywhere along the tract from the hypothalamus through the infundibulum, when there is an intrasellar mass obstructing the flow of the hormonal granules, or if the infundibulum is disrupted/transected (**Fig. 10**).[11,12]

## INTRASELLAR LESIONS
### Microadenomas

The most common indication for pituitary imaging is hormonal dysfunction, especially hyperprolactinemia. Additional common indications include an abnormal appearance of the pituitary or sella turcicia/parasellar region on MRI or CT studies performed to evaluate symptoms that are often unrelated.

Most prolactinomas are diagnosed when they are less than 1 cm in size (microadenomas) (**Fig. 11**). These lesions rarely result in chiasmatic compression, but on occasion can invade the cavernous sinus. Imaging can exclude both of these important issues but cannot completely exclude an adenoma itself. Additionally, imaging can detect infundibular displacement by an intrasellar or suprasellar mass that may be

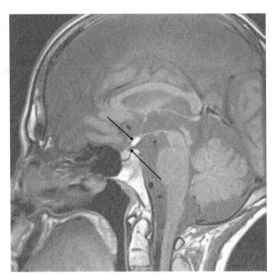

**Fig. 10.** T1-weighted noncontrast sagittal image. Thin infundibulum (*long arrow*). Ectopic high signal posterior pituitary in the upper infundibulum (*short arrow*).

causing elevated prolactin levels by impressing on or distorting the infundibulum (stalk effect) (**Fig. 12**).

By definition a microadenoma is an intrapituitary tumor of 10 mm or less in maximum diameter. Their detection is exceptionally important in cases of adrenocorticotropic hormone (ACTH) or growth hormone–producing tumors because surgery is often the therapeutic procedure of choice, and therefore exact localization is crucial. With prolactin-producing microadenomas, the imaging detection is less crucial

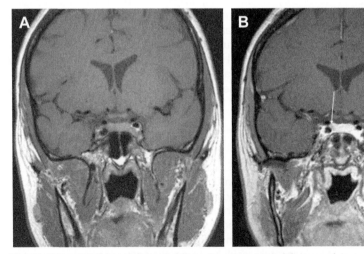

**Fig. 11.** T1-weighted precontrast (*A*) and postcontrast (*B*) coronal images. The pituitary gland appears normal on the noncontrast images. A small hypoenhancing lesion (*arrow*) is present in the far right lateral aspect of the gland on the postcontrast image. This extends between the limbs of the carotid arteries reaching the mid-intercarotid line (Knosp 2).

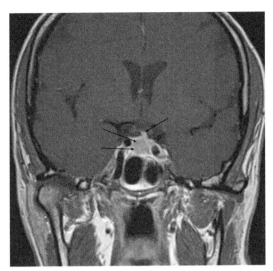

**Fig. 12.** T1-weighted postcontrast coronal image. A mass in the right side of the gland is hypoenhancing (*double arrows*). The infundibulum (*single arrow*) is thickened in appearance, elevated, and displaced to the left.

because they rarely threaten the chiasm. However, with visible lesions imaging is useful to follow therapeutic response and to localize the lesion in patients who require surgery because of medical therapeutic failures.

Excellent imaging technique is the key to detection of microadenomas. Most microadenomas are mildly hypointense on noncontrast T1-weighted images and hypoenhancing relative to normal pituitary tissue on postcontrast T1-weighted images. However, isointensity (equal intensity) to normal tissue on noncontrast scans is not uncommon (**Fig. 13**). Isointensity on postcontrast images may also occur, especially if the imaging is delayed after the contrast administration (allowing for the slower-enhancing tumor to become isointense with the remainder of the normal gland). Postcontrast hyperintensity relative to the normal gland is unusual (**Fig. 14**). T2-weighted images should be performed in patients to whom contrast may not be safely administered (eg, renal compromise). In such instances the T2 images may be helpful in delineating a lesion that is poorly or not visible on noncontrast studies (**Fig. 15**).

Typically prolactinomas develop in the posterolateral pars anterior (see **Fig. 11**; **Fig. 16**). Because they are rarely central in location, visualization of a central lesion should raise the possibility of a pars intermedia cyst or Rathke's pouch cyst (see **Fig. 16**). Pars intermedia cysts have the same MRI signal characteristics as CSF: hypointense on noncontrast T1-weighted images and nonenhancing, although the wall may enhance. This is in contrast to Rathke cysts, which are most often hyperintense on precontrast images because of the nature of the cystic fluid. T2-weighted images may help to further evaluate possible cysts because the lesion is homogeneous and hyperintense, and less commonly hypointense, depending on the nature of the contained fluid. On occasion microadenomas may be multiple or coexist with a cyst (see **Fig. 16**). Growth hormone– and ACTH-producing microadenomas may occur throughout the pars anterior and are best differentiated from cysts by the patient's hormonal status.[13,14]

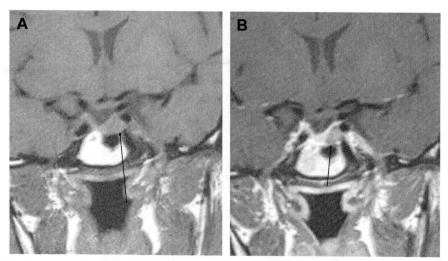

**Fig. 13.** T1-weighted noncontrast (*A*) and postcontrast (*B*) coronal images. On the noncontrast image there is an ill-defined questionable area of abnormality (*arrow*), which is clearly defined on the postcontrast image as a hypoenhancing lesion (*arrow*).

Unusually, microadenomas involve the cavernous sinus, but more often this is a specious appearance (see **Fig. 11**). This misinterpretation can result from the tumor impinging on the medial wall of the cavernous sinus but not actually violating it (discussed later in the section on Knosp criteria for cavernous sinus invasion.)

### Macroadenomas

Imaging interpretation of macroadenomas adds several levels of complexity compared with that of microadenomas. These lesions often extend into the suprasellar

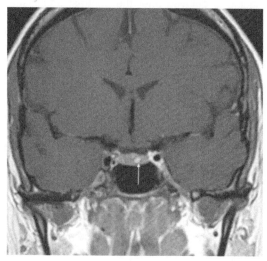

**Fig. 14.** T1-weighted postcontrast coronal image with a hyperenhancing pituitary microadenoma (*arrow*).

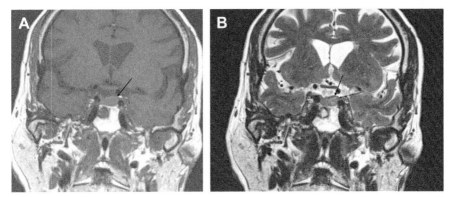

**Fig. 15.** (*A*) T1-weighted noncontrast coronal image. The arrow points to the asymmetrically enlarged left side of the gland with no definable mass. (*B*) The T2-weighted coronal image clearly shows a hyperintense lesion (*arrows*).

space, involve or seem to involve the cavernous sinus, may be cystic, and may contain hemorrhage (**Fig. 17**). Suprasellar extension is generally obvious. Intrasellar masses narrow as they pass through the diaphragma sella into the suprasellar space (**Fig. 18**). Pituitary tumors may grow laterally into the cavernous sinuses. Occasionally they grow preferentially or exclusively inferiorly into the sphenoid sinus and/or clivus, but they rarely cross the spheno-occipital synchondrosis (**Fig. 19**).

Detection of compression and elevation of the optic chiasm are key elements in understanding the critical presentation of visual deficits, and for surgical planning. On occasion, macroadenomas also extend to, and invade, the hypothalamus. T2-weighted imaging is particularly helpful in fully evaluating such lesions because they may more clearly demonstrate tumor margins and brain invasion. That is also true for the rarer tumor that extends through or around the cavernous sinus into the temporal fossa and temporal lobe (**Fig. 20**).

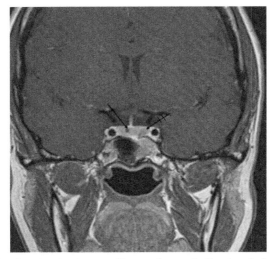

**Fig. 16.** T1-weighted postcontrast coronal image demonstrating two lesions: a hypoenhancing microadenoma (*crosshatched arrow*) and a nonenhancing pars media cyst (*long arrow*).

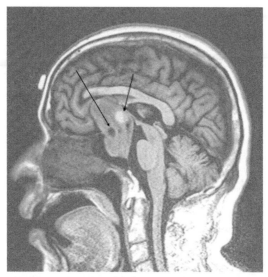

**Fig. 17.** T1-weighted noncontrast sagittal image. A large macroadenoma expands the sella turcica and extends into the suprasellar space almost reaching the corpus callosum. There is a hyperintense hemorrhagic (*short arrow*) and a hypointense cystic area (*long arrow*).

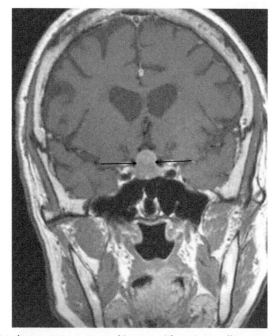

**Fig. 18.** T1-weighted postcontrast coronal image with an intrasellar mass extending into the suprasellar space. Note the narrowing of the tumor as it extends through the diaphragmatic sellae (*arrows*).

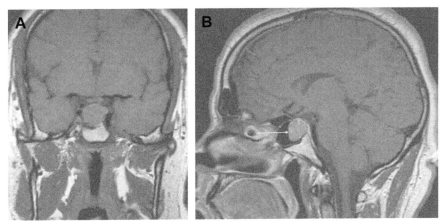

**Fig. 19.** T1-weighted noncontrast coronal (*A*) and sagittal (*B*) images demonstrating an intrasellar mass with growth primarily downward into the sphenoid sinus (*arrow*).

Malignancy, such as pituitary carcinoma and metastases, do occur infrequently. Carcinomas grow more quickly and aggressively infiltrate rather remodel the bony margins of the sella turcica. They may extend through the cavernous sinus into the temporal lobe, or inferiorly within the sinus to the foramen ovale and into the upper deep neck. Metastases from numerous primary sites have been reported and unless they grow rapidly it may be difficult to differentiate from a primary pituitary macroadenoma.

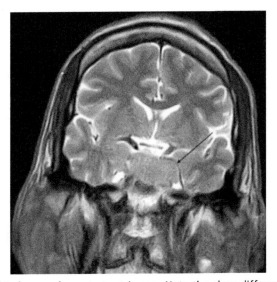

**Fig. 20.** T2-weighted coronal noncontrast image. Note the clear differentiation between the margin of the large pituitary tumor extending from the sella turcica mass impinging on the temporal lobe (*arrow*). There is no edema in the temporal lobe indicating that the mass is not invading the temporal lobe parenchyma.

Radiation cerebritis and radiation necrosis of the temporal lobe may be consequences of pituitary tumor radiation. Edema associated with these conditions is best recognized on T2-weighted images. Contrast enhancement, which is a hallmark of radiation necrosis, is visualized on T1-weighted postcontrast images (**Fig. 21**).

Bleeding may occur as a response to drug therapy (bromocriptine, cabergoline) but may also be spontaneous (pituitary apoplexy). It is recognized as hyperintensity on noncontrast T1-weighted images, but must be differentiated from a Rathke cleft cyst, which most commonly are also hyperintense on T1-weighted images (**Fig. 22**). Hemorrhage into the cystic component of a macroadenoma often demonstrates a blood fluid level because in the supine patient the heavier hyperintense red blood cells sink to the dependent portion of the cyst with the more hypointense serum layered anteriorly (**Fig. 23**). If a pituitary abscess is suspected diffusion-weighted images, best performed in the axial plane, usually are positive (**Fig. 24**).

Cavernous sinus involvement is important to detect for surgical and prognostic considerations. Knosp has developed a grading system that helps to rate the likelihood of cavernous sinus invasion versus medial wall compression and distortion of the cavernous sinus (**Fig. 25**).[15] A Knosp 0 is a lesion that is clearly not involving the cavernous sinus. Knosp 1 lesions reach the medial intercarotid line (between the superior and inferior loops of the carotid artery). Knosp 2 lesions reach the mid-carotid line, and Knosp 3 the lateral intercarotid line. When the carotid artery is encased by the mass, the lesion is considered a Knosp 4 (**Fig. 26**).

The statistical likelihood of cavernous sinus invasion based on the Knosp criteria was recently reported by Micko and colleagues[16]:

- Knosp 0 = 0%
- Knosp 1 = 1.5%
- Knosp 2 = 9.9%
- Knosp 3 = 37.9%
- Knosp 4 = 100%

Although these percentages likely vary in different series, they offer an excellent approximation of the relative risk based on the imaging findings.

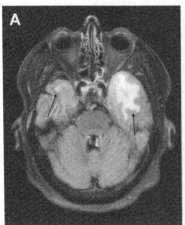 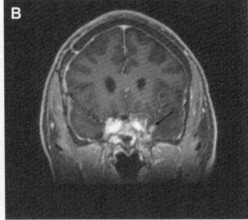

**Fig. 21.** T2-weighted axial image (*A*), bilateral, left greater than right, temporal lobe edema (*arrows*) in this patient who has undergone radiotherapy for recurring pituitary neoplasm. (*B*) T1-weighted postcontrast coronal image-contrast enhancement in the deep left temporal lobe (*arrow*), indicative of radiation necrosis.

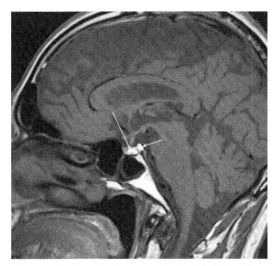

**Fig. 22.** T1-weighted noncontrast sagittal image. Rathke cleft cyst (*long arrow*) and posterior pituitary (*short arrow*) are both hyperintense.

## INFUNDIBULAR LESIONS

The infundibulum is a midline structure passing through the suprasellar space into the sella turcica. If the infundibulum is displaced from the midline one must exclude a contiguous mass, whether intrasellar or suprasellar in origin (**Fig. 27**). Cystic tumors may be detectable only by such infundibular displacement because they may otherwise be mistaken for CSF.

The normal infundibulum enhances avidly with contrast because of the absence of a blood-brain barrier. It should be no more than 2 mm to 3 mm in thickness. Thickening

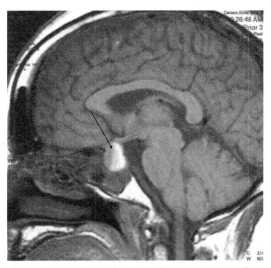

**Fig. 23.** T1-weighted noncontrast sagittal image. There is an intrasellar mass with suprasellar extension, and a fluid level (*arrow*) demarcating the hyperintense dependent red cell component and the ventral isotense serum component in this supine patient (hematocrit).

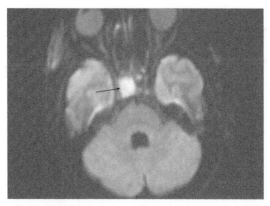

**Fig. 24.** Axial diffusion-weighted image. The intrasellar lesion is hyperintense (*arrow*) indicative of diffusion restriction, which is typical of abscesses.

raises the likelihood of infundibular pathology, particularly infundibulitis, especially if the margins appear shaggy. Elevation/buckling of the infundibulum by an intrasellar mass may result in an appearance suggesting stalk thickening. Differential considerations for stalk lesions include neoplasm, such as pituicytomas (astrocytoma) and chordoid gliomas, and inflammatory infundibulitis (lymphocydic, lymphomatous, granulomatous, and infectious). Infundibulitis and neoplasm may be quite similar in appearance with enhancement and expansion of the infundibulum (**Fig. 28**). In addition, the pituitary gland and the hypothalamus are not infrequently also involved with infundibulitis.

## PARASELLAR AND SUPRASELLAR MASSES

Craniopharyngiomas are the most common of the suprasellar tumor masses. They may also have an intrasellar component or even be entirely intrasellar. They have a bimodal age distribution with the adamantimous form most typical in childhood and the much less common papillary form seen primarily in later adulthood. The

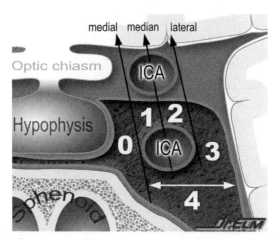

**Fig. 25.** Knosp classification. ICA, internal carotid artery. (*Case courtesy of* Dr Elnur Mehdi, Radiopaedia.org, rID: 29524.)

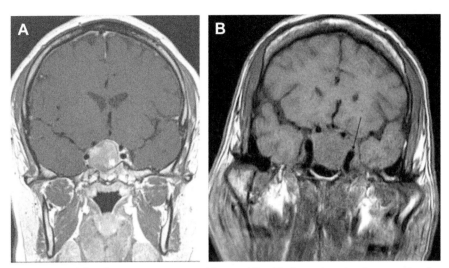

**Fig. 26.** T1-weighted postcontrast coronal image (*A*) with the enhancing tumor extending to the intercarotid line or slightly beyond, consistent with a Knosp 2/3 classification. (*B*) A T1-weighted noncontrast coronal image with the carotid artery (*arrow*) engulfed by tumor constituting a Knosp 4 lesion.

adamantimous form frequently contains cystic cavities, cholesterol, and calcifications, whereas papillary forms are more solid. On MRI examination, adamantimous cranio-pharyngiomas are therefore heterogeneous in signal with areas of T1 hyperintensity related to the cholesterol and blood content, T1 hypointensity secondary to cysts,

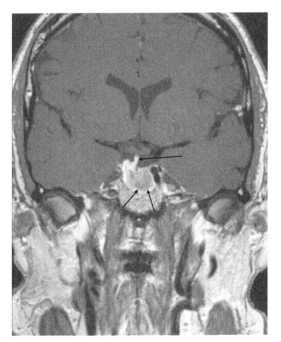

**Fig. 27.** T1-weighted postcontrast coronal image. The long arrow demonstrates the infun-dibulum, which is displaced to the right as a result of the intrasellar tumor (*short arrows*).

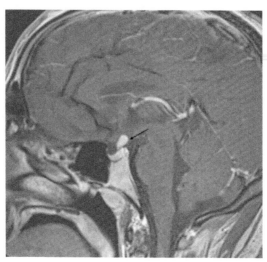

**Fig. 28.** T1-weighted postcontrast sagittal image. The infundibulum (*arrow*) is bulbus because of infundibulitis. This same appearance could be seen with tumors, such as pituicytomas.

and T1 and/or T2 hypointensity secondary to the presence of calcium. Calcium on occasion may also appear hyperintense on T1-weighted images. CT with its improved ability to detect calcifications may be useful to further characterize a suprasellar mass (**Fig. 29**).

Large suprasellar/parasellar aneurysms are usually obvious secondary to a signal void (loss of signal) in the lumen, related to the flowing blood. Flowing blood has no signal or markedly reduced signal and can therefore be detected by MRI. In addition, motion, such as blood flow, may result in a well-known phase-encoded artifact that is helpful in detecting aneurysms and other vascular abnormalities. The margins of

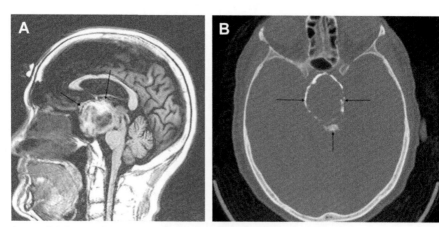

**Fig. 29.** (*A*) T1-weighted noncontrast sagittal image with arrows pointing to a complex mass in the intrasellar and suprasellar space containing areas of hyperintensity and hypointensity. Note that the mass has grown into the interpeduncular space and is displacing the mesencephalon dorsally. (*B*) Axial CT image of the same patient with heavy calcification (*arrows*) along the margins of the craniopharyngioma.

aneurysms may be calcified so, once again, CT may be helpful if MRI and magnetic resonance angiography do not clarify the diagnosis.

There are a multitude of additional suprasellar and parasellar masses. Meningiomas of the tuberculum sellae may extend into the sella turcica. They enhance avidly with contrast and often have what is known as a dural tail, that is, dural thickening or tumor extending beyond the margins of the lesions along the dural surface. Careful attention should be paid to determining if the mass is arising separately from the pituitary. Intrasellar meningiomas are typically difficult to differentiate from the pituitary gland on noncontrast images because they are both approximately isointense to brain on noncontrast T1 images. However, with contrast the meningioma usually enhances to a greater extent and the differential can be made (**Fig. 30**).

Meningiomas of the lateral wall of the cavernous sinus widen the contrast enhancement associated with the sinus and may be indistinguishable from intrinsic cavernous sinus tumor, inflammatory conditions, and thrombosis of the sinus (**Fig. 31**). Paracavernous lymphoma, sarcoidosis, and Tolosa-Hunt syndrome also may be difficult to differentiate from primary cavernous sinus disease because they also may widen the profile of the cavernous sinus.

Suprasellar Langerhans cell histiocytosis usually involves the infundibulum and may involve the hypothalamus. Optic gliomas are usually apparent because they expand the optic chiasm and, especially in cases of neurofibromatosis type I, extend into the orbital optic nerve (**Fig. 32**). Optic gliomas not infrequently extend along the optic tracts. Axial T2-weighted images are best to evaluate this possibility (**Fig. 33**). Extension along the optic tracts helps to differentiate an optic glioma from a primary hypothoramic neoplasm, which usually do not involve the optic tracts. Germ cell tumors enhance markedly and are often associated with pineal tumors, which may be recognized on the sagittal images of the pituitary MRI examination. Hamartomas of the tuber cinereum at the floor of the hypothalamus are isointense to brain and do not enhance.

## RATHKE CLEFT CYST

Rathke cleft cysts are a vestige of the Rathke pouch. They may be found within the pituitary and/or in the suprasellar space. These lesions are well defined and most often hyperintense on T1-weighted images and do not enhance with contrast. Therefore they may appear hypointense relative to the normally enhancing gland on postcontrast images. On occasion they may be isointense, or even hypointense, on noncontrast T1-weighted images, depending on the contents of the cysts (**Fig. 34**).

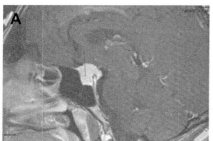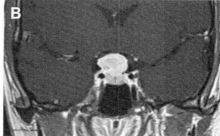

**Fig. 30.** T1-weighted postcontrast sagittal (*A*) and coronal (*B*) images in a patient with a tuberculum sellae meningioma growing into the sella turcica. Note the demarcation between the more brightly enhancing superior meningioma and the less brightly enhancing intrasellar normal pituitary (*arrows*).

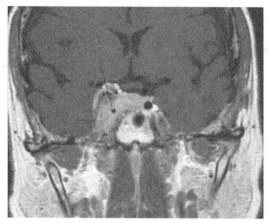

**Fig. 31.** T1-weighted postcontrast coronal image in a patient with a large meningioma (*short arrow*) along the margin of the right cavernous sinus. This tumor has also apparently invaded the cavernous sinus and is encasing and narrowing the carotid artery (*long arrow*).

Some reports indicate that 77% of Rathke cleft cysts demonstrate an intracystic nodule, although that has not been my experience.[17,18] These nonneoplastic benign processes are usually followed clinically unless they are associated with symptoms, such as headache, stalk effect with elevated prolactin, or pressure on the optic chiasm with associated visual deficits.

## PRIMARY CAVERNOUS SINUS DISEASE

The cavernous sinus is a two-way conduit for venous blood from the face and orbits to the intracranial cavity. Diseases of the cavernous sinus can result in carotid artery occlusion, intracranial infection, distended orbital veins, and ophthalmoplegia.

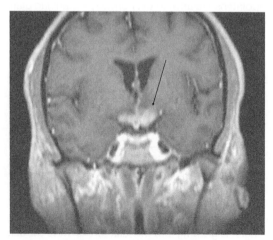

**Fig. 32.** T1-weighted postcontrast coronal image. The optic chiasm is enlarged bilaterally and particularly so on the left (*arrow*) by a diffuse optic glioma.

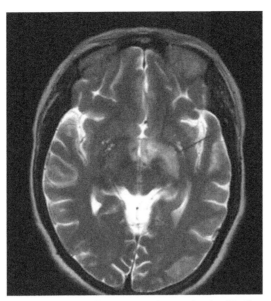

**Fig. 33.** T2-weighted axial image in the same patient as in **Fig. 32.** The optic glioma is extending along the optic tract resulting in edema (*arrows*).

The cavernous sinus may be intrinsically affected by schwannomas of the cranial nerves, especially numbers 3 and 5, which pass through the sinus. Meningiomas, lymphoma, sarcoid, and metastatic disease all generally present contiguous to the sinus along its lateral wall, but may cause symptoms from sinus compression and thrombosis (see **Fig. 31**).

Cavernous sinus thrombosis is often secondary to infection. Such infections most typically extend into the cavernous sinus from the orbit or from the sphenoid sinuses.

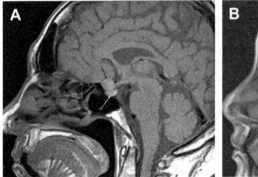
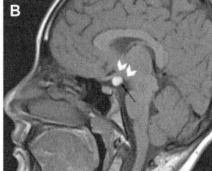

**Fig. 34.** T1-weighted noncontrast sagittal images. (*A*) An isointense suprasellar and intrasellar Rathke cleft cyst (*black arrow*) impinging on the superior surface of the pituitary gland (*white arrow*). (*B*) Suprasellar Rathke cleft cyst is hyperintense (*arrow*), and is impinging on the undersurface of the hypothalamus at the tuber cinereum (*arrowheads*). This young patient presented with precocious puberty similar to the symptoms seen with hamartomas of the tuber cinereum.

Inflammatory conditions, such as Tolosa-Hunt syndrome, may also occlude the sinus. Sinus occlusion can cause proptosis secondary to dilatation of the intraorbital venous structures and/or orbital edema.

Dural arteriovenous malformations and caroticocavernous arteriovenous fistulas (a direct communication between the carotid artery and the cavernous sinus) may distend the sinus and appear similar to sinus thrombosis. Also these conditions distend the orbital veins and cause proptosis and pain. The venous changes often help to differentiate these entities from paracavernous tumors.

Intracavernous carotid aneurysms are usually seen as distinct masses associated with the carotid artery. However, when they are large, and especially when thrombosed, they may be a challenge to differentiate from tumor.

## SURGICAL CONSIDERATIONS

There are several anatomic issues to be considered by the surgeon anticipating transsphenoidal or open pituitary surgery. The location of the tumor is of foremost importance in the case of small microadenomas. The size, shape, and septation of the sphenoid sinus are important to consider in planning the approach. If there is a thick nonpneumatized bony plate between the sphenoid sinus and the sella turcica, transsphenoidal surgery may not be possible or may require special instrumentation and planning. When the sphenoid septum deviates sharply to one side, the surgeon should be alerted to avoid having their instruments inadvertently directed too far laterally if they use the septum as a surgical landmark.

Medially placed cavernous carotid arteries make transphenoidal surgery more difficult and potentially dangerous, and the surgeon should be alerted to this condition (**Fig. 35**). The location and extent of intracavernous extension of a pituitary tumor also affects surgical planning and approach, and affects prognosis because complete excision may not be possible.

If there is any suggestion that the suprasellar extension of a pituitary tumor is adherent to the chiasm or to the hypothalamus, or invading the hypothalamus, T2-weighted images are valuable to detect associated parenchymal edema.

Transphenoidal postsurgical changes including inflammatory changes in the sphenoid sinsuses, a defect in sella floor, and fat grafts are well demonstrated on T1-weighted noncontrast images. Fat grafts are hyperintense on such images and occasionally may be mistaken for hemorrhage (**Fig. 36**). In such instances T2-weighted images may clarify the diagnosis because subacute and chronic hemorrhage is hyperintense on T2-weighted images, whereas fat is more isointense.

Differentiation of recurrent tumor from postoperative fibrosis is challenging. Scar most often does not enhance, whereas tumor usually shows some enhancement and progressive growth. Therefore, interval follow-up may be necessary before a definitive differentiation is possible (**Fig. 37**).

### Cavernous Sinus Sampling

The accurate diagnosis of the source of elevated ACTH is crucial in the diagnosis of patients with hypercortisolemia. Although most are secondary to pituitary microadenomas (Cushing disease), ectopic sources occur in up to 10% in some series.[19]

When MRI is diagnostic of a microadenoma, a higher level of certainty may be attached to the efficacy of surgical removal. However, ACTH-producing microadenomas are notoriously small with up to 50% reported to be not detectable even with excellent MRI technique, including dynamic imaging.[20] In such cases, an additional level of support and precision for surgical intervention may be obtained from

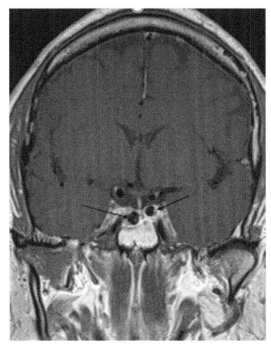

**Fig. 35.** T1-weighted postcontrast coronal image. Bilateral medially placed (kissing) carotid arteries (*arrows*) extending into the sella turcica. This makes transsphenoidal surgery exceptionally difficult and dangerous.

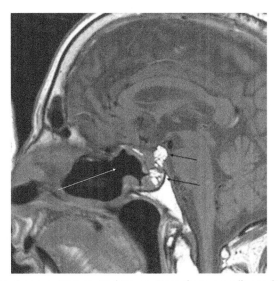

**Fig. 36.** T1-weighted noncontrast sagittal image. Note the suprasellar and intrasellar hyperintensity caused by fat grafts (*short arrows*) placed during transsphenoidal surgery. Notice the large defect in the sphenoid sinus related to this surgical procedure (*long arrow*).

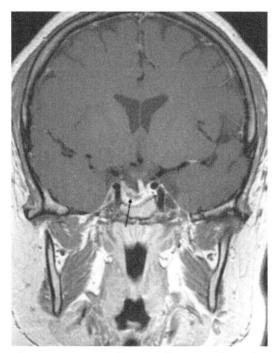

**Fig. 37.** T1-weighted postcontrast coronal image. This patient has undergone transsphenoidal surgery. The infundibulum is angled toward the left where the normal pituitary remains. Nonenhancing postoperative fibrous tissue is present in the right side of the sella turcica (*arrow*).

cavernous sinus or IPS venous sampling. This procedure has been reported to be exceptionally accurate, with one report of 93 cases demonstrating 100% accuracy.[21]

The anterior pituitary drains via small veins into the cavernous sinuses on either side of the sella turcica. Drainage from the cavernous sinuses is via the IPS, which joins the jugular vein. The drainage is symmetric in approximately 60% of patients.[22] Asymmetrical ACTH levels in the cavernous sinuses may clearly localize the side of a lesion producing the hormone. However, in those patients with asymmetrical flow, an asymmetrical gradient between the two cavernous sinuses or IPSs may be falsely localizing. A cavernous sinus/peripheral venous gradient, however, may still help to localize the lesion to the pituitary gland (**Fig. 38**).

The technique of IPS retrograde catheterization from the femoral veins to the internal jugular vein is straightforward, but not without risk. On usual occasions brainstem hemorrhage can be induced.[23] Further advancing the catheter into the cavernous sinuses improves specificity of the sampling, but it is often more challenging.

The technique involves placing catheters into the bilateral IPS, but preferably the cavernous sinuses. Proper placement is confirmed with the gentle and careful administration of contrast to avoid retrograde venous pressure that could result in brainstem hemorrhage. Additionally, a peripheral venous catheter in the femoral vein or lower inferior vena cava is also placed. Multiple blood samples are obtained simultaneously from the two sides and the peripheral catheter over 10 to 15 minutes. corticotropin-releasing hormone (CRH) (100 µg) is then administered intravenously as a bolus. Blood samples are again immediately obtained at rapid intervals over the next 15 minutes.

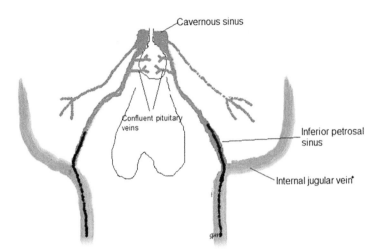

**Fig. 38.** Sketch of the venous drainage of the pituitary gland. Note that the drainage is via small veins into the cavernous sinuses, which then drain into the inferior petrosal sinus and then into the internal jugular vein. (*Image reprinted with permission from* Gauri Mankekar, MBBS, PhD, published by Medscape Drugs & Diseases (http://emedicine.medscape.com/), 2017, Available at: http://emedicine.medscape.com/article/2114270-overview.)

A central to peripheral gradient of 2/1 in the pre-CRH samples and 3/1 in the post-CRH samples is generally considered diagnostic.[20,24] In the absence of a gradient, more attention must be paid to the possibility of an ectopic ACTH-producing tumor. If none is detected with imaging, pituitary surgical exploration may still be indicated but with a lower likelihood of success than in those cases with a detectable gradient.

## REFERENCES

1. Elster AD. High-resolution, dynamic pituitary MR imaging: standard of care or academic pastime? AJR Am J Roentgenol 1994;163:680–2.
2. Kucharczyk W, Bishop JE, Plewes DB, et al. Detection of pituitary microademomas: comparison of dynamic keyhole fast spin echo, unenenhanced, and conventional contrast-enhanced MR imaging. AJR Am J Roentgenol 1994;163:671–9.
3. Stadnik T, Spruyt D, van Binst A, et al. Pituitary microadenomas: diagnosis with dynamic serial CT, conventional CT and T1-weighted MR imaging before and after injection of gadolinium. Eur J Radiol 1994;18:191–8.
4. Tabarin A, Laurent F, Catargi B, et al. Comparative evaluation of conventional and dynamic magnetic resonance imaging of the pituitary gland for the diagnosis of Cushing's disease. Clin Endocrinol (Oxf) 1998;49:293–300.
5. Wiener SN, Rzeszotarski MS, Droege RT, et al. Measurement of pituitary gland height with MR imaging. AJNR Am J Neuroradiol 1985;6:717–22.
6. Roppolo HMN, Latchaw RE, Meyer JD, et al. 1 Normal pituitary gland. Macroscopic anatomy-CT correlation. AJNR Am J Neuroradiol 1983;4:927–35.
7. Peyster RG, Adler LP, Viscarello RR, et al. CT of the normal pituitary gland. Neuroradiology 1986;28:161–5.
8. Wolpert SM, Molitch ME, Goldman JA, et al. Size, shape and appearance of the normal female pituitary gland. AJR Am J Roentgenol 1984;143:377–81.

9. Chanson P, Daujat F, Young J, et al. Normal pituitary hypertrophy as a frequent cause of pituitary incidentaloma: a follow-up study. J Clin Endocrinol Metab 2001;86:3009–15.

10. Colombo N, Berry I, Kucharczyk J, et al. Posterior pituitary gland: appearance on MR images in normal and pathologic states. Radiology 1987;165:481–5.

11. Brooks BS, Gammal TE, Allison JD, et al. Frequency and variation of the posterior pituitary bright signal on MR images. AJNR Am J Neuroradiol 1989;10:943–8.

12. El Gammal T, Brooks BS, Hoffman WH. MR imaging of the ectopic bright signal of posterior pituitary regeneration. AJNR Am J Neuroradiol 1989;10:323–8.

13. Martin MC, Schrlock ED, Jaffe RB. Prolactin-secreting pituitary ademomas. West J Med 1983;139:663–72.

14. Podlas H. Diagnosis of pituitary microadenomas by computed tomography. Medicamundi 1981;26:20–2.

15. Knosp E, Steiner E, Kitz K, et al. Pituitary adenomas with invasion of the cavernous sinus space: a magnetic resonance imaging classification compared with surgical findings. Neurosurgery 1993;33:610–8.

16. Micko ASG, Wohrer A, Wolfsberger S, et al. Invasion of the cavernous sinus space in pituitary adenomas: endoscopic verification and its correlation with an MRI-based classification. J Neurosurg 2015;122:803–11.

17. Kucharczyk W, Peck WW, Kelly WM, et al. Rathke cleft cysts: CT, MR imaging and pathologic features. Radiology 1987;165:491–5.

18. Byun WM, Kim OL, Kim D. MR imaging findings of Rathke's cleft cysts: significance of intracystic nodules. AJNR Am J Neuroradiol 2000;21:485–8.

19. Corsello SM, Senes P, Lezzi R, et al. Cushing's syndrome due to a bronchial ACTH-secreting carcinoid successfully treated with radiofrequency ablation (RFA). J Clin Endocrinol Metab 2014;99(5):E862–5. Available at: http://press. endocrine.org/doi/full/10.1210/jc.2013-4359. Accessed November 7, 2016.

20. Gandhi CD, Meyer SA, Patel AB, et al. Neurologic complications of inferior petrosal sinus sampling. AJNR Am J Neuroradiol 2008;29(4):760–5. Available at: http://www.ajnr.org/content/29/4/760.full. Accessed November 7, 2016.

21. Graham KE, Samuels MH, Nesbit GM, et al. Cavernous sinus sampling is highly accurate in distinguishing Cushing's disease from the ectopic adrenocorticotropin syndrome and in predicting intrapituitary tumor location. J Clin Endocrinol Metab 1999;84(5):1602–10. Available at: http://press.endocrine.org/doi/full/10. 1210/jcem.84.5.5654. Accessed November 7, 2016.

22. Mankekar G. Petrosal sinus sampling. 2015. Available at: http://emedicine. medscape.com/article/2114270-overview. Accessed November 17, 2016.

23. Burkhardt T, Flitsch J, van Leyen P, et al. Cavernous sinus sampling in patients with Cushing's disease. Neurosurg Focus 2015;38(2):E6.

24. Zampetti B, Grossrubatscher E, Ciaramella PD, et al. Bilateral inferior petrosal sinus sampling. Endocr Connect 2016;5(4):R12–25. Available at: https://www.ncbi. nlm.nih.gov/pmc/articles/PMC5002953. Accessed November 7, 2016.

# Adrenal Imaging

N. Reed Dunnick, MD[a],*, Anca Avram, MD[b],
Mishal Mendiratta-Lala, MD[c], Adina F. Turcu, MD[d]

## KEYWORDS

- Adrenal imaging • Pheochromocytomas • Adrenal venous sampling
- Adrenal incidentaloma

## KEY POINTS

- Cross-sectional imaging can make a specific diagnosis in lesions, such as myelolipomas, cysts, and hemorrhage, and is often sufficient to distinguish benign from malignant adrenal processes.
- CT and MRI are also useful studies to identify pheochromocytomas and cortisol-secreting or androgen-secreting tumors.
- In patients with primary aldosteronism, adrenal venous sampling (AVS), remains the most accurate localizing study and should be performed in all patients older than 35 years of age, even if an adenoma is detected by CT or MRI.
- Radiolabeled isotope studies serve as second-line diagnostic tests for malignant adrenal tumors, either primary or metastatic, as well as for pheochromocytoma.
- Nuclear imaging studies should always follow a robust hormonal diagnosis and be correlated with findings on cross-sectional imaging.

## INTRODUCTION

Medical imaging plays an increasingly prominent role in patients with endocrine diseases.[1] In patients with either a cortisol-secreting adrenal tumor or pheochromocytoma, the degree of hormonal excess correlates directly with the size of the secreting tumor,[2–4] and CT is highly accurate in localizing the tumor. Conversely, cross-sectional imaging is not as accurate in localizing aldosterone-producing adenomas due to their small size. Furthermore, an adrenal nodule found on imaging may not be secreting aldosterone. AVS, which measures the hormone level coming

The author has nothing to disclose.

[a] Department of Radiology, University of Michigan Health System, 1500 East Medical Center Drive, B1 G503, Ann Arbor, MI 48109-5030, USA; [b] Department of Radiology, University of Michigan Health System, 1500 East Medical Center Drive, B1 G505, Ann Arbor, MI 48109-5030, USA; [c] Department of Radiology, University of Michigan Health System, 1500 East Medical Center Drive, B1D502, Ann Arbor, MI 48109-5030, USA; [d] Department of Internal Medicine, University of Michigan Health System, Cancer Center, 1500 East Medical Center Drive, Ann Arbor, MI 48109-5911, USA
* Corresponding author.
E-mail address: rdunnick@med.umich.edu

endo.theclinics.com

from each gland, may identify adenomas too small to be confidently diagnosed on CT or MRI. The concordance between CT or MRI and AVS varies from 50% to 76% and decreases with age.[5–7] Thus, AVS is often used in the subclassification of patients with primary aldosteronism.[7,8]

Although CT and MRI are valuable in localizing hormone-producing tumors, incidental findings are often detected in organs other than the one for which the examination was designed. Adrenal nodules are common incidental findings, and the frequency with which these adrenal incidentalomas (AIs) are found has increased, probably due to advances in imaging technology. In a study of 61,054 patients undergoing CT scans between 1985 and 1989, only 259 (0.4%) patients were found to have incidental adrenal nodules larger than 1 cm.[9] In more recent years, AIs have been reported in more than 4% of patients.[10,11] The prevalence of AI increases with age, to as high as 10%, as suggested by both imaging and autopsy studies.[12] AIs are most commonly unilateral, but up to 15% of patients may have bilateral nodules.[13,14] When an AI is found, 2 aspects are relevant in their clinical assessment: (1) their etiology and malignant potential and (2) their hormonal status. Contemporary imaging studies can assist in addressing both questions.

Cross-sectional imaging dedicated to the adrenal gland is second only to surgical pathology in determining the malignant potential of adrenal masses. The physiologic nature of radionuclide studies, such as PET/CT and metaiodobenzylguanidine (MIBG), is also useful in clarifying the diagnosis of suspicious adrenal nodules. When correlated with the clinical context, imaging can often diagnose the specific cause of an adrenal mass.

If the cause of an adrenal lesion is uncertain, imaging may direct a percutaneous adrenal biopsy. This is most often performed with ultrasound guidance, but CT may be used, especially in deep lesions where the ultrasound images are degraded by intervening fat. Biopsy performs poorly, however, in differentiating benign adenomas from adrenocortical carcinomas (ACCs). A meta-analysis of 8 studies (240 biopsies) found that the sensitivity of biopsy for detecting adrenal cortical carcinoma was only 70%.[15] Thus, adrenal biopsy is only rarely indicated for indeterminate adrenal nodules and must be performed only after hormonal testing to exclude pheochromocytoma. Image-guided biopsy can be offered to patients with suspected metastases from an extra-adrenal malignancy if confirmation of the metastases will change therapy. Longitudinal imaging of AI remains a topic of debate. For lipid-rich adrenal nodules smaller than 4 cm, follow-up imaging may not be necessary.[12,16] Conversely, surveillance CT or MRI is recommended for patients with larger lesions and those with indeterminate findings on the initial assessment.[12,17]

## IMAGING FINDINGS

The adrenal glands are seen on all CT and MRI scans of the abdomen. On cross-sectional imaging, the normal adrenal glands appear as an inverted V shape or Y shape, lying anterior and superior to the kidneys, within Gerota fascia. The 2 limbs converge to form the apex of the gland. The mean thickness of the gland is between 5 mm and 10 mm.[18,19] Adrenal cysts, hematomas, and myelolipomas are often easily characterized. Other lesions, however, usually require dedicated imaging techniques. In the absence of a known malignancy, a lesion larger than 1 cm usually undergoes further investigation.

### Benign Adrenal Lesions

#### Adrenal adenoma
A majority of adrenal adenomas are nonhyperfunctioning; however, contralateral adrenal atrophy suggests a hyperfunctioning lesion.[20,21] Adenomas are usually

homogeneous, are less than 3 cm in size, and have well-defined margins.[22,23] Approximately 70% of adrenal adenomas contain a large amount of cytoplasmic fat (lipid rich) and are easy to characterize by CT or MRI. Those with little cytoplasmic fat are considered lipid poor (30%) and are more difficult to distinguish from other adrenal lesions, such as metastases (**Table 1**).[23,24]

A lipid-rich adrenal adenoma can be characterized with either unenhanced CT or chemical shift MRI. On unenhanced CT, a region of interest is placed on one-half to one-third of the surface area of the adrenal lesion to obtain a density measurement. CT attenuation below 10 Hounsfield units (HUs) is diagnostic for a lipid-rich adrenal adenoma (**Fig. 1**).[24-26] Chemical shift imaging uses resonant frequencies of fat and water protons to evaluate intracellular fat content. In-phase imaging uses an echo time, in which the fat and water proton signal are additive, whereas out-of-phase imaging uses an echo time in which the fat and water proton signals are 180° opposed, thus resulting in signal cancellation. Therefore, lesions that contain a high intracellular fat content show a drop in signal on the out-of-phase imaging. Most lipid-rich adenomas demonstrate loss of signal on out-of-phase imaging (**Fig. 2**). Some studies report that a 20% decrease in signal intensity is diagnostic for an adrenal adenoma.[25,26]

Neither unenhanced CT nor chemical shift MRI can characterize lipid-poor adenomas. They measure greater than 10 HUs on noncontrast CT, and there is no loss of signal on out-of-phase MRI. Measuring CT contrast washout, however, can differentiate benign adrenal adenomas from other lesions. The high vascular density and permeability of metastases is related to disorganized angiogenesis in malignant lesions and thus leads to prolonged contrast accumulation compared with benign adrenal adenomas.[27] Both lipid-rich and lipid-poor adenomas demonstrate rapid washout, which can be calculated by relative or absolute washout kinetics.[23,27-29] Absolute washout is determined by (enhancement HU value − delayed enhancement HU value)/(enhanced HU value − unenhanced HU value) × 100. When no unenhanced CT scan is available, relative washout is determined by (enhanced HU value − delayed HU value)/(enhanced HU value) × 100.[28] An adenoma that demonstrates 60% absolute washout or 40% relative washout is considered a benign adenoma (**Fig. 3**).[28] Limitations to this method exist. Hypervascular metastatic lesions, such as hepatocellular carcinoma and neuroendocrine tumors, may occasionally demonstrate washout characteristics, which mimic benign adrenal adenomas. Thus, in the setting of a known primary malignancy, washout values must be interpreted with caution. Some investigators suggest that an unenhanced HU value greater than 43 HUs should be considered a malignant lesion regardless of washout characteristics.[29]

Rarely, adrenal adenomas may contain areas of altered attenuation or signal characteristics secondary to hemorrhage or cystic changes.

**Table 1**
**Imaging findings of adrenal adenomas**

|  | Lipid-rich Adrenal Adenoma | Lipid-poor Adrenal Adenoma |
|---|---|---|
| CT | <10 HUs on noncontrast<br>>60% absolute washout[a]<br>>40% relative washout[b] | >10 HUs on noncontrast<br>>60% absolute washout[a]<br>>40% relative washout[b] |
| MRI | Loss of signal intensity on out-of-phase imaging (at least 20%) | No loss of signal intensity on out-of-phase imaging |

[a] Absolute washout: (enhanced HU value − delayed HU value)/(enhanced HU value − unenhanced HU value) × 100.
[b] Relative washout: (enhanced HU value − delayed HU value)/(enhanced HU value) × 100.

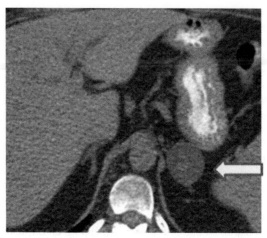

**Fig. 1.** This left adrenal nodule measures −4 HUs on unenhanced imaging and is diagnostic of a lipid-rich adenoma.

### Myelolipoma

A myelolipoma is a benign tumor of the adrenal gland composed of bone marrow elements, which is primarily fatty tissue with hematopoietic cells. It is usually discovered incidentally.[30] The incidence of myelolipomas ranges from 2.6% to 6% of primary adrenal lesions.[31] It is a nonfunctioning tumor and patients usually become symptomatic only when there is mass effect on adjacent structures, hemorrhage, or tumor necrosis.

On CT, myelolipomas have large areas of macroscopic fat with negative HU values intermixed with denser myeloid tissue (**Fig. 4**). On MRI, the fatty portion of the tumor is hyperintense on non–fat-suppressed T1-weighted images, with loss of signal intensity within the fatty component on T1 fat-suppressed images (**Fig. 5**). An India ink artifact along the border between the lesion and the adrenal gland seen on in-phase and out-of-phase MRI suggests a myelolipoma.

### Adrenal cysts

Adrenal cysts are rare lesions that are easily diagnosed by their imaging features. On CT, they have a homogeneous water density, and on MRI they tend to be T2

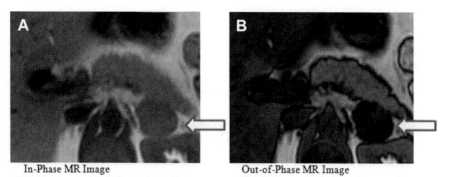

In-Phase MR Image                    Out-of-Phase MR Image

**Fig. 2.** Large left adrenal nodule demonstrates (*A*) diffuse loss of signal on (*B*) out-of-phase imaging, consistent with a lipid-rich adrenal adenoma.

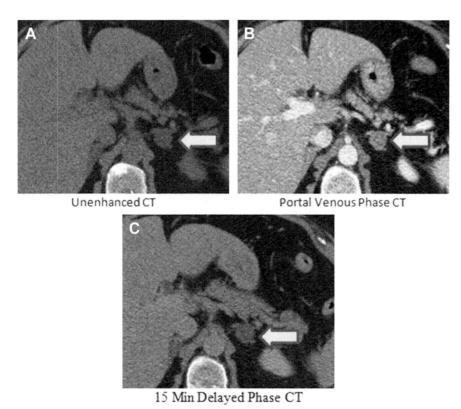

**Fig. 3.** A 46-year-old woman with incidentally discovered left adrenal mass, which measured (A) 12 HUs on unenhanced imaging, (B) 69 HUs on portal venous phase imaging, and (C) 21 HUs on 15-minute delayed imaging. The 85% absolute washout and 70% relative washout are diagnostic of a lipid-poor adrenal adenoma.

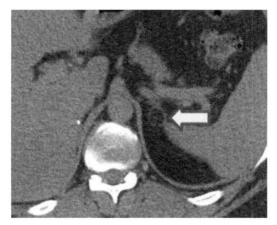

**Fig. 4.** Well-circumscribed low-attenuation lesion within the left adrenal gland is consistent with an adrenal myelolipoma.

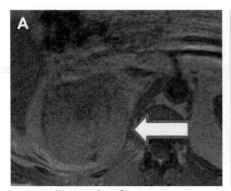
T1 Weighted Image

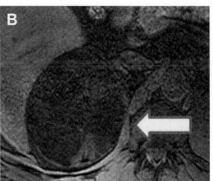
T1 Pre-Contrast Fat Saturated
Sequence

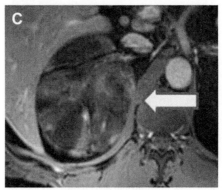
T1 Post-Contrast

**Fig. 5.** Myelolipoma. This right adrenal mass is hyperintense on (*A*) T1-weighted imaging and (*B*) shows a diffuse low signal intensity with fat saturation. (*C*) After contrast administration, there is heterogeneous enhancement of the lesion.

hyperintense, T1 hypointense, and without enhancement. Peripheral calcification is common in pseudocysts but seldom found in true endothelial cysts.[32]

Endothelial cysts are the most common type, accounting for 45% of adrenal cysts, with classic fluid characteristics on MRI and CT.[33–35] Pseudocysts usually result from prior hemorrhage and account for approximately 40% of adrenal cysts. They have a complex MR appearance, with septations, residual blood products, thicker walls, and often central hypointensity.[36] If the cyst demonstrates soft tissue components, other causes, such as a cystic metastasis and cystic pheocromocytoma, could be considered.

### Adrenal infections

Most infections of the adrenal gland are due to granulomatous diseases, such as tuberculosis and histoplasmosis. The imaging findings are usually bilateral but nonspecific and include enlargement of the glands, cystic changes or calcifications.

### Adrenal hemorrhage

On CT, adrenal hemorrhage is seen as a round to ovoid mass that often measures more than 50 HUs in the acute phase (**Fig. 6**). The hematoma may resorb or form a pseudocapsule, with decreasing density as the red cells lyse, eventually becoming a calcified pseudocyst.[37]

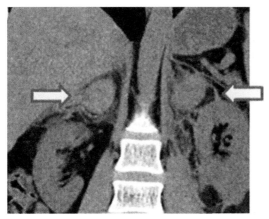

**Fig. 6.** Coronal unenhanced CT demonstrates bilateral adrenal masses measuring 42 HUs and stranding, which extends into the pararenal space consistent with bilateral adrenal hemorrhage.

MRI characteristics vary with evolution of the hematoma. In the acute phase, the hematoma is mildly T1 hypointense with marked T2 hypointensity. As the hematoma matures, in the subacute phase there is T1 and T2 hyperintense signal. Finally, in the chronic phase, there is a hypointense rim around the hematoma, which is known as blooming artifact. When adrenal hemorrhage is identified, it is important to exclude an underlying malignancy.

### Malignant Adrenal Lesions

#### Adrenocortical carcinoma
ACCs are rare, and only approximately half are hormonally active. On CT, they are heterogeneous due to areas of necrosis and hemorrhage (**Fig. 7**). They can contain lipid,

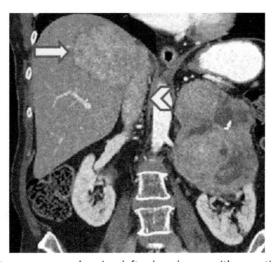

**Fig. 7.** Large, heterogeneous, enhancing left adrenal mass with necrotic areas and thick dystrophic calcifications. There is extension into the IVC (*arrowhead*) and a hepatic metastatic lesion (*arrow*).

which is intracellular and not macroscopic, because they may have cortisol and other fatty precursors in the hormonally active portions of the tumor. There is frequently a peripheral rim of enhancement. Occasionally, these lesions demonstrate relative washout characteristics similar to that of an adenoma; however, the large size and heterogeneity seen in these lesions indicates a malignant process.[38] On MRI, there is heterogeneous T1-weighted and T2-weighted signal intensity, with heterogeneous contrast enhancement.[39] There are often areas of increased T1-weighted signal secondary to different ages of hemorrhage within the mass (**Fig. 8**). Furthermore, there may be areas of signal loss on out-of-phase imaging from cytoplasmic lipid. ACC is often metastatic when diagnosed, and invasion of the IVC is common.

### Pheochromocytoma

Because pheochromocytomas are functional tumors, they are often small at diagnosis. On CT, the attenuation varies from homogenous to heterogeneous with solid

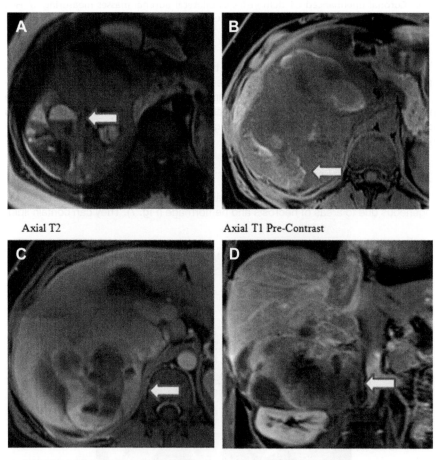

Axial T2

Axial T1 Pre-Contrast

Axial T1 Post-Contrast Portal Venous Phase      Coronal T1 Post-Contrast

**Fig. 8.** MRI demonstrates a large heterogeneous mass within the right adrenal gland with fluid-fluid levels on the (*A*) axial T2-weighted images and hyperintense signal on the (*B*) T1 precontrast images, consistent with hemorrhage. There are (*C*) heterogeneous enhancement images with (*D*) tumor thrombus in the IVC.

and cystic components, hemorrhage, calcification, and occasionally macroscopic fat.[40] Most pheochromocytomas have an attenuation greater than 10 HUs, because the fat tends to be macroscopic. Pheochromocytomas demonstrate avid contrast enhancement secondary to the rich capillary network of the tumor, although enhancement can be heterogenous due to cystic changes or hemorrhage (**Fig. 9**).[40] The contrast washout characteristics are variable, although they typically retain contrast on delayed images. Thus, biochemical and clinical evaluation is critical.

On MRI, these masses demonstrate low signal intensity on T1-weighted images and are often extremely bright on T2-weighted images. Pheochromocytomas do not contain a significant amount of cytoplasmic fat and thus do not lose signal on out-of-phase imaging. There is intense contrast enhancement on T1 sequences, often with areas of heterogeneity depending on the presence of cystic changes and hemorrhage (**Fig. 10**).[41]

### Adrenal lymphoma

Primary adrenal lymphoma is rare, and secondary involvement is found more often in patients with non-Hodgkin lymphoma than Hodgkin lymphoma. On CT, there is homogeneous enlargement of the adrenal gland, with variable enhancement.[42,43] On MRI, lymphoma is characterized as low signal intensity on T1-weighted images with heterogeneous high signal intensity on T2-weighted images and minimal contrast enhancement.[42]

### Adrenal metastases

The adrenal gland is the fourth most common site of metastatic disease, after lung, liver, and bone.[44] Adrenal metastases can present as nodular masses or enlargement of the entire gland. They tend to be heterogeneous, measuring greater than 10 HUs on unenhanced CT images, with variable enhancement patterns. Hypervascular metastases, such as those from renal cell carcinoma and melanoma, may enhance similarly to pheochromocytomas. Washout characteristics of metastases differ from adenomas, with absolute washout less than 60% and relative washout less than 40%.[29] Tumors that

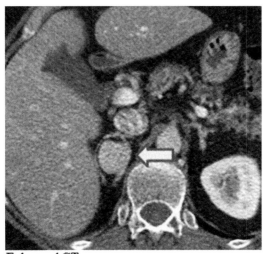

Enhanced CT

**Fig. 9.** Pheochromocytoma. An enhanced CT demonstrates a 2.4-cm homogeneous, avidly enhancing lesion.

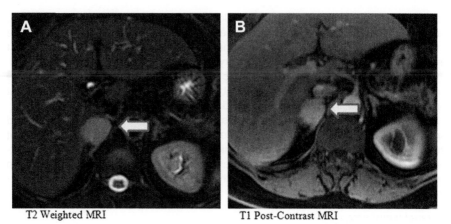

T2 Weighted MRI                    T1 Post-Contrast MRI

**Fig. 10.** Pheochromocytoma. A hyperintense, right adrenal mass is seen on (A) T2-weighted MRI, with (B) avid enhancement.

demonstrate rapid enhancement and washout, however, such as hepatocellular carcinomas, may mimic adenomas. On MRI, adrenal metastases have low signal intensity on T1-weighted images, variable high signal intensity on T2-weighted images, and progressive contrast enhancement. There is rarely cytoplasmic lipid; thus, there is no loss of signal on out-of-phase images.[26] Rarely, tumors that contain cytoplasmic fat, such as clear cell renal carcinoma and hepatocellular carcinoma, can be diagnostic dilemmas, because they may demonstrate loss of signal on out-of-phase imaging.

## FUNCTIONAL ADRENAL IMAGING

Functional imaging permits evaluation of different aspects of pathophysiology (metabolism, receptor density, enzyme activity, and proliferation) using radiotracers dedicated to specific metabolic and synthetic processes within the adrenal gland. Adrenal functional imaging has evolved from planar scintigraphy to single-photon emission CT (SPECT) and positron emission tomography (PET) using molecules labeled with either gamma-emitting radionuclides (eg, 123-I, 131-I, and 111-In) or positron-emitting radionuclides (eg, 18-F, 11-C, and 68-Ga). The physiologic basis of adrenal molecular imaging is based on the metabolic processes within the 2 functionally distinct units of the adrenal gland: the adrenal cortex, which is of mesodermal origin and secretes steroid hormones, and the medulla, which is of neural crest origin and secretes catecholamines.[45]

### Adrenal Cortex

Adrenal cortex–specific molecular imaging probes have been developed using metomidate (MTO) and etomidate (ETO), which are potent inhibitors of the 2 cytochrome P450 (CYP) 11B enzymes, 11β-hydroxylase (CYP11B1) and aldosterone synthase (CYP11B2), that catalyze the last step of cortisol and aldosterone formation, respectively. 11C-MTO PET has been used to demonstrate high uptake in normal adrenal tissue and all adrenocortical tumors, with no significant difference between benign and malignant etiologies and distinguished aldosterone-producing adenomas from bilateral adrenal hyperplasia. The principal uses of MTO and its analogs are to distinguish cortical from noncortical adrenal lesions, which is particularly helpful in patients with nonsecreting adrenal masses and inconclusive CT or MRI findings, and to detect metastatic lesions in patients with ACC.[46] Alternative radiotracers for the CYP11B1 and CYP11B2 enzymatic pathways include [18F]-fluoro-ETO 123I-MTO and 18F-CDP2230.[47]

### Adrenal Medulla

MIBG is a guanethidine analog structurally similar to norepinephrine, which is accumulated in the adrenal medulla; 123-I MIBG scintigraphy has demonstrated 87% sensitivity and 99% specificity for the detection of pheochromocytomas.[48] It has been particularly useful in identifying metastases from malignant pheochromocytomas (**Fig. 11**) and for the localization of paragangliomas.

Most pheochromocytomas, whether benign or malignant, are metabolically active and can be imaged with fludeoxyglucose F 18 (FDG) PET, although uptake is more common in malignant than benign pheochromocytomas.[49]

In a series of 29 patients with pheochromocytoma, focal FDG uptake was demonstrated in 76% of tumors. Some pheochromocytomas that concentrated MIBG poorly were well visualized on FDG PET/CT imaging; thus, 18F-FDG PET/CT imaging is indicated for MIBG-negative tumors. All FDG-negative pheochromocytomas were detected on MIBG scintigraphy.[50]

Somatostatin receptors are expressed in tumors of neural crest origin, and somatostatin receptor analogs labeled with either gamma-emitting (eg, 111-In pentetreotide) or positron-emitting radionuclides, such as 68Ga-DOTA(0)-Tyr(3)-octreotate (68Ga DOTATATE), have been useful for the detection of MIBG-negative tumors, such as paragangliomas of parasympathetic origin (eg, head and neck paragangliomas) and metastatic pheochromocytomas. Recent clinical studies have demonstrated the superiority of 68Ga-DOTATATE PET/CT compared with all other functional and anatomic imaging modalities for the detection of both sporadic and succinate dehydrogenase subunit B (SDHB)-associated metastatic pheochromocytoma and paraganglioma. For sporadic metastatic medullary tumors, 68Ga-DOTATATE PET/CT showed superior lesion detection rates (97.6%), compared with 18F-FDG PET/CT (49.2%), 18F-fluorodihydroxyphenylalanine (FDOPA) PET/CT (74.8%), 18F-fluorodopamine PET/CT (77.7%), and CT/MRI (81.6%).[51] For localization of SDHB-associated metastatic pheochromocytomas and paragangliomas, 68Ga-DOTATATE PET/CT demonstrated superior lesion detection rates (98.6%) compared with 18F-FDG PET/CT (85.8%), 18F-FDOPA PET/CT (61.4%), 18F-fluorodopamine PET/CT (51.9%), and CT/MRI (84.8%).[52]

### Incidentalomas

Clinical studies demonstrated the ability of 18-F FDG PET to accurately differentiate benign AI from malignant adrenal tumors and adrenal metastases, with a sensitivity of 100%, specificity of 94%, and accuracy of 96% for the diagnosis of malignancy.[53] In a series of 105 patients with AIs, 49 lesions (46%) were characterized as primary adrenal tumors, of which all 8 malignant lesions (3 ACCs and 5 neuroblastomas) demonstrated focally increased FDG uptake. Most benign adrenal lesions (83%) were PET negative; however, 7 benign tumors (17%) were PET positive. Functional benign adrenal nodules demonstrated variable FDG activity, with 2 of 4 aldosterone-secreting adenomas and 2 of 3 pheochromocytomas PET positive.[54] A prospective study evaluating 18F-FDG PET/CT imaging for characterization of 41 AIs considered indeterminate on cross-sectional anatomic imaging and without biochemical evidence of hormonal hypersecretion found that 4 of 29 (14%) benign lesions, demonstrated elevated FDG uptake (false positives); all 12 malignant lesions (3 ACCs and 9 adrenal metastases) demonstrated focally increased FDG

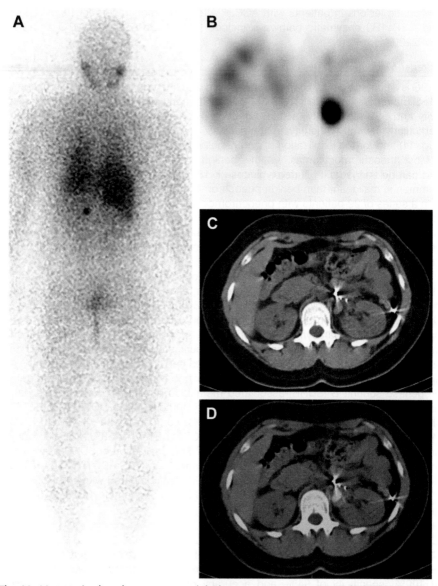

**Fig. 11.** Metastatic pheochromocytoma. (*A*) Planar scan, posterior view demonstrates focal intense MIBG uptake in the left posterior abdomen; there is physiologic radiotracer activity in the liver, heart, salivary glands, and bladder. (*B*) SPECT, (*C*) CT, and (*D*) fused SPECT/CT demonstrate MIBG-avid left paravertebral soft tissue nodule in close proximity to surgical clips.

activity (no false-negative results). The investigators concluded that a negative FDG PET-CT is a valid predictor of benign behavior, and that visual qualitative interpretation (adrenal lesion activity > liver activity) is more accurate than semiquantitative assessment based on SUV$_{max}$ alone, resulting in a sensitivity of 100%, a specificity of 86%, and a negative predictive value of 100%.[55] Benign adrenal lesions with false-positive PET results include adrenal nodular cortical hyperplasia, adrenal endothelial cysts, and inflammatory/infectious adrenal lesions.[50,54,56–58] Caoili and colleagues[59] found that 5 of 47 (10%) adrenal adenomas demonstrated FDG activity greater than liver, and Vikram and colleagues[60] found that 12 of 82 (15%) benign adrenal nodules had false positive PET results, demonstrating focal FDG activity greater than liver.

FDG PET is useful to characterize metastatic adrenal lesions in patients with extra-adrenal malignancies. Boland and colleagues[61] demonstrated a statistically significant difference between mean tumor-to-background ratios for malignant versus benign adrenal lesions. Particularly useful for evaluation of indeterminate adrenal lesions, 18-FDG PET/CT imaging has demonstrated improved characterization of adrenal masses in patients with cancer: sensitivity of 100%, specificity of 99%, positive predictive value of 93%, negative predictive value of 100%, and an accuracy of 99% for detection of malignancy.[62] Malignant adrenal lesions that may produce false-negative PET results have been reported in patients with adrenal metastases secondary to pulmonary carcinoid[63] and bronchioloalveolar lung carcinoma.[64] Hemorrhage and necrosis within a metastatic adrenal lesion and small metastatic lesions ($\leq$10 mm) are other causes of false-negative PET results.[63–66]

### Adrenal Cortical Carcinoma

ACC has consistently demonstrated high metabolic activity on 18F-FDG PET imaging.[54,55] Due to the high incidence of disseminated disease (50% of patients) at presentation,[67] and the high rate of recurrence after initial resection (73%–86% at 2 years), patients with ACC require serial imaging evaluation for restaging.[68] 18-F-FDG PET/CT plays an important role in both staging and surveillance. The intensity of FDG uptake (maximum standardized uptake value [$SUV_{max}$] >10) and the volume of FDG uptake (>150 mL) were significant prognostic factors for survival.[69]

In conjunction with anatomic cross-sectional imaging, F-18 FDG PET/CT has become an important imaging modality for initial staging and follow-up evaluation of patients with ACC (**Fig. 12**).

## ADRENAL VENOUS SAMPLING
### Technique

Successful AVS requires inosculation of the right and left adrenal veins. Because the left adrenal vein drains into the inferior phrenic vein, it is often possible to obtain a satisfactory sample from blood in the inferior phrenic vein just distal to the entrance of the adrenal vein. The technical challenge is usually successful catheterization of the right adrenal vein as it enters into the inferior vena cava (IVC).[70]

The right adrenal vein is variable in length and usually 3.5 mm to 5.0 mm in diameter. It enters the posterior wall of the IVC and may be confused with small hepatic veins draining into the IVC at nearly the same location. CT scanning may be helpful, because the adrenal vein can often be detected on thin, reconstructed images.[71]

Although the left adrenal vein is easier to identify and catheterize, approximately 10% of patients have an anomaly of the left renal vein (LRV), such as retroaortic LRV, circumaortic LRV, or duplicated IVC. Knowledge of these anatomic variants facilitates cannulation of the adrenal vein.

Small catheters, usually 5 French, are used; the preformed C2 Cobra catheter (Cook Medical, Bloomington, Indiana) is often successful for catheterizing the right adrenal vein whereas a reversed Cobra or MK1B catheter (Cook, Bloomington, Indiana) is often used for the left adrenal vein. A side hole is placed near the end of the catheter

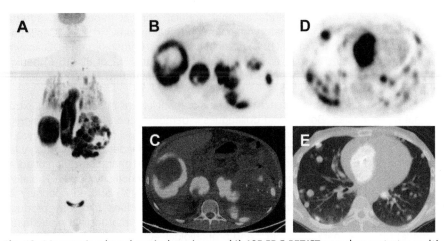

**Fig. 12.** Metastatic adrenal cortical carcinoma. (*A*) 18F-FDG PET/CT scan demonstrates multifocal bilateral lung activity, multiple hypermetabolic foci throughout the abdomen and extending across the diaphragm. (*B*) Abdomen transaxial PET and (*C*) fused PET/CT demonstrate a heterogeneous hypermetabolic left adrenal mass with central necrosis and calcifications, retroperitoneal lymphadenopathy; centrally necrotic liver metastasis and tumor thrombus within the IVC. (*D*) Chest transaxial PET and (*E*) fused PET/CT demonstrate innumerable hypermetabolic bilateral pulmonary nodules.

to facilitate sample collection.[71,72] Heparinization is used to prevent clotting of blood during the slow collection process.

Peripheral blood samples are also obtained at the time of AVS to demonstrate the higher cortisol levels in the adrenal venous samples.[73] It is expected that the cortisol level in the adrenal vein is at least 3 times that of the peripheral vein. Cortisol serves as an excellent measure of the dilution of the blood from the adrenal vein by blood from the left inferior phrenic vein, renal vein, or IVC. Thus, the ratio of aldosterone to cortisol corrects for venous dilution. Some endocrinologists prefer to collect samples both before and after intravenous infusions of corticotropin, which stimulates cortisol and aldosterone release.

### Complications

To verify the location of the catheter in the adrenal vein, a small amount of contrast is injected. Complications of AVS include thrombus formation, hemorrhage, contrast extravasation, and adrenal infarction. With the more frequent use of CT and MRI, the need for adrenal venography is diminished and contrast is injected only to verify the location of the catheter, not to diagnose a tumor. Thus, only small contrast injections are needed. Furthermore, the use of heparin has made venous thrombus formation and adrenal infarction an uncommon complication. In major centers in which AVS is commonly performed, complications are now found in fewer than 1% of patients.[70]

### Results

In tertiary referral centers, successful AVS is performed in more than 90% of cases. The level of cortisol in the adrenal vein is compared with a peripheral vein or the IVC below the adrenal and renal veins. The cortisol level in the adrenal vein is often 10 times or more that of the peripheral vein but at least 2 to 3 times as great to confirm adequate sampling. Accurate sampling is accomplished in more than 85% of cases in the right adrenal vein and 95% of cases for the left adrenal vein.[71] The hormone levels in venous samples from an adrenal gland containing an aldosterone-producing adenoma are usually dramatically higher than the contralateral gland.[74–76] In practice, a level of at least 4 times the unaffected side is sufficient for a confident diagnosis and localization of the APA.[72]

## SUMMARY

Cross-sectional imaging can make a specific diagnosis in lesions, such as myelolipomas, cysts, or hemorrhage, and is often sufficient to distinguish benign from malignant adrenal processes. CT and MRI are also useful studies to identify pheochromocytomas and cortisol-secreting or androgen-secreting tumors. In patients with primary aldosteronism, AVS remains the most accurate localizing study and should be performed in all patients older than 35 years of age, even if an adenoma is detected by CT or MRI. Radiolabeled isotope studies serve as second-line diagnostic tests for malignant adrenal tumors, either primary or metastatic, as well as for pheochromocytoma. Nuclear imaging studies should always follow a robust hormonal diagnosis and be correlated with findings on cross-sectional imaging. Ongoing research that uses CYP11B2-specific radiotracers may localize autonomous aldosterone synthesis and replace invasive AVS.

## REFERENCES

1. Debillon E, Velayoudom-Cephise FL, Salenave S, et al. Unilateral adrenalectomy as a first-line treatment of Cushing's Syndrome in patients with primary bilateral macronodular adrenal hyperplasia. J Clin Endocrinol Metab 2015;100(12): 4417–24.

2. Perogamvros I, Vassiliadi DA, Karapanou O, et al. Biochemical and clinical benefits of unilateral adrenalectomy in patients with subclinical hypercortisolism and bilateral adrenal incidentalomas. Eur J Endocrinol 2015;173(6):719–25.

3. Lenders JW, Duh QY, Eisenhofer G, et al, Endocrine Society. Pheochromocytoma and paraganglioma: an endocrine society clinical practice guideline. J Clin Endocrinol Metab 2014;99(6):1915–42.

4. Dunnick NR, Doppman JL, Mills SR, et al. Preoperative diagnosis and localization of aldosteronomas by measurement of corticosteroids in adrenal venous blood. Radiology 1979;133:331–3.

5. Zhu L, Zhang Y, Zhang H, et al. Comparison between adrenal venous sampling and computed tomography in the diagnosis of primary aldosteronism and in the guidance of adrenalectomy. Medicine 2016;95(39):e4986.

6. Kempers MJ, Lenders JW, van Outheusden L, et al. Systematic review: diagnostic procedures to differentiate unilateral from bilateral adrenal abnormality in primary aldosteronism. Ann Intern Med 2009;151(5):329–37.

7. Funder JW, Carey RM, Mantero F, et al. The management of primary aldosteronism: case detection, diagnosis, and treatment: an Endocrine Society clinical practice guideline. J Clin Endocrinol Metab 2016;101(5):1889–916.

8. Rossi GP, Auchus RJ, Brown M, et al. An expert consensus statement on use of adrenal vein sampling for the subtyping of primary aldosteronism. Hypertension 2014;63(1):151–60.

9. Herrera MF, Grant CS, van Heerden JA, et al. Incidentally discovered adrenal tumors: an institutional perspective. Surgery 1991;110(6):1014–21.

10. Bovio S, Cataldi A, Reimondo G, et al. Prevalence of adrenal incidentaloma in a contemporary computerized tomography series. J Endocrinol Invest 2006;29(4): 298–302.

11. Song JH, Chaudhry FS, Mayo-Smith WW. The incidental adrenal mass on CT: prevalence of adrenal disease in 1,049 csonsecutive adrenal masses in patients with no known malignancy. AJR Am J Roentgenol 2008;190(5):1163–8.

12. Fassnacht M, Arlt W, Bancos I, et al. Management of adrenal incidentalomas: European Society of Endocrinology Clinical Practice Guideline in collaboration with the European Network for the Study of Adrenal Tumors. Eur J Endocrinol 2016; 175(2):G1–34.

13. Angeli A, Osella G, Ali A, et al. Adrenal incidentaloma: an overview of clinical and epidemiological data from the National Italian Study Group. Horm Res 1997; 47(4–6):279–83.

14. Barzon L, Scaroni C, Sonino N, et al. Incidentally discovered adrenal tumors: endocrine and scintigraphic correlates. J Clin Endocrinol Metab 1998;83(1): 55–62.

15. Bancos I, Tamhane S, Shah M, et al. Diagnosis of endocrine disease: the diagnostic performance of adrenal biopsy: a systematic review and meta-analysis. Eur J Endocrinol 2016;175(2):R65–80.

16. Schalin-Jantti C, Raade M, Hamalainen E, et al. 5-year prospective follow-up study of lipid-rich adrenal incidentalomas: no tumor growth or development of hormonal hypersecretion. Endocrinol Metab 2015;30(4):481–7.

17. Ozsari L, Kutahyalioglu M, Elsayes KM, et al. Preexisting adrenal masses in patients with adrenocortical carcinoma: clinical and radiological factors contributing to delayed diagnosis. Endocrine 2016;51(2):351–9.

18. Dunnick NR, Korobkin M, Francis I. Adrenal radiology: distinguishing benign from malignant adrenal masses. AJR Am J Roentgenol 1996;167(4):861–7.

19. Johnson PT, Horton KM, Fishman EK. Adrenal mass imaging with multidetector CT: pathologic conditions, pearls, and pitfalls. Radiographics 2009;29(5): 1333–51.

20. Reznek RH, Armstrong P. The adrenal gland. Clin Endocrinol (Oxf) 1994;40(5): 561–76.

21. Chaudhary V, Bano S. Anatomical and functional imaging in endocrine hypertension. J Comput Assist Tomogr 2012;16(5):713–21.

22. Dunnick NR, Leight GS, Roubidoux MA, et al. CT in the diagnosis of primary aldosteronism: sensitivity in 29 patients. Am J Roentgenol 1993;160(2):321–4.

23. Sohaib SA, Peppercorn PD, Allan C, et al. Primary hyperaldosteronism (Conn Syndrome): MR imaging findings. Radiology 2000;214(2):527–31.

24. Lee MJ, Hahn PF, Papanicolaou N, et al. Benign and malignant adrenal masses: CT distinction with attenuation coefficients, size, and observer analysis. Radiology 1991;179(2):415–8.

25. Korobkin M, Brodeur FJ, Francis IR, et al. CT time-attenuation washout curves of adrenal adenomas and nonadenomas. AJR Am J Roentgenol 1998;170(3): 747–52.

26. Korobkin M, Giordano TJ, Brodeur FJ, et al. Adrenal adenomas: relationship between histologic lipid and CT and MR findings. Radiology 1996;200(3):743–7.

27. Namimoto T, Yamashita Y, Mitsuzaki K, et al. Adrenal masses: quantification of fat content with double-echo chemical shift in-phase and opposed-phase FLASH MR images for differentiation of adrenal adenomas. Radiology 2001;218(3): 642–6.

28. Mayo-Smith WW, Lee MJ, McNicholas MM, et al. Characterization of adrenal masses (<5 cm) by use of chemical shift MR imaging: observer performance versus quantitative measures. AJR Am J Roentgenol 1995;165(1):91–5.

29. Caoili EM, Korobkin M, Francis IR, et al. Delayed enhanced CT of lipid-poor adrenal adenomas. AJR Am J Roentgenol 2000;175(5):1411–5.

30. Caoili EM, Korobkin M, Francis IR, et al. Adrenal masses: characterization with combined unenhanced and delayed enhanced CT. Radiology 2002;222(3): 629–33.

31. Blake MA, Kalra MK, Sweeney AT, et al. Distinguishing benign from malignant adrenal masses: multi-detector row CT protocol with 10-minute delay. Radiology 2006;238(2):578–85.

32. Itani M, Wasnik AP, Platt JP. Radiologic-pathologic correlation in extra-adrenal myelolipoma. Abdom Radiol 2013;39:394–7.

33. Lam KY, Lo CY. Adrenal lipomatous tumours: a 30 year clinicopathological experience at a single institution. J Clin Pathol 2001;54(9):707–12.

34. Rozenblit A, Morehouse HT, Amis ES Jr. Cystic adrenal lesions: CT features. Radiology 1996;201(2):541–8.

35. Johnson CD, Baker ME, Dunnick NR. CT demonstration of an adrenal pseudocyst. J Comput Assist Tomogr 1984;9(4):817–9.

36. Ricci Z, Chernyak V, Hsu K, et al. Adrenal cysts: natural history by long-term imaging follow-up. AJR Am J Roentgenol 2013;201:1009–16.

37. Dunnick NR. Hanson lecture. Adrenal imaging: current status. AJR Am J Roentgenol 1990;154(5):927–36.

38. Dunnick NR, Heaston D, Halvorsen R, et al. CT appearance of adrenal cortical carcinoma. J Comput Assist Tomogr 1982;5:978–82.

39. Schlund JF, Kenney PJ, Brown ED, et al. Adrenocortical carcinoma: MR imaging appearance with current techniques. J Magn Reson Imaging 1995;5(2):171–4.

40. Blake MA, Kalra MK, Maher MM, et al. Pheochromocytoma: an imaging chameleon. Radiographics 2004;24(Suppl 1):S87–99.

41. Francis IR, Korobkin M. Pheochromocytoma. Radiol Clin North Am 1996;34(6): 1101–12.

42. Paling MR, Williamson BRJ. Adrenal involvement in non-hodgkin lymphoma. AJR Am J Roentgenol 1983;141:303–5.

43. Lee FT Jr, Thornbury JR, Grist TM, et al. MR imaging of adrenal lymphoma. Abdom Imaging 1993;18(1):95–6.

44. Abrams HL, Spiro R, Goldstein N. Metastases in carcinoma: analysis of 1,000 autopsied cases. Cancer 1950;3:74–85.

45. Avram AM, Fig LM, Gross MD. Adrenal gland scintigraphy. Semin Nucl Med 2006;36(3):212–27.

46. Hahner S, Sundin A. Metomidate-based imaging of adrenal masses. Horm Cancer 2011;2(6):348–53.

47. Abe T, Naruse M, Young WF Jr, et al. A novel CYP11B2-specific imaging agent for detection of unilateral subtypes of primary aldosteronism. J Clin Endocrinol Metab 2016;101(3):1008–15.

48. Rubello D, Bui C, Casara D, et al. Functional scintigraphy of the adrenal gland. Eur J Endocrinol 2002;147(1):13–28.

49. Timmers HJ, Chen CC, Carrasquillo JA, et al. Staging and functional characterization of pheochromocytoma and paraganglioma by 18F-fluorodeoxyglucose (18F-FDG) positron emission tomography. J Natl Cancer Inst 2012;104(9):700–8.

50. Shulkin BL, Thompson NW, Shapiro B, et al. Pheochromocytomas: imaging with 2-[fluorine-18]fluoro-2-deoxy-D-glucose PET. Radiology 1999;212(1):35–41.

51. Janssen I, Chen CC, Millo CM, et al. PET/CT comparing (68)Ga-DOTATATE and other radiopharmaceuticals and in comparison with CT/MRI for the localization of sporadic metastatic pheochromocytoma and paraganglioma. Eur J Nucl Med Mol Imaging 2016;43(10):1784–91.

52. Janssen I, Blanchet EM, Adams K, et al. Superiority of [68Ga]-DOTATATE PET/CT to Other Functional Imaging Modalities in the Localization of SDHB-Associated Metastatic Pheochromocytoma and Paraganglioma. Clin Cancer Res 2015; 21(17):3888–95.

53. Yun M, Kim W, Alnafisi N, et al. 18F-FDG PET in characterizing adrenal lesions detected on CT or MRI. J Nucl Med 2001;42(12):1795–9.

54. Han SJ, Kim TS, Jeon SW, et al. Analysis of adrenal masses by 18F-FDG positron emission tomography scanning. Int J Clin Pract 2007;61(5):802–9.

55. Tessonnier L, Sebag F, Palazzo FF, et al. Does 18F-FDG PET/CT add diagnostic accuracy in incidentally identified non-secreting adrenal tumours? Eur J Nucl Med Mol Imaging 2008;35(11):2018–25.

56. Blake MA, Slattery JM, Kalra MK, et al. Adrenal lesions: characterization with fused PET/CT image in patients with proved or suspected malignancy–initial experience. Radiology 2006;238(3):970–7.

57. Shimizu A, Oriuchi N, Tsushima Y, et al. High [18F] 2-fluoro-2-deoxy-D-glucose (FDG) uptake of adrenocortical adenoma showing subclinical Cushing's syndrome. Ann Nucl Med 2003;17(5):403–6.

58. Rao SK, Caride VJ, Ponn R, et al. F-18 fluorodeoxyglucose positron emission tomography-positive benign adrenal cortical adenoma: imaging features and pathologic correlation. Clin Nucl Med 2004;29(5):300–2.

59. Caoili EM, Korobkin M, Brown RK, et al. Differentiating adrenal adenomas from nonadenomas using (18)F-FDG PET/CT: quantitative and qualitative evaluation. Acad Radiol 2007;14(4):468–75.

60. Vikram R, Yeung HD, Macapinlac HA, et al. Utility of PET/CT in differentiating benign from malignant adrenal nodules in patients with cancer. Am J Roentgenol 2008;191(5):1545–51.

61. Boland GW, Goldberg MA, Lee MJ, et al. Indeterminate adrenal mass in patients with cancer: evaluation at PET with 2-[F-18]-fluoro-2-deoxy-D-glucose. Radiology 1995;194(1):131–4.

62. Boland GW, Blake MA, Holalkere NS, et al. PET/CT for the characterization of adrenal masses in patients with cancer: qualitative versus quantitative accuracy in 150 consecutive patients. Am J Roentgenol 2009;192(4):956–62.

63. Jana S, Zhang T, Milstein DM, et al. FDG-PET and CT characterization of adrenal lesions in cancer patients. Eur J Nucl Med Mol Imaging 2006;33(1):29–35.

64. Chong S, Lee KS, Kim HY, et al. Integrated PET-CT for the characterization of adrenal gland lesions in cancer patients: diagnostic efficacy and interpretation pitfalls. Radiographics 2006;26(6):1811–24 [discussion: 24–6].

65. Kumar R, Xiu Y, Yu JQ, et al. 18F-FDG PET in evaluation of adrenal lesions in patients with lung cancer. J Nucl Med 2004;45(12):2058–62.

66. Metser U, Miller E, Lerman H, et al. 18F-FDG PET/CT in the evaluation of adrenal masses. J Nucl Med 2006;47(1):32–7.

67. Luton JP, Cerdas S, Billaud L, et al. Clinical features of adrenocortical carcinoma, prognostic factors, and the effect of mitotane therapy. N Engl J Med 1990; 322(17):1195–201.

68. Icard P, Goudet P, Charpenay C, et al. Adrenocortical carcinomas: surgical trends and results of a 253-patient series from the French Association of Endocrine Surgeons study group. World J Surg 2001;25(7):891–7.

69. Leboulleux S, Dromain C, Bonniaud G, et al. Diagnostic and Prognostic Value of 18-fluorodeoxyglucose positron emission tomography in adrenocortical carcinoma: a prospective comparison with computed tomography. J Clin Endocrinol Metab 2006;91(3):920–5.
70. Daunt N. Adrenal vein sampling: how to make it quick, easy, and successful. Radiographics 2005;25(Suppl 1):S143–58.
71. Ota H, Seiji K, Kawabata M, et al. Dynamic multidetector CT and non-contrast-enhanced MR for right adrenal vein imaging: comparison with catheter venography in adrenal venous sampling. Eur Radiol 2015;26(3):622–30.
72. Kahn SL, Angle JF. Adrenal vein sampling. Tech Vasc Interv Radiol 2010;13(2): 110–25.
73. Mailhot J, Traistaru M, Soulez G, et al. Adrenal vein sampling in primary aldosteronism: sensitivity and specificity of basal adrenal vein to peripheral vein cortisol and aldosterone ratios to confirm catheterization of the adrenal vein. Radiology 2015;277(3):887–94.
74. Dunnick NR, Doppman JL, Gill JR, et al. Localization of functional adrenal tumors by computed tomography and venous sampling. Radiology 1982;142(2):429–33.
75. Patel SM, Lingam RK, Beaconsfield TI, et al. Role of radiology in the management of primary aldosteronism. Radiographics 2007;27(4):1145–57.
76. Rossi GP, Bernini G, Caliumi C, et al. A prospective study of the prevalence of primary aldosteronism in 1,125 hypertensive patients. J Am Coll Cardiol 2006; 48(11):2293–300.

# Pancreatic Imaging

Mark Masciocchi, MD

## KEYWORDS

- Neuroendocrine tumor • Islet cell tumor • Insulinoma • Gastrinoma • MEN1 • VHL
- TSC • NF1

## KEY POINTS

- Most pancreatic neuroendocrine tumors are not "hyperfunctioning."
- Imaging alone is not reliable for subtyping neuroendocrine tumors.
- Pancreatic neuroendocrine tumors are seen in genetic syndromes including multiple endocrine neoplasia I, Von Hippel-Lindau disease, tuberous sclerosis complex, and neurofibramatosis-1.
- There are numerous imaging mimics of pancreatic neuroendocrine tumors.
- Imaging may play a role in the future for predicting patients at risk for diabetes mellitus.

## INTRODUCTION

The pancreas is composed of both exocrine and endocrine tissue. Although exocrine tissue predominates in the overall mass of the gland, the physiology of the islets of Langerhans is no less essential and imaging plays a critical role in the diagnosis and evaluation of entities involving both components. From an endocrine standpoint, the subject of pancreatic imaging is dominated by pancreatic endocrine neoplasms. The usefulness of different modalities depends in great deal on the particular clinical scenario. This article examines the advantages and disadvantages of different imaging methods in pancreatic endocrine imaging with attention to the best modalities for referring physicians in common situations. In addition to a detailed discussion of pancreatic neuroendocrine tumors, common imaging mimics, associated genetic syndromes, and endocrine insufficiency are examined.

## MODALITIES
### Ultrasound Imaging

Transabdominal ultrasound is low yield in pancreatic tumor detection owing to its limited sensitivity and specificity.[1,2] This is likely due to the depth of the organ, variable patient body habitus, and frequent obscuration by air within the stomach and bowel.

The author has nothing to disclose.
Department of Radiology, UMass Memorial Medical Center, University of Massachusetts Medical School, 55 Lake Avenue North, Worcester, MA 01655, USA
E-mail address: mark.masciocchi@umassmemorial.org

Endocrinol Metab Clin N Am 46 (2017) 761–781
http://dx.doi.org/10.1016/j.ecl.2017.04.006
0889-8529/17/© 2017 Elsevier Inc. All rights reserved.

Despite these limitations, incidental lesions may be detected on routine imaging for nonpancreatic indications and further characterization beyond solid or cystic components is usually not possible. In contrast, pancreas transplants are better assessed owing to a more superficial location, allowing for better penetration with high frequency transducers as well as the usefulness of Doppler evaluation to interrogate graft vessels (**Fig. 1**).

Unlike transabdominal ultrasound imaging, endoscopic ultrasound (EUS) imaging has excellent sensitivity, including small lesions measuring less than 3 cm thanks to higher spatial resolution.[1–5] However, sensitivity decreases precipitously toward the pancreatic tail.[6] Unfortunately, certain pancreatic endocrine neoplasms such as insulinoma have a higher incidence in the regions that are difficult to visualize on either endoscopic or transabdominal ultrasound imaging.[7] Regardless, for suspected lesions on other imaging modalities, EUS imaging allows for tissue diagnosis at the same time as imaging, an advantage that none of the other modalities offer.

### Computed Tomography Scans

Cross-sectional imaging (computed tomography [CT] or MRI) is usually required to completely image the gland. Further, multiphasic imaging is usually appropriate in the case of neuroendocrine tumors[8–12] (**Fig. 2**). This is especially important when there is high suspicion for a lesion and combining with EUS imaging improves sensitivity.[13] Although it confers a considerable radiation dose, CT has the advantage of high

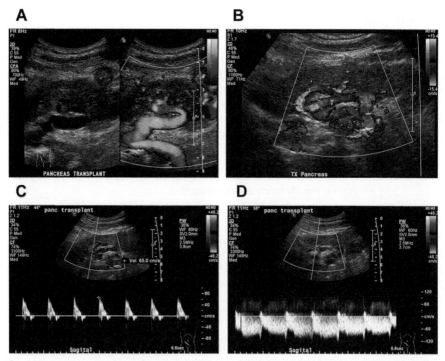

**Fig. 1.** Pancreas transplant ultrasound imaging. (*A*) Grayscale and power Doppler imaging showing the graft and anastomosis to the iliac vessels. (*B*) Color Doppler image displaying directional flow. Individual vessels are interrogated using spectral Doppler imaging to show (*C*) arterial and (*D*) venous waveforms.

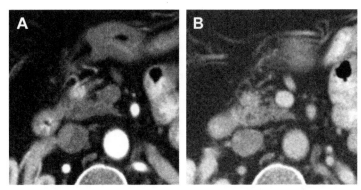

**Fig. 2.** Axial computed tomography images through the head of the pancreas during the (*A*) arterial and (*B*) venous phases. Note how the small lesion is only visible during the arterial phase.

contrast and spatial resolution, making it excellent for the preoperative assessment of pancreatic tumors owing to noninvasiveness, delineation of vascular involvement, and evaluation for metastasis.[8,14] Radiation dosage becomes an even greater concern because pancreas CT protocols often require multiple postcontrast phases. This can be somewhat mitigated with dual-energy CT, but use of this technique is variable among institutions and long-term benefits from relatively small reductions in radiation dosage are not yet proven.

## MRI

The pancreas has unique signal characteristics on MRI, allowing for superior tissue characterization as well as beautiful depiction of ductal anatomy. MRI is especially helpful for lesions with indeterminate imaging features on other modalities (**Fig. 3**). In the case of pancreatic neuroendocrine tumors, the imaging appearance can be variable and MRI allows for both lesion characterization and metastasis detection.[15] Similar to CT scanning, there is a benefit to multiphasic imaging, but without the disadvantage of increasing radiation dose.[12,16]

The superiority of CT versus MRI in lesion detection is subject to debate. When deciding between the two modalities, it is worth considering that MRI is more susceptible to motion artifacts and contraindications from metallic foreign bodies are not uncommon. Multiple breath holds in a confined space over the course of 20 to 45 minutes may disqualify many otherwise suitable patients with diminished respiratory status and claustrophobia. Regardless of which modality may be ideal for the particular clinical question, it is always critical to consider the patient's ability to complete the examination.

## Nuclear Medicine

Although lacking spatial resolution, nuclear medicine studies offer an unparalleled ability to identify tissues based on the presence of specific cell receptors. Octreotide scans take advantage of the somatostatin receptor types expressed by neuroendocrine cells, allowing for localization of well-differentiated neuroendocrine tumors.[17] However, tracer uptake is also normal in the liver, spleen, and kidneys, which can make finding a new pancreatic tumor difficult owing to overlapping structures. This can partially be solved with the use of single-photon emission computed tomography (SPECT)-CT scans, which allows for cross-sectional imaging (**Fig. 4**).

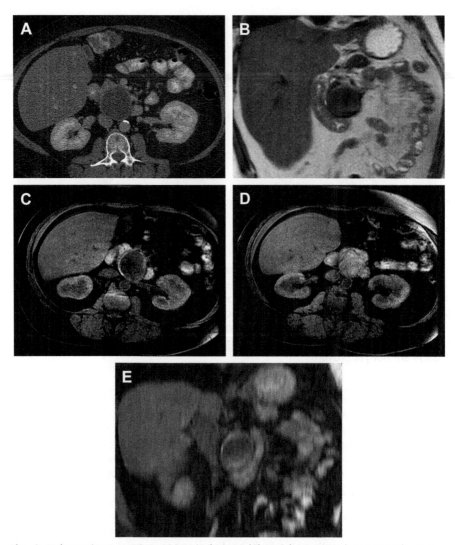

**Fig. 3.** Indeterminate cystic pancreatic lesion. (*A*) Axial computed tomography image showing a large cystic lesion within the uncinate process of the pancreas. (*B*) T2-weighted MRI image shows markedly low signal, inconsistent with simple fluid that would be expected with a cystic lesion. T1-weighted axial MRI images at the (*C*) superior and (*D*) inferior aspects of the lesion showing different signal intensities. (*E*) Coronal reformation showing layering T1 hyperintense material. Endoscopic ultrasound imaging with fine-needle aspiration was performed and fluid analysis was consistent with a pseudocyst. The patient had no recent history of pancreatitis.

## NEUROENDOCRINE TUMORS

Neuroendocrine tumors are found in many different organs. In the pancreas, these tumors are classically associated with clinical syndromes at presentation, but now are increasingly diagnosed as an incidental lesion.[18–21] Often referred to as islet cell tumors, the term is somewhat misleading because it implies that tumors arise de

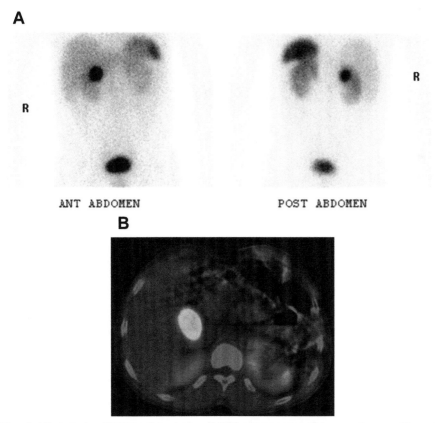

A

R

ANT ABDOMEN

R

POST ABDOMEN

B

Fig. 4. (A) Anterior (ANT) and posterior (POST) planar octreotide scan images. There is normal background uptake within the liver, spleen, and kidneys along with excreted tracer in the bladder. Focal increased uptake overlies the upper pole of the right kidney. (B) Single photon emission computed tomography (SPECT)-CT allows for more accurate localization, revealing the lesion to be within the second portion of the duodenum/pancreatic head.

novo from the islets of Langerhans. This nomenclature would also imply that these tumors are α, β, or δ cells gone awry, when in fact most neuroendocrine tumors are not hyperfunctioning.[19,22,23] In reality, they more likely originate from ductal–acinar stem cells.[24–26] With this perspective, it is easier to see why pancreatic neuroendocrine tumors should not be thought of as adenomas that can be treated medically, but rather surgical lesions with malignant potential. The World Health Organization classification system is used to classify tumors according to their malignant potential based on features such as mitotic and Ki-67 index[27] (**Fig. 5**).

Histologically, neuroendocrine tumors are distinguished by positive staining for chromogranin A and synaptophysin among several other markers[20,28] (**Fig. 6**). Most secrete one or multiple hormones but are considered "functioning" or "nonfunctioning" based on whether there are clinical symptoms from hormone hypersecretion.[29–31] A more accurate term would be "hyperfunctioning" versus "nonhyperfunctioning." Hyperfunctioning tumors in order of decreasing incidence are insulinoma, gastrinoma, and glucagonoma.[28] VIPoma, somatostatinoma, ACTHoma, and other subtypes are exceedingly rare (**Fig. 7**). Although the imaging

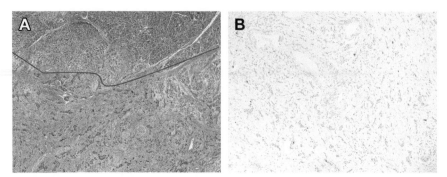

**Fig. 5.** (A) Hematoxylin & eosin staining of a pancreatic neuroendocrine tumor at the bottom of the image with normal pancreatic tissue at the top for comparison. (B) Ki-67 staining of the same tumor showing a low proliferation index.

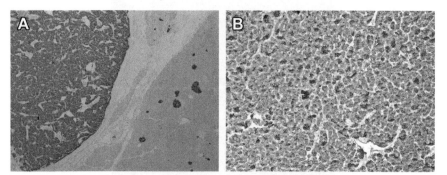

**Fig. 6.** (A) Well-differentiated neuroendocrine tumor staining positive for synaptophysin on the left side of the image. Note normal islets of Langerhans scattered throughout the right side of the image. (B) Diffuse positive chromogranin staining for a different, well-differentiated tumor.

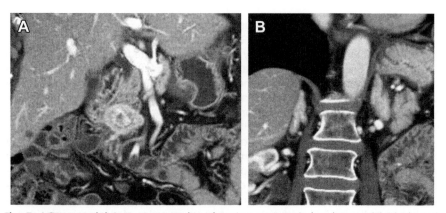

**Fig. 7.** ACTHoma. (A) Heterogeneously enhancing pancreatic head mass. (B) Thickened, enhancing adrenal glands. The patient also had elevated cortisol levels and the tumor stained grossly positive for adrenocorticotropic hormone (ACTH).

features cannot reliably differentiate types of hyperfunctioning neuroendocrine tumors, there are distinctive features compared with other focal pancreatic lesions. The classic CT/MRI appearance is that of a solid arterially hyperenhancing lesion. With the exception of poorly differentiated tumors, these lesions also tend to be discrete and do not cause ductal dilatation in contrast with pancreatic adenocarcinoma, although there are always exceptions (**Fig. 8**). Other focal lesions that can commonly be mistaken for neuroendocrine tumors are discussed elsewhere in this article.

Insulinomas are the most common hyperfunctioning tumor and are usually small, benign lesions.[28,32,33] Similar to the distribution of the islets of Langerhans, these lesions are also more common in the pancreatic body or tail[7] (**Figs. 9** and **10**). The lower incidence of somatostatin type 2 receptors makes octreotide scans less reliable compared with other tumor subtypes.[34,35] Aside from location and size, there is little imaging can provide to solidify the diagnosis without coexisting endogenous hyperinsulinemia (elevated C-peptide). More importantly, cross-sectional imaging allows for the noninvasive delineation of surrounding structures, making patients potential candidates for enucleation rather than a more extensive resection.

Unlike insulinomas, gastrinomas are much more common in the pancreatic head, which lies within the "gastrinoma triangle" bounded by the junctions of the cystic

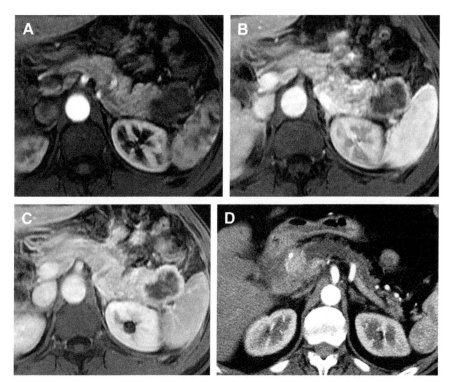

**Fig. 8.** Pancreatic tail mass during (*A*) arterial, (*B*) venous, and (*C*) delayed postcontrast phases. The mass is arterially hypoenhancing and shows progressive peripheral enhancement. This mass proved to be pancreatic adenocarcinoma. The location prevents using ductal dilatation as supporting evidence. (*D*) Enhancing pancreatic head mass in a different patient with a dilated duct and parenchymal atrophy. This proved to be a neuroendocrine tumor.

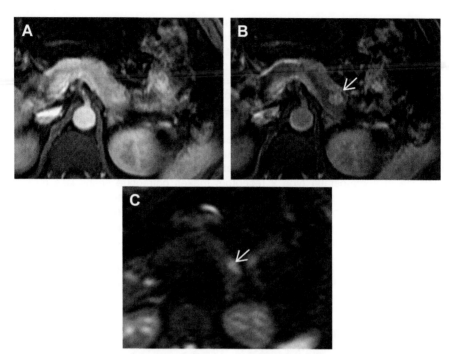

**Fig. 9.** Insulinoma. (*A*) The tumor is difficult to visualize on postcontrast MRI images, but much better seen (*arrow*) with (*B*) subtraction of precontrast from postcontrast images as well as (*C*) diffusion-weighted images.

and common bile ducts, second and third portions of the duodenum, and pancreatic head and neck.[36] Extrapancreatic tumors within the triangle and malignant histology are common. There is also a strong association with multiple endocrine neoplasia I (MEN1).[28,32,33,37] This specific diagnosis can only be strongly suggested on imaging when there is coexisting evidence of gastritis or peptic ulcer disease. The need for endoscopic evaluation along with the common periampullary location of these tumors makes EUS imaging especially useful. Ultimately, cross-sectional imaging is usually

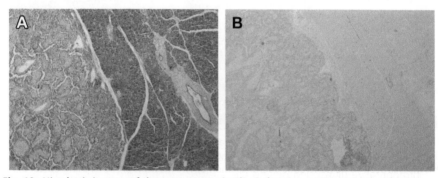

**Fig. 10.** Histologic images of the same tumor in **Fig. 9** showing positive staining for (*A*) amyloid using congo red within tumor stroma and (*B*) positive insulin immunohistochemistry.

indicated owing to the higher incidence of malignancy, making preoperative delineation of anatomy essential (**Fig. 11**).

Glucagonomas are known for the associated dermatologic syndrome of necrolytic migratory erythema. Unlike insulinomas and gastrinomas, these tumors are usually both large and malignant.[28,38] When considering this rare diagnosis owing to unexpected hyperglycemia or an unusual rash, it is often simplest to review whether the patient has had a recent CT or MRI examination of the abdomen before proceeding to new imaging because an occult tumor is unlikely to be the etiology.

When defined as tumors without clinical symptoms of hormone hypersecretion, nonhyperfunctioning tumors are the most common type of pancreatic neuroendocrine tumor and are increasingly diagnosed as an incidental finding.[19–21] Although neuroendocrine tumors can have several atypical imaging features, cystic neuroendocrine tumors deserve attention owing to their frequency and the potential to be mistaken for other lesions (**Fig. 12**). Most are nonhyperfunctioning tumors and tend to be larger.[39,40] One possible explanation is that these tumors grow silently for longer, allowing time for cystic degeneration or necrosis. However, there is a counterargument that they are actually more likely to be benign.[41] For cystic pancreatic lesions where the diagnosis is not known, MRI is especially useful owing to its ability to evaluate for other differentiating features, such as ductal communication, encapsulation, and enhancement pattern.[16]

## Metastasis

The liver is by far the most common site of metastasis in the case of pancreatic neuroendocrine tumors. Detection of metastatic disease is critical to staging and therefore affects treatment. Therefore, imaging modalities with higher sensitivity for metastatic disease have become especially helpful. Owing to the smaller size of neuroendocrine metastases, imaging has shown disappointing accuracy across modalities, but with MRI leading the group.[42,43]

Similar to the primary tumor, neuroendocrine metastases are often identified as hypervascular liver masses[44,45] (**Fig. 13**). However, this requires masses to be large enough to show macroscopic evidence of neovascularity. Smaller metastases may not have these histologic features and so other distinguishing characteristics must be visible with imaging. Hypercellularity and lack of hepatocytes are two features that can be identified with diffusion-weighted imaging and the use of hepatobiliary contrast, respectively.

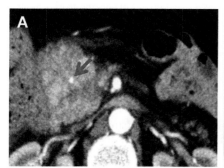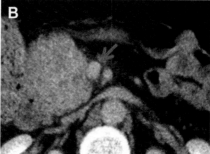

**Fig. 11.** Computed tomography images acquired during the (A) arterial and (B) venous phases depicting a hyperenhancing pancreatic head mass partially abutting the superior mesenteric vein (blue arrow) and encasing the gastroduodenal artery (red arrow).

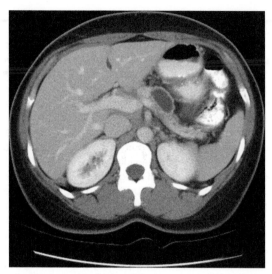

**Fig. 12.** Axial computed tomography image showing a cystic lesion in the pancreatic body in a patient with abdominal pain. Originally thought to be a pseudocyst, this proved to be a well-differentiated neuroendocrine tumor when resected.

The underlying physics of diffusion-weighted imaging are complex and beyond the scope of this article. Simply put, diffusion-weighted imaging can detect hypercellularity, a feature common but not always present in malignancy. This technique has been shown by d'Assignies and colleagues[46] to have a higher sensitivity for detection of neuroendocrine metastases including those less than 1 cm compared with gadolinium-enhanced MRI. Diffusion-weighted imaging is a fast imaging technique that does not require intravenous (IV) contrast. Although sensitivity improves further by combining techniques together in the imaging protocol, this study showed that patients with contraindications to IV contrast owing to a low glomerular filtration rate can still benefit from an unenhanced MRI for staging purposes.

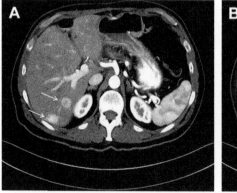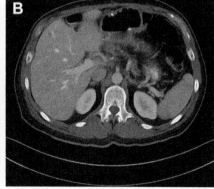

**Fig. 13.** Axial computed tomography images in a patient with a large pancreatic neuroendocrine tumor showing multiple hepatic masses that are much more conspicuous during the (A) arterial (*arrows*) than (B) venous phases.

Gadoxetate (Eovist, Bayer HealthCare) is a gadolinium-based IV contrast agent that is taken up by hepatocytes and excreted into the bile ducts. Metastases replace hepatocytes in normal liver tissue, resulting in a focus of low signal on a background of a bright liver (**Fig. 14**). It should be noted that these imaging features are not unique to neuroendocrine tumors or even malignancies and so the specificity is limited. Nevertheless, gadoxetate-enhanced MRI has shown improved detection of metastases and focal liver lesions in general.[47,48] However, large-scale studies showing a benefit in the case of neuroendocrine metastases are lacking. Unlike diffusion-weighted imaging, which takes only a short amount of time in additional scanning, gadoxetate imaging requires using a different IV contrast agent, necessitating either a request by the ordering clinician or preference by the protocoling radiologist.

### Syndromes

There are four genetic syndromes associated with pancreatic neuroendocrine tumors: MEN1, Von Hippel-Lindau disease, tuberous sclerosis complex, and neurofibromatosis type I.[37,49] Imaging is indispensable for the numerous types of lesions throughout the body associated with these syndromes. However, these fall into different radiology subspecialties and so making the unifying diagnosis for multiple lesions may be difficult without the proper clinical context for the radiologist. Although the diagnosis may already be established, the provided history of one of these syndromes can also alter the differential diagnosis provided by the radiologist for a new lesion (**Fig. 15**).

MEN1 is the most closely associated genetic syndrome with pancreatic neuroendocrine tumors. Traditionally, most of these tumors have been thought to be hyperfunctioning, but there likely are many more occult nonhyperfunctioning tumors that go undetected.[37,50,51] It should be noted that MEN1 is not limited to only the three "P's" (pituitary, parathyroid, and pancreas) and other organs are frequently involved, potentially aiding in the diagnosis if not already made[52] (**Fig. 16**).

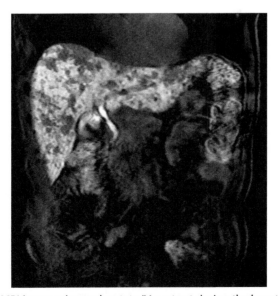

**Fig. 14.** Coronal MRI image using gadoxetate IV contrast during the hepatobiliary phase in a patient with metastatic pancreatic neuroendocrine cancer. Metastases lack hepatocytes and therefore appear hypointense. Note the normal excretion of contrast into the common bile duct.

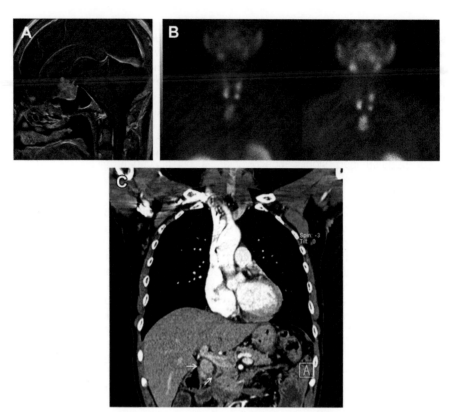

**Fig. 15.** Multiple endocrine neoplasia I. (*A*) Sagittal MRI brain postcontrast image showing a pituitary macroadenoma. (*B*) $^{99m}$Tc-Sestamibi scan showing multiple foci of retained tracer on delayed image (*right*), consistent with multiple parathyroid adenomas. (*C*) Coronal computed tomography image demonstrating a well-circumscribed tumor (*yellow arrow*) near the confluence of the common bile duct and pancreatic duct (*white arrow*). These three studies would fall into neuroradiology, nuclear medicine, and abdominal imaging subspecialties. When interpreted in the context of the other studies, the correct diagnosis is clear.

Unlike MEN1, pancreatic neuroendocrine tumors associated with Von Hippel-Lindau disease are not hyperfunctioning.[37,49,50] Instead, the diagnostic dilemma lies in the multitude of pancreatic lesions that may occur including lymphoepithelial cysts and serous microcystadenomas.[53] Fortunately, imaging features are often distinctive, allowing differentiation of neuroendocrine tumors from benign lesions that would require no additional management.

Tuberous sclerosis complex and neurofibromatosis type I are both phakomatoses that along with several other syndromes carry an increased risk of endocrine tumors, possibly from converging metabolic effects of the culprit genes.[54] Tumors can be both hyperfunctioning and nonhyperfunctioning.[37,49] Therefore, the appearance of a pancreatic lesion in a patient with tuberous sclerosis complex who otherwise is being screened for renal angiomyolipomas should raise suspicion for a neuroendocrine tumor (**Fig. 17**). Ampullary somatostatinomas are associated with neurofibromatosis type I, but this is not the only tumor in the differential diagnosis[37,49,55] (**Fig. 18**).

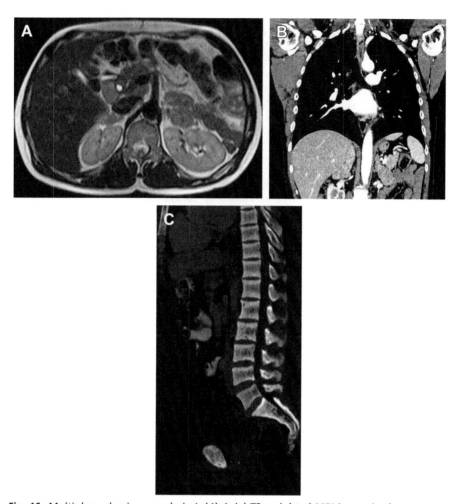

**Fig. 16.** Multiple endocrine neoplasia I. (*A*) Axial T2-weighted MRI image in the same patient from **Fig. 15** showing a hyperintense pancreatic head/duodenal tumor that proved to be a gastrinoma. (*B*) Computed tomography images show the patient had bilateral adrenal masses and (*C*) osseous changes from hyperparathyroidism.

## *Mimics*

Commonly referred to as splenules, accessory spleens are a common incidental finding on imaging, occurring in 16% of patients.[56] They are easily recognizable as small perisplenic masses with well-defined margins and identical imaging characteristics to the spleen.[57] The diagnosis becomes less obvious when splenic tissue lies within the adjacent pancreatic tail. With a rounded shape and different enhancement pattern compared to pancreatic parenchyma, this benign entity will simulate a hypervascular mass, such as a neuroendocrine tumor. This can lead to an unnecessary biopsy, which carries the risk of periprocedural complications and nondiagnostic samples (**Fig. 19**). The key is to consider this as a possibility in an incidentally detected pancreatic lesion without symptoms from hormone hypersecretion. Several imaging options can noninvasively aid in the diagnosis. Multiphasic CT or MRI scans

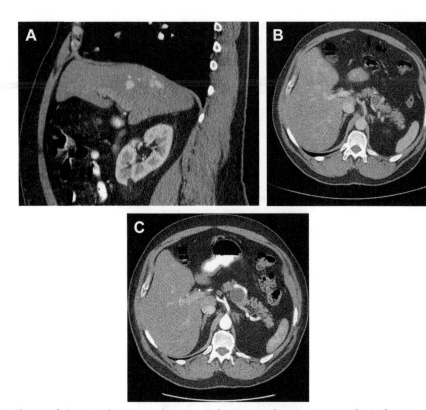

**Fig. 17.** (*A*) Sagittal computed tomography image showing an exophytic fat-containing lesion arising from the right kidney, consistent with an angiomyolipoma. (*B*,*C*) Axial images of the pancreas showing a cystic lesion that enlarged over the course of 2.5 years and required resection, proving to be a low-grade neuroendocrine tumor. The patient did not carry a history of tuberous sclerosis, but genetic testing has not been performed.

can show the lesion following the enhancement pattern of the spleen over time. Additionally, MRI can use diffusion-weighted sequences, which can detect restricted diffusion in normal lymphoid organs, such as the spleen and lymph nodes. It should be noted that this is by no means definitive of splenic tissue and malignancies can show the same feature. The most specific imaging test for splenic tissue is a [99m]Tc heat-damaged red blood cell nuclear medicine study, which relies on the physiologic action of the spleen in removing senescent red blood cells from the circulation. However, this is no longer widely available owing to pharmacy regulations. Instead, [99m]Tc sulfur-colloid scans detect uptake throughout the reticuloendothelial system (liver, spleen, and bone marrow), although resulting in less sensitivity and specificity[58] (**Fig. 20**).

Following the same principal as the case of an accessory spleen, recognizing an aneurysm or pseudoaneurysm requires noticing that a pancreatic hyperenhancing mass follows the same enhancement pattern as the aorta. The importance of distinguishing this entity cannot be understated, because a biopsy could have catastrophic results. Usually, multiphasic postcontrast imaging is not necessary if a communication with the arterial tree can be visualized. In cases when the lesion arises from a small branch of the pancreaticoduodenal arcade, homogenous enhancement and mural thrombus may be the most important features (**Fig. 21**).

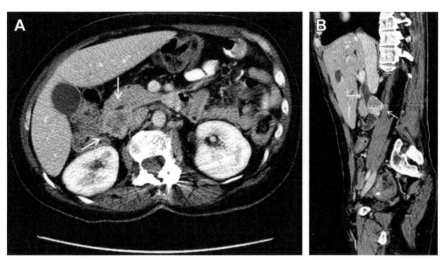

**Fig. 18.** Neurofibromatosis I (NF-1). (*A*) Axial and (*B*) sagittal computed tomography images in a patient with NF-1 showing a periampullary mass (*white arrow*) adjacent to the common bile duct (*yellow arrow*). The mass was resected and proved to be a gastrointestinal stromal tumor.

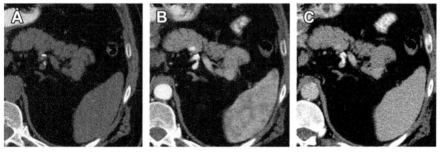

**Fig. 19.** Intrapancreatic accessory spleen. Enhancing pancreatic tail mass during the (*A*) non-contrast, (*B*) arterial, and (*C*) venous phases. The mass shows similar density in Hounsfield units to the spleen. Multiple biopsies were performed with endoscopic ultrasound guidance before the diagnosis could be made.

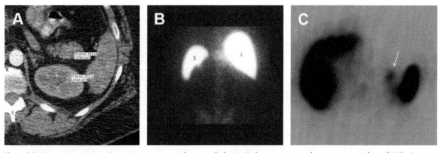

**Fig. 20.** Intrapancreatic accessory spleen. (*A*) Axial computed tomography (CT) image showing an arterially enhancing solid lesion in the pancreatic tail. (*B*) Posterior projection $^{99m}$Tc sulfur-colloid scan showing expected uptake in the liver (*L*), spleen (*S*), and bone marrow (*M*). (*C*) Axial single-photon emission CT image in the same patient showing a focus of tracer uptake in the expected location of the pancreatic lesion (*arrow*).

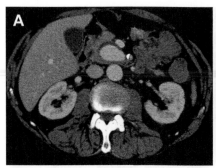
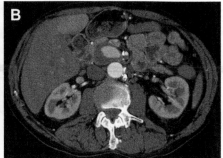

**Fig. 21.** Pancreatic pseudoaneurysm. (*A*) Single-phase axial computed tomography (CT) image in a patient more than one month after an episode of acute pancreatitis shows an enhancing lesion in the pancreatic head with a thick hypodense wall. No communication with the arterial tree could be demonstrated on this study or at angiography. (*B*) Follow-up CT angiography obtained nearly two weeks later showing increased mural thrombus, but different enhancement from the aorta.

The pancreas is not a common site of metastatic disease, but it is not exceedingly rare either. The most common primary tumors are renal cell carcinoma and lung cancer, which can present as hyperenhancing tumors that can easily have the same appearance as a neuroendocrine tumor[59] (**Fig. 22**). Knowledge of a coexisting renal mass or previous treatment for renal cell carcinoma is the key to making the differentiation, even in the case of patients with Von Hippel-Lindau disease, who are at increased risk for both tumors.

A rare tumor, solid pseudopapillary tumor (also known as solid pseudopapillary epithelial neoplasm) is another hypervascular pancreatic tumor. This lesion is most commonly seen in young females as a large pancreatic tumor, commonly with hemorrhage or cystic elements (**Fig. 23**). The diagnosis is not always possible before resection, but awareness of this entity in a young female with a hypervascular pancreatic mass is essential.

### Endocrine Insufficiency

Because insulin is made exclusively in the pancreas, repeated insults from entities such as chronic pancreatitis, cystic fibrosis, or pancreatic resection can predispose

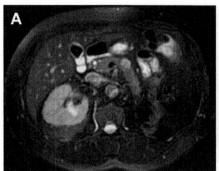
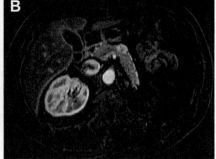

**Fig. 22.** Pancreatic metastasis. (*A*) Axial T2-weighted and (*B*) postcontrast arterial subtraction MRI images showing a discrete enhancing lesion in the pancreatic body in a patient with a history renal cell carcinoma (note absent left kidney).

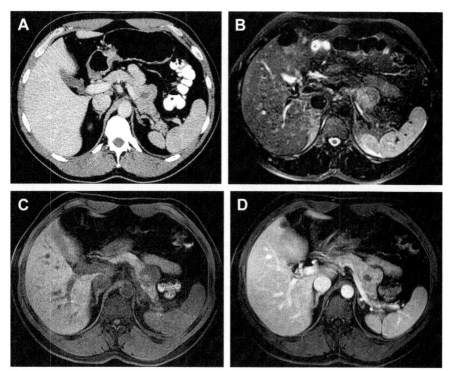

**Fig. 23.** Solid pseudopapillary tumor. (A) Axial computed tomography (CT) image showing a heterogeneously enhancing lesion in the pancreatic body/tail. (B) Axial T2-weighted MRI image showing the mass is hyperintense, but not fluid intensity. (C) Precontrast axial T1-weighted image showing a focus of high signal compatible with hemorrhage. (D) Postcontrast image showing similar enhancement pattern as demonstrated on CT.

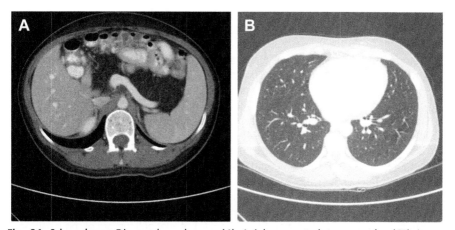

**Fig. 24.** Schwachman-Diamond syndrome. (A) Axial computed tomography (CT) image showing complete fatty replacement of the pancreas. Although the patient did have exocrine insufficiency, the patient had no history of diabetes or endocrine insufficiency. (B) CT image through the lung bases shows no evidence of bronchiectasis, as might be seen in a patient with cystic fibrosis.

a patient to the development of a unique form diabetes mellitus.[60] Pancreatic atrophy is a common finding on imaging, but is much better correlated with exocrine insufficiency[61,62] (**Fig. 24**). However, there is evidence of imaging signs such as pancreatic calcifications and distal pancreatectomy predicting the development of diabetes mellitus and abnormal pancreatic imaging has been proposed as a diagnostic criterion.[63,64] Unfortunately, the diagnosis of diabetes mellitus is simpler than identifying the etiology. Ultimately, imaging will never be the sole basis of the diagnosis, but may aid in recognizing patients at risk for developing diabetes mellitus, which could have substantial effects on their long-term outcomes.

## SUMMARY

Pancreatic neuroendocrine tumors are a diverse group of neoplasms with many different appearances clinically and at imaging that can range from an incidental finding to a correctable endocrine syndrome to an aggressive malignancy. Understanding the wide array of imaging modalities available to clinicians is important in both making the diagnosis and determining treatment. Imaging may also play a greater role in the future for the evaluation of endocrine insufficiency. Radiologists are available as consultants for many of these clinical questions, but referring clinicians are greatly empowered by understanding the essentials of pancreatic imaging.

## REFERENCES

1. Rösch T, Lorenz R, Braig C, et al. Endoscopic ultrasound in pancreatic tumor diagnosis. Gastrointest Endosc 1991;37(3):347–52.
2. Rösch T, Lightdale CJ, Botet JF, et al. Localization of pancreatic endocrine tumors by endoscopic ultrasonography. N Engl J Med 1992;326(26):1721–6.
3. Müller MF, Meyenberger C, Bertschinger P, et al. Pancreatic tumors: evaluation with endoscopic US, CT, and MR imaging. Radiology 1994;190(3):745–51.
4. Anderson MA, Carpenter S, Thompson NW, et al. Endoscopic ultrasound is highly accurate and directs management in patients with neuroendocrine tumors of the pancreas. Am J Gastroenterol 2000;95(9):2271–7.
5. Pais SA, Al-Haddad M, Mohamadnejad M, et al. EUS for pancreatic neuroendocrine tumors: a single-center, 11-year experience. Gastrointest Endosc 2010; 71(7):1185–93.
6. Sotoudehmanesh R, Hedayat A, Shirazian N, et al. Endoscopic ultrasonography (EUS) in the localization of insulinoma. Endocrine 2007;31(3):238–41.
7. Howard TJ, Stabile BE, Zinner MJ, et al. Anatomic distribution of pancreatic endocrine tumors. Am J Surg 1990;159(2):258–64.
8. Tan EH, Tan CH. Imaging of gastroenteropancreatic neuroendocrine tumors. World J Clin Oncol 2011;2(1):28–43.
9. Stafford-Johnson DB, Francis IR, Eckhauser FE, et al. Dual-phase helical CT of nonfunctioning islet cell tumors. J Comput Assist Tomogr 1998;22(2):335–9.
10. Van Hoe L, Gryspeerdt S, Marchal G, et al. Helical CT for the preoperative localization of islet cell tumors of the pancreas: value of arterial and parenchymal phase images. Am J Roentgenol 1995;165(6):1437–9.
11. Sheth S, Hruban RK, Fishman EK. Helical CT of islet cell tumors of the pancreas: typical and atypical manifestations. Am J Roentgenol 2002;179(3):725–30.
12. Ichikawa T, Peterson MS, Federle MP, et al. Islet cell tumor of the pancreas: biphasic CT versus MR imaging in tumor detection. Radiology 2000;216(1): 163–71.

13. Gouya H, Vignaux O, Augui J, et al. CT, endoscopic sonography, and a combined protocol for preoperative evaluation of pancreatic insulinomas. Am J Roentgenol 2003;181(4):987–92.

14. Horton KM, Hruban RH, Yeo C, et al. Multi-detector row CT of pancreatic islet cell tumors. Radiographics 2006;26(2):453–64.

15. Herwick S, Miller FH, Keppke AL. MRI of islet cell tumors of the pancreas. Am J Roentgenol 2006;187(5):W472–80.

16. Dewhurst CE, Mortele KJ. Cystic tumors of the pancreas: imaging and management. Radiol Clin 2012;50(3):467–86.

17. Rufini V, Calcagni ML, Baum RP. Imaging of neuroendocrine tumors. Semin Nucl Med 2006;36(3):228–47.

18. Cheema A, Weber J, Strosberg JR. Incidental detection of pancreatic neuroendocrine tumors: an analysis of incidence and outcomes. Ann Surg Oncol 2012; 19(9):2932–6.

19. Vagefi PA, Razo O, Deshpande V, et al. Evolving patterns in the detection and outcomes of pancreatic neuroendocrine neoplasms. Arch Surg 2007;142(4):347–54.

20. Kuo JH, Lee JA, Chabot JA. Nonfunctional pancreatic neuroendocrine tumors. Surg Clin North Am 2014;94(3):689–708.

21. Lawrence B, Gustafsson BI, Chan A, et al. The epidemiology of gastroenteropancreatic neuroendocrine tumors. Endocrinol Metab Clin North Am 2011; 40(1):1–18, vii.

22. Halfdanarson TR, Rabe KG, Rubin J, et al. Pancreatic neuroendocrine tumors (PNETs): incidence, prognosis and recent trend toward improved survival. Ann Oncol 2008;19(10):1727–33.

23. Classification, epidemiology, clinical presentation, localization, and staging of pancreatic neuroendocrine tumors (islet-cell tumors). Available at: http://www.uptodate.com/contents/classification-epidemiology-clinical-presentation-localization-and-staging-of-pancreatic-neuroendocrine-tumors-islet-cell-tumors. Accessed December 4, 2016.

24. Vortmeyer AO, Huang S, Lubensky I, et al. Non-Islet origin of pancreatic islet cell tumors. J Clin Endocrinol Metab 2004;89(4):1934–8.

25. Kimura W, Kuroda A, Morioka Y. Clinical pathology of endocrine tumors of the pancreas. Dig Dis Sci 1991;36(7):933–42.

26. Asa SL. Pancreatic endocrine tumors. Mod Pathol 2011;24(S2):S66–77.

27. Rindi G, Arnold R, Bosman FT, et al. WHO classification of tumours of the digestive system. 4th edition. Lyon: IARC Press; 2010.

28. Lewis RB, Lattin GE, Paal E. Pancreatic endocrine tumors: radiologic-clinicopathologic correlation. Radiographics 2010;30(6):1445–64.

29. Buetow PC, Miller DL, Parrino TV, et al. Islet cell tumors of the pancreas: clinical, radiologic, and pathologic correlation in diagnosis and localization. Radiographics 1997;17(2):453–72.

30. Le Bodic MF, Heymann MF, Lecomte M, et al. Immunohistochemical study of 100 pancreatic tumors in 28 patients with multiple endocrine neoplasia, type I. Am J Surg Pathol 1996;20(11):1378–84.

31. Heitz PU, Kasper M, Polak JM, et al. Pancreatic endocrine tumors. Hum Pathol 1982;13(3):263–71.

32. Halfdanarson TR, Rubin J, Farnell MB, et al. Pancreatic endocrine neoplasms: epidemiology and prognosis of pancreatic endocrine tumors. Endocr Relat Cancer 2008;15(2):409–27.

33. Öberg K, Eriksson B. Endocrine tumours of the pancreas. Best Pract Res Clin Gastroenterol 2005;19(5):753–81.

34. Reubi JC. Somatostatin and other peptide receptors as tools for tumor diagnosis and treatment. Neuroendocrinology 2004;80(Suppl 1):51–6.
35. Gibril F, Jensen RT. Diagnostic uses of radiolabelled somatostatin receptor analogues in gastroenteropancreatic endocrine tumours. Dig Liver Dis 2004; 36(Suppl 1):S106–20.
36. Stabile BE, Morrow DJ, Passaro E. The gastrinoma triangle: operative implications. Am J Surg 1984;147(1):25–31.
37. Jensen RT, Berna MJ, Bingham DB, et al. Inherited pancreatic endocrine tumor syndromes: advances in molecular pathogenesis, diagnosis, management and controversies. Cancer 2008;113(7 Suppl):1807–43.
38. Mansour JC, Chen H. Pancreatic endocrine tumors. J Surg Res 2004;120(1): 139–61.
39. Buetow PC, Parrino TV, Buck JL, et al. Islet cell tumors of the pancreas: pathologic-imaging correlation among size, necrosis and cysts, calcification, malignant behavior, and functional status. Am J Roentgenol 1995;165(5):1175–9.
40. Noone TC, Hosey J, Firat Z, et al. Imaging and localization of islet-cell tumours of the pancreas on CT and MRI. Best Pract Res Clin Endocrinol Metab 2005;19(2): 195–211.
41. Boninsegna L, Partelli S, D'Innocenzio MM, et al. Pancreatic cystic endocrine tumors: a different morphological entity associated with a less aggressive behavior. Neuroendocrinology 2010;92(4):246–51.
42. Elias D, Lefevre JH, Duvillard P, et al. Hepatic metastases from neuroendocrine tumors with a "thin slice" pathological examination: they are many more than you think. Ann Surg 2010;251(2):307–10.
43. Dromain C, de Baere T, Lumbroso J, et al. Detection of liver metastases from endocrine tumors: a prospective comparison of somatostatin receptor scintigraphy, computed tomography, and magnetic resonance imaging. J Clin Oncol 2005;23(1):70–8.
44. Paulson EK, McDermott VG, Keogan MT, et al. Carcinoid metastases to the liver: role of triple-phase helical CT. Radiology 1998;206(1):143–50.
45. Dromain C, de Baere T, Baudin E, et al. MR imaging of hepatic metastases caused by neuroendocrine tumors: comparing four techniques. Am J Roentgenol 2003;180(1):121–8.
46. d'Assignies G, Fina P, Bruno O, et al. High sensitivity of diffusion-weighted MR imaging for the detection of liver metastases from neuroendocrine tumors: comparison with T2-weighted and dynamic gadolinium-enhanced MR imaging. Radiology 2013;268(2):390–9.
47. Huppertz A, Balzer T, Blakeborough A, et al. Improved detection of focal liver lesions at MR imaging: multicenter comparison of gadoxetic acid-enhanced MR images with intraoperative findings. Radiology 2004;230(1):266–75.
48. Chen L, Zhang J, Zhang L, et al. Meta-analysis of gadoxetic acid disodium (Gd-EOB-DTPA)-enhanced magnetic resonance imaging for the detection of liver metastases. PLoS One 2012;7(11):e48681.
49. Philips S, Shah SN, Vikram R, et al. Pancreatic endocrine neoplasms: a current update on genetics and imaging. Br J Radiol 2012;85(1014):682–96.
50. Jensen RT. Pancreatic endocrine tumors: recent advances. Ann Oncol 1999; 10(Suppl 4):S170–6.
51. Thomas-Marques L, Murat A, Delemer B, et al. Prospective endoscopic ultrasonographic evaluation of the frequency of nonfunctioning pancreaticoduodenal endocrine tumors in patients with multiple endocrine neoplasia type 1. Am J Gastroenterol 2006;101(2):266–73.

52. Scarsbrook AF, Thakker RV, Wass JAH, et al. Multiple endocrine neoplasia: spectrum of radiologic appearances and discussion of a multitechnique imaging approach. Radiographics 2006;26(2):433–51.
53. Leung RS, Biswas SV, Duncan M, et al. Imaging features of von Hippel–Lindau disease. Radiographics 2008;28(1):65–79.
54. Lodish MB, Stratakis CA. Endocrine tumours in neurofibromatosis type 1, tuberous sclerosis and related syndromes. Best Pract Res Clin Endocrinol Metab 2010;24(3):439–49.
55. Hoffmann KM, Furukawa M, Jensen RT. Duodenal neuroendocrine tumors: classification, functional syndromes, diagnosis and medical treatment. Best Pract Res Clin Gastroenterol 2005;19(5):675–97.
56. Mortelé KJ, Mortelé B, Silverman SG. CT features of the accessory spleen. Am J Roentgenol 2004;183(6):1653–7.
57. Hayward I, Mindelzun RE, Jeffrey RB. Intrapancreatic accessory spleen mimicking pancreatic mass on CT. J Comput Assist Tomogr 1992;16(6):984–5.
58. MacDonald A, Burrell S. Infrequently performed studies in nuclear medicine: part 1. J Nucl Med Technol 2008;36(3):132–43.
59. Klein KA, Stephens DH, Welch TJ. CT characteristics of metastatic disease of the pancreas. Radiographics 1998;18(2):369–78.
60. Gudipaty L, Rickels MR. Pancreatogenic (Type 3c) diabetes. Pancreapedia: Exocrine Pancreas Knowledge Base. 2015. http://dx.doi.org/10.3998/panc. 2015.35.
61. Domínguez-Muñoz JE, Alvarez-Castro A, Lariño-Noia J, et al. Endoscopic ultrasonography of the pancreas as an indirect method to predict pancreatic exocrine insufficiency in patients with chronic pancreatitis. Pancreas 2012;41(5):724–8.
62. Schneider ARJ, Hammerstingl R, Heller M, et al. Does secretin-stimulated MRCP predict exocrine pancreatic insufficiency? A comparison with noninvasive exocrine pancreatic function tests. J Clin Gastroenterol 2006;40(9):851–5.
63. Malka D, Hammel P, Sauvanet A, et al. Risk factors for diabetes mellitus in chronic pancreatitis. Gastroenterology 2000;119(5):1324–32.
64. Ewald N, Bretzel RG. Diabetes mellitus secondary to pancreatic diseases (Type 3c)–are we neglecting an important disease? Eur J Intern Med 2013;24(3):203–6.

# Selected Controversies of Radioiodine Imaging and Therapy in Differentiated Thyroid Cancer

Douglas Van Nostrand, MD

## KEYWORDS

- Thyroid cancer • Radioiodine scanning • I-131 • Remnant ablation
- I-131 adjuvant treatment • Radioiodine refractory disease

## KEY POINTS

- Radioiodine isotopes of iodine-123 and iodine-131 (I-131) remain valuable diagnostic staging tools, and I-131 remains a valuable therapy for differentiated thyroid cancer.
- Properly performed radioiodine scans are valuable diagnostic staging tools.
- Before patients are considered radioiodine refractory, which thereby eliminates an I-131 treatment that may be potentially beneficial to patients, the physician must confirm patients are truly radioiodine refractory; the classification of radioiodine refractory is rapidly changing with new research developments.
- The classification of differentiated thyroid cancer as radioiodine refractory warrants reassessment and reclassification.

## INTRODUCTION

Radioiodine is important in the diagnostic and therapeutic armamentarium of differentiated thyroid cancer (DTC); however, many controversies persist. This article addresses some of these controversies, namely, the utility of pretherapy staging radioiodine scans; the prescribed activity for iodine-131 (I-131) remnant ablation, adjuvant treatment, and distant metastases; preparation with thyroid hormone withdrawal (THW) versus recombinant human thyroid-stimulating hormone (rhTSH); and the classification of radioiodine refractory DTC. Discussion of these controversies requires definitions of selected terms in the first section.

Disclosure statement: Dr D. Van Nostrand is a speaker and advisor for Genzyme and Jubilant Draximage. This article was funded by donations from grateful patients.
Nuclear Medicine Research, Division of Nuclear Medicine, MedStar Health Research Institute, MedStar Washington Hospital Center, Georgetown University School of Medicine, Suite GA60F, 110 Irving Street, Northwest, Washington, DC 20010, USA
E-mail addresses: douglas.van.nostrand@medstar.net; douglasvannostrand@gmail.com

## TERMINOLOGY

*Remnant ablation* is the use of I-131 to destroy normal thyroid tissue with the objective of improving serum thyroglobulin (Tg) levels to be a better tumor marker. Additional secondary objectives of *remnant ablation* are potentially to improve the quality of future radioiodine imaging studies and/or therapies. As defined by the American Thyroid Association's (ATA) guidelines from 2009 and 2015, remnant ablation does not have any objectives to reduce recurrences or to increase survival or progression-free survival.[1,2] *Adjuvant treatment* is the use of I-131 to treat suspected but unproven residual DTC with the objective of reducing recurrence, increasing survival, or increasing progression-free survival. *Treatment* is the use of I-131 to treat known residual locoregional disease and/or distant metastases having goals such as progression-free survival, overall survival, or even cure. *Therapy* is the generic use of I-131 for remnant ablation, adjuvant treatment, or treatment of known locoregional or distant metastases. These definitions are different from the 2015 guidelines from the ATA in the use of the words *treatment* and *therapy*,[1,2] but this author submits that the usage of these terms herein is more consistent with the usage of the terms in oncology of *chemotherapy* and *chemo treatment* and the terms in radiation therapy for *radiation therapy* and *radiation treatment*.

Two additional terms, *dose* and *dosage*, require distinction and definition herein. The term *dose* is frequently used with competing and, therefore, confusing definitions. In the specialty of nuclear medicine and radiation therapy, *dose* refers to absorbed dose of radiation to an organ or tumor. This value is measured in *radiation absorbed dose* (rad) or gray. Unfortunately, some individuals use the term *dose* to mean the amount of prescribed activity of I-131 administered to a patient. We measure such amounts in millicuries or megabecquerels (MBq). Millicurie and becquerel are not interchangeable with rad or gray, respectively. Although the amount of millicuries or becquerels administered will be a factor that affects how many rad or grays are delivered to normal tissue or a tumor, there are many other factors that affect the absorbed dose, such as I-131 uptake, dose rate, and residence time. As alternatives to using the same word to mean to 2 different measurements, the term *dosage* is frequently used to indicate prescribed activity administered. An additional alternative is using the term *prescribed activity* itself.

## UTILITY OF RADIOIODINE SCANS

The utility of radioiodine scans remains one of the more frequently debated controversies. However, in order to better understand the arguments for and against radioiodine scanning, radioiodine scanning must be subdivided; this author proposes the following subdivisions (1) pre–I-131 therapy staging scans performed after patients' first surgery, (2) post-therapy scans performed 3 to 10 days after an I-131 therapy, (3) follow-up surveillance/baseline scans performed 6 to 18 months after the initial I-131 therapy, and (4) restaging scans performed when recurrence and/or progression of DTC is suspected.

### Postoperative Pretherapy (Iodine-131) Staging Scans

In regard to postoperative pretherapy (I-131) staging scans, **Table 1** (column 1) lists many of the arguments presented against performing these scans, with the counter arguments in **Table 1** (column 2). However, with the development of single-photon emission computed tomography (SPECT) imaging, the literature overwhelmingly supports the utility of such scans (**Table 2**).[3–17] **Table 3** shows the ATA's 2015 guidelines. This author thinks that one of the reasons that there is such widespread difference of

**Table 1**
**Arguments against the utility of pretherapy staging scans**

| Arguments Against the Performance of Pretherapy Staging Scan | Counter Arguments |
|---|---|
| • Everything I need to know, I learn on the post-therapy scan. | • The literature demonstrates that significant findings are frequently found on the pretherapy staging scan that alters management before any I-131 therapy.[18] |
| • It is expensive. | • It is less than the cost of 2 serum Tg and Tg antibody levels. And<br>• It is less than the cost of 2 ultrasounds in the United States. |
| • It is inconvenient. | • This author thinks that the potential benefits and information warrants the inconveniences. |
| • It may cause stunning. | • Use I-123. Or<br>• Use a lower the prescribed activity of I-131 of 1–2 mCi. |
| • There is unnecessary radiation exposure. | • There is reasonable radiation exposure for the information obtained. And<br>• There is inconsequential radiation exposure if I-131 is to be administered for a therapy. |
| • There is no evidence-based literature. | • See **Table 4**. |

**Table 2**
**Evidence-based literature supporting utility of single-photon emission computed tomography–computed tomography radioiodine scans[a]**

| Author | Altered Staging, Indeterminate, Management, and/or Outcomes (%) |
|---|---|
| Aide et al,[3] 2009 | 22 |
| Barwick et al,[4] 2010 | 42 |
| Ciappuccini et al,[5] 2011 | Sole prognostic variable |
| Geerlings et al,[6] 2010 | 27 |
| Grewal et al,[7] 2010 | 20 |
| Kohlfuerst et al,[8] 2009 | 36 |
| Maruoka et al,[9] 2012 | 22 |
| Mustafa et al,[10] 2010 | 25 |
| Ruf et al,[11] 2004 | 25 |
| Schmidt et al,[12] 2009 | 35 |
| Spanu et al,[13] 2009 | 36 |
| Tharp et al,[14] 2004 | 41 |
| Wang et al,[15] 2009 | 23 |
| Yamamato et al,[16] 2003 | 88 |
| Avram et al,[17] 2015 | 29 |

[a] Some of these studies are a combination of pretherapy staging and post-therapy SPECT-CT scans.

| | | |
|---|---|---|
| **Table 3** | | |
| **2015 ATA guidelines for post-operative pretherapy (iodine-131) staging scans** | | |
| American Thyroid Association[1] | "Post-operative diagnostic radioiodine whole-body scans may be useful when the extent of the thyroid remnant or residual disease cannot be accurately ascertained from the surgical report or neck ultrasonography, and when the results may alter the decision to treat, or the activity of RAI that is to be administered. Identification and localization of uptake foci may be enhanced by concomitant SPECT/CT. When performed, pretherapy diagnostic scans should utilize 123I (1.5–3 mCi) or a low activity of 131I (1–3 mCi), with the therapeutic activity optimally administered within 72 h of the diagnostic activity" | Weak recommendation, low-quality evidence |

opinion vis-à-vis the utility of radioiodine scans stems from the technique used. As with ultrasound, not all practitioners perform radioiodine scans equally well. However, a discussion of the techniques that maximize the information from radioiodine scans is beyond the scope of this article, but further reading is available.[18]

### Post-Therapy (Iodine-131) Scans

The literature again overwhelming supports the utility of post–I-131 therapy scans, and there is little to no controversy apropos the performance of these scans.[19–25] The utility of post–I-131 therapy scans is a result of the higher therapeutic prescribed activity of I-131 administered, which in turn allows delayed imaging with better clearance of patients' background activity relative to the clearance of patients' normal tissue or sites of metastases. This delayed imaging in turn increases the contrast of the normal tissue or metastases relative to background. The ATA's 2015 guidelines recommend the following: "A posttherapy WBS (whole body scan) (with or without SPECT/CT). . . after RAI (radioactive iodine) remnant ablation or treatment, to inform disease staging and document the RAI avidity of any structural disease (Recommendation 58)."[2]

### Surveillance/Baseline Scans

Presently, the ATA's 2015 guidelines state,

*After the first post-treatment WBS performed following RAI remnant ablation or adjuvant therapy, low-risk and intermediate-risk patients with an undetectable Tg (thyroglobulin) on thyroid hormone with negative anti-Tg antibodies and a negative US (ultrasound) do not require routine diagnostic WBS during follow-up (Recommendation 66).[2]*

If the objective of this scan is to screen (surveillance) for metastatic disease, then this author agrees with this statement. However, if any I-131 therapy has been performed, then this author recommends that a scan be performed at 6 to 18 months to establish a new baseline scan for future comparison. The logic here is that should a patient subsequently develop an elevated serum Tg level or a rapidly increasing serum Tg level, one will typically perform multiple additional studies to localize the source of the elevated and/or increasing Tg level, and one of these studies would most likely be a radioiodine scan. If this scan shows a focus of uptake in the thyroid bed, then a comparison of that scan with a prior follow-up baseline scan may help determine whether that focus of uptake represents persistent thyroid tissue that was not completely ablated or a metastasis. A radioiodine scan at 6 to 18 months is a reasonable and inexpensive scan to perform to establish a new baseline after any previous I-131 therapy. Although data are not presently published documenting the utility of these baseline scans, this author submits that this is a reasonable empirical approach until such data are published clarifying the outcomes of a baseline scan in various patient populations.

### Restaging Scans

A restaging radioiodine scan is a reasonable diagnostic study to perform in those patients suspected of local recurrence or distant metastases in whom I-131 therapy may be a potential therapeutic option.

## PRESCRIBED ACTIVITY FOR REMNANT ABLATION, ADJUVANT TREATMENT, AND DISTANT METASTASES

The amount of prescribed activity of I-131 for remnant ablation as defined earlier has been decreasing, and presently 30 to 50 mCi is recommended.[2] The ATA's guidelines state,

> If RAI remnant ablation is performed after total thyroidectomy for ATA low-risk thyroid cancer or intermediate-risk disease with lower risk features (ie, low volume central neck nodal metastases with no other known gross residual disease or any other adverse features), a low administered activity of approximately of 30 mCi is generally favored over higher administered activities (Recommendation 55).[2]

However, it bears emphasis that remnant ablation does not presuppose an objective of reducing recurrence or increasing progression-free survival or overall survival. These objectives are for I-131 adjuvant treatment of suspected but unproven residual locoregional disease or I-131 treatment of known locoregional or distant metastases.

The spectrum of the amount of prescribed activity of I-131 for adjuvant treatment with the aforementioned objectives remains controversial, ranging from 30 to 150 mCi.[26] However, in our frequent pursuit of "less is more,"[27] Ross McDougall has quoted the first Roman emperor, Augustus Caesar, who stated "festina lente" (hurry slowly), which may be excellent advice.[28] An evaluation of Castagna and colleagues'[29] valuable article provides an example of hurrying slowly. These investigators published a peer-reviewed study evaluating the effectiveness of 30 mCi versus ≥100 mCi of I-131 for the treatment of DTC with end points of remission, biochemical disease, metastatic disease after first initial therapy and for remission, recurrent disease, persistent disease, and death for final outcome. **Table 4** tabulates a distillation

| Table 4<br>Festina lente | | | |
|---|---|---|---|
| **Recurrent Disease, Biochemical Disease,<br>Metastasis, Persistent Disease, or Death** | **30 mCi** | **100 mCi** | **P** |
| All patients | 40.0% (20) | 40.0% (39) | NS |
| T3N0-X | 25.6% | 27.8% | NS |
| T1-2N1 and T1-2N0 | 47.4% | 40.0% | NS |

*Abbreviation:* NS, not significant.

of some of the data from their article. Although a full discussion of this article is outside the scope of this article, the article concluded, "Our study provides the first evidence that in DTC patients at intermediate risk, high RAI activities [≥100 mCi] at ablation have no major advantage over low activities [30 mCi]."[29] The author would submit that this is an acceptable statement by the investigators from their data. However, a problem emerges when other individuals conclude from this statement that "[30 mCi] is equally effective as 100 mCi" in the treatment of intermediate-risk patients with DTC. If an individual does conclude such, then that individual may in fact be making a less-is-more mistake and demonstrating a bias toward *less is more*. Instead, with the percentages reported in **Table 4** for the various categories, why could not one have concluded that 100 mCi is equally as *ineffective* as 30 mCi in the treatment of intermediate-risk patients with DTC and that in fact one needs to administer higher prescribed activity of I-131. This author submits that our rush to *less is more* needs to be tempered by festina lente; as previously noted, fallacious reasoning is one of the major reasons calling for festina lente in medicine.[28]

For the amount of prescribed activity for I-131 treatment of known locoregional or distant metastases, the controversy frequently revolves around empirically versus dosimetrically guided prescribed activity. The most frequent argument submitted in favor of empirically prescribed activities is that until outcome data are published demonstrating that dosimetrically guided prescribed activities result in better outcomes, one should administer empirically prescribed activity. On further analysis, however, this argument is not only specious but also is not based in any fundamentals of radiation therapy. First, if one argues for using empirically prescribed activity until dosimetrically guided prescribed activity has better outcomes, then how does one select between the various empirically prescribed activities that represent the preference of one individual or the policy of an institution for treating locoregional or distant metastases. Based on the original argument, one would have to have outcome data regarding which empirical approach had the best outcomes before one selected any empirical approach. Second, there is a retrospective study from Klubo-Gwiezdzinska and colleagues[30] that reports better outcomes for locoregional disease with dosimetrically guided prescribed activity than empirically prescribed activity for lymph node metastases. Third, as already noted, empirically prescribed activities have their origins based either on physician preference or institutional preference for prescribed activity for treating known locoregional disease or distant metastases. It is not based on either one of the two fundamentals of radiation therapy to deliver enough absorbed dose to the tumor to achieve the planned objective (eg, cure, progression-free survival, palliation, and so forth) and to minimize the absorbed dose to normal tissues. Empirical approaches are not based on either one of these; they are based on empiricism. Dosimetrically guided prescribed activities are based on at least one of these two fundamentals, and this author submits that until data demonstrate that empirically prescribed activities are equal or superior to dosimetrically guided prescribed activities, the latter should be the preferred method. Finally, a frequent argument against dosimetry-guided prescribed activity is the process itself. Dosimetry takes time; the number of facilities performing dosimetry is limited; third-party payers do not adequately compensate it. The third reason may be one of the most covert reasons for not using dosimetrically guided prescribed activities. However, simplified dosimetric methods have been published by Van Nostrand and colleagues,[31] Hanscheid and colleagues,[32] and Jentzen and colleagues,[33]; these can be performed by almost any nuclear medicine facility. Whether the practitioner selects an empirically or dosimetrically guided prescribed activity of I-131 for treatment of known locoregional disease or distant metastases, this author thinks it is important and appropriate for patients to be knowledgeable regarding the benefits and risks of the options for determining their prescribed activity as well as the locations where patients may obtain the dosimetrically guided prescribed activity.

## THYROID HORMONE WITHDRAWAL VERSUS RECOMBINANT HUMAN THYROID-STIMULATING HORMONE

For diagnostic radioiodine (eg, I-123, I-131) imaging or I-131 therapy, patients must be prepared with either THW or injections of rhTSH to stimulate normal thyroid tissue and/or functioning DTC to take up the administered radioiodine. The recommendations for the method of THW, the injections of rhTSH, and the subsequent protocols for radioiodine imaging or therapies are beyond the scope of this section; however, this section discusses the indications for the use of THW or rhTSH in low-, intermediate-, and high-risk patients.

The *New England Journal of Medicine* published the important publications of Schlumberger and colleagues[34] and Mallick and colleagues[35] together; both were prospective, noninferiority studies demonstrating that there was no statistical difference in the success of I-131 remnant ablation when patients were prepared with THW versus rhTSH. Subsequently, the US Food and Drug Administration (FDA) approved and expanded the use of rhTSH (Thyrogen®); the 2015 guidelines from the ATA stated in Recommendation 54 that "in patients with ATA low-risk and ATA intermediate-risk DTC without extensive lymph node involvement (ie, T1–T3, N0/Nx/N1a, M0), in whom RAI remnant ablation or adjuvant therapy is planned, preparation with rhTSH stimulation is an acceptable alternative to thyroid hormone withdrawal for achieving remnant ablation...."[2] "In patients with ATA intermediate-risk DTC who have extensive lymph node disease (multiple clinically involved LN) in the absence of distant metastases, preparation with rhTSH stimulation may be considered as an alternative to thyroid hormone withdrawal prior to adjuvant RAI treatment."[2]

A frequent controversy is the use of THW versus rhTSH in patients with ATA high-risk disease or distant metastases. Currently, rhTSH (Thyrogen®) is not approved by the FDA for preparation of I-131 for treatment of distant metastases. The ATA's 2015 guidelines suggest that additional controlled studies with long-term outcome are warranted. However, and until those studies are published, physicians and patients must still make a decision. In those patients whose comorbidities make THW an unacceptable option, preparation with rhTSH is a reasonable alternative. The ATA's 2015 guidelines give examples of significant comorbidities that may exclude THW, and these include "(a) a significant medical or psychiatric condition that could be acutely exacerbated with hypothyroidism, leading to a serious adverse event, or (b) inability to mount an adequate endogenous TSH response with thyroid hormone withdrawal."[2] In those patients for whom THW is an option, this author submits that practitioners should offer both options to patients with as little bias as possible of the benefits, risks, and limited availability of comparison data of the two options. It has been this author's experience that most such patients will decide based on their priorities rather than their doctors' priorities or bias.

## RADIOIODINE REFRACTORY DISEASE

The ATA's recent 2015 guidelines included recommendations regarding radioiodine refractory disease. Recommendation 91 states, "When a patient with DTC is classified as refractory to radioiodine, there is no indication for further treatment."[2] This author would submit that there will be little disagreement with this recommendation. However, the problem is as follows: When is a patient classified as radioiodine refractory?

The ATA's 2015 guidelines have 4 criteria. The first criterion asserts, "[T]he malignant/metastatic tissue does not ever concentrate radioiodine (no uptake outside the thyroid bed at the first therapeutic WBS)."[2] Now, if a patient with either postoperative pretherapy staging scan and/or post-therapy scan that has no uptake outside the thyroid bed subsequently develops a lesion 2 years later on CT strongly suggestive of a bone metastases and confirmed histologically, then is that DTC bone metastases to be considered radioiodine refractory because it did not show up on the *first* therapeutic WBS 2 years earlier? Perhaps the metastases were too small to see or occurred after the first pretherapy staging scan and/or post-therapy scan. Patients should not be considered radioiodine refractory based on no uptake outside the thyroid bed seen on the first therapeutic WBS. Furthermore, especially with the development of redifferentiation agents, such as selumetinib, absence of uptake on a post-therapy scan may not indicate radioiodine refractory disease.[36]

The second ATA criterion states, "The tumor tissue loses the ability to concentrate RAI after previous evidence of RAI-avid disease (in the absence of stable iodine contamination)."[2] Is this on a diagnostic or therapeutic scan? If it was seen earlier on a diagnostic scan but is now not seen on the diagnostic scan, then that patient should not necessarily be classified as radioiodine refractory. Admittedly, the likelihood that the patient has radioiodine refractory disease increases, but that is not prima facie evidence that the patient is radioiodine refractory. A tabulation of the literature shows that 20% to 64% of patients may have a positive post–I-131 therapy scan after a treatment of I-131 despite the diagnostic scan being negative (eg, "a blind treatment").[37] However, by classifying that patient as having radioiodine refractory disease, one is inappropriately eliminating a potential therapeutic option for a patient who is running out of options. Again, approval of redifferentiation agents, such as selumetinib, would also alter this criterion.

The third ATA criterion is the following: "Radioiodine is concentrated in some lesions but not in others."[2] By this criterion, if a patient has 3 bone lesions, and 2 bone lesions have radioiodine uptake but one lesion does not, then this patient is classified as radioiodine refractory and I-131 is not an option. This author would submit that this patient is not necessarily radioiodine refractory; one could treat the nonfunctioning bone metastases with radiofrequency ablation, cryotherapy, embolization, external radiation therapy, and so forth and then treat the other two lesions with I-131.

The fourth ATA criterion asserts, "Metastatic disease progresses despite significant concentration of radioiodine."[2] This assertion is problematic from 2 standpoints. First, if patients have progressive disease after I-131 therapies of 100 mCi prescribed activity every 3 or 6 months, then that could be a result of insufficient prescribed activity of I-131 for each administration and not a result of refractory disease. Second, if metastatic disease progresses despite significant concentration of radioiodine but the patients' metastases responded for a significant period (eg, 12 months) after the last I-131 therapy, then why are those patients' diseases considered radioiodine refractory? Rather, one should consider another therapeutic administration of I-131. Progression after a single therapy of I-131 should not necessarily be considered a failure without consideration of whether or not there was a response, the significance of that response, and the duration of that response. One does not give a single dose of a tyrosine kinase inhibitor (TKI) but rather gives daily doses of TKIs. If progression-free survival with lenvatinib of 12 months may be considered a positive response, then why would not progression-free survival after a therapy of I-131 of 12 months be considered a positive response and warrant consideration of another therapy with I-131?

These criteria are presently the 4 criteria in the ATA's 2015 guidelines. Although this author applauds the efforts of those who first classified radioiodine refractory disease, it is time to reassess these classifications.

## SUMMARY

Radioiodine isotopes of I-123 and I-131 remain valuable diagnostic staging tools, and I-131 remains a valuable therapy for differentiated thyroid cancer. In our discussion of radioiodine theragnostics (ie, therapy and diagnosis using radioiodine), it is important to define the terms and clarify the objectives of I-131 remnant ablation, adjuvant treatment, treatment, and therapy as well as to use the terms *dose*, *dosage*, *rad*, *gray*, and prescribed activity to articulate our intended message accurately.

Properly performed radioiodine scans are valuable diagnostic staging tools when performed before first-time I-131 therapy, 3 to 10 days after all I-131 therapies, approximately 12 months after any I-131 therapy to establish a new baseline scan, and when used to restage patients with evidence of progressing disease for which I-131 therapy is a potential option.

The amount of prescribed activities for remnant ablation, adjuvant treatment, and treatment of distant metastases will remain controversial; but this author favors lower prescribed activities (eg, 30–50 mCi) for remnant ablation, 100 to 150 mCi for adjuvant treatment, and full or simplified dosimetrically guided prescribed activity for I-131 treatment of known locoregional or distant metastases.

Before patients are considered radioiodine refractory, which thereby eliminates an I-131 treatment that is potentially beneficial to patients, the physician must confirm patients are truly radioiodine refractory; the classification of radioiodine refractory is rapidly changing with new research developments. The classification of DTC as radioiodine refractory warrants reassessment and reclassification.

## ACKNOWLEDGMENTS

I would like to thank Dr Di Wu for clerical and technical assistance.

## REFERENCES

1. Cooper DS, Doherty GM, Haugen BR, et al. Revised American Thyroid Association management guidelines for patients with thyroid nodules and differentiated thyroid cancer. Thyroid 2009;19:1167–214.
2. Haugen BR, Alexander EK, Bible KC, et al. 2015 American Thyroid Association management guidelines for adult patients with thyroid nodules and differentiated thyroid cancer: the American Thyroid Association Guidelines Task Force on Thyroid Nodules and Differentiated Thyroid Cancer. Thyroid 2016; 26:1–133.
3. Aide N, Heutte N, Rame JP, et al. Clinical relevance of single-photon emission computed tomography/computed tomography of the neck and thorax in postablation (131) I scintigraphy for thyroid cancer. J Clin Endocrinol Metab 2009; 94:2075–84.
4. Barwick T, Murray I, Megadmi H, et al. Single photon emission computed tomography (SPECT)/computed tomography using iodine-123 in patients with differentiated thyroid cancer: additional value over whole body planar imaging and SPECT. Eur J Endocrinol 2010;162:1131–9.
5. Ciappuccini R, Heutte N, Trzepla G, et al. Postablation (131) I scintigraphy with neck and thorax SPECT-CT and stimulated serum thyroglobulin level predict the

outcome of patients with differentiated thyroid cancer. Eur J Endocrinol 2011;164: 961–9.

6. Geerlings JA, van Zuijlen A, Lohmann EM, et al. The value of I-131 SPECT in the detection of recurrent differentiated thyroid cancer. Nucl Med Commun 2010;31: 417–22.

7. Grewal RK, Tuttle RM, Fox J, et al. The effect of posttherapy 131I SPECT/CT on risk classification and management of patients with differentiated thyroid cancer. J Nucl Med 2010;51:1361–7.

8. Kohlfuerst S, Igerc I, Lobnig M, et al. Posttherapeutic (131) I SPECT-CT offers high diagnostic accuracy when the findings on conventional planar imaging are inconclusive and allows a tailored patient treatment regimen. Eur J Nucl Med Mol Imaging 2009;36:886–93.

9. Maruoka Y, Abe K, Baba S, et al. Incremental diagnostic value of SPECT/CT with 131I scintigraphy after radioiodine therapy in patients with well-differentiated thyroid carcinoma. Radiology 2012;265:902–9.

10. Mustafa M, Kuwert T, Weber K, et al. Regional lymph node involvement in T1 papillary thyroid carcinoma: a bicentric prospective SPECT/CT study. Eur J Nucl Med Mol Imaging 2010;37:1462–6.

11. Ruf J, Lehmkuhl L, Bertram H, et al. Impact of SPECT and integrated low-dose CT after radioiodine therapy on the management of patients with thyroid carcinoma. Nucl Med Commun 2004;25:1177–82.

12. Schmidt D, Szikszai A, Linke R, et al. Impact of 131I SPECT/spiral CT on nodal staging of differentiated thyroid carcinoma at the first radioablation. J Nucl Med 2009;50:18–23.

13. Spanu A, Solinas ME, Chessa F, et al. 131I SPECT/CT in the follow-up of differentiated thyroid carcinoma: incremental value versus planar imaging. J Nucl Med 2009;50:184–90.

14. Tharp K, Israel O, Hausmann J, et al. Impact of 131I-SPECT/CT images obtained with an integrated system in the follow-up of patients with thyroid carcinoma. Eur J Nucl Med Mol Imaging 2004;31:1435–42.

15. Wang H, Fu HL, Li JN, et al. The role of single-photon emission computed tomography/computed tomography for precise localization of metastases in patients with differentiated thyroid cancer. Clin Imaging 2009;33:49–54.

16. Yamamoto Y, Nishiyama Y, Monden T, et al. Clinical usefulness of fusion of 131I SPECT and CT images in patients with differentiated thyroid carcinoma. J Nucl Med 2003;44:1905–10.

17. Avram AM, Esfandiari NH, Wong KK. Preablation 131-I scans with SPECT/CT contribute to thyroid cancer risk stratification and 131-I therapy planning. J Clin Endocrinol Metab 2015;100:1895–902.

18. Van Nostrand D. To perform or not to perform radioiodine scans prior to 131I remnant ablation? PRO. In: Wartofsky L, Van Nostrand D, editors. Thyroid cancer: a comprehensive guide to clinical management. New York: Springer New York; 2016. p. 245–54.

19. Nemec J, Rohling S, Zamrazil V, et al. Comparison of the distribution of diagnostic and thyroablative I-131 in the evaluation of differentiated thyroid cancers. J Nucl Med 1979;20:92–7.

20. Balachandran S, Sayle BA. Value of thyroid carcinoma imaging after therapeutic doses of radioiodine. Clin Nucl Med 1981;6:162–7.

21. Sherman SI, Tielens ET, Sostre S, et al. Clinical utility of posttreatment radioiodine scans in the management of patients with thyroid carcinoma. J Clin Endocrinol Metab 1994;78:629–34.

22. Spies WG, Wojtowicz CH, Spies SM, et al. Value of post-therapy whole-body I-131 imaging in the evaluation of patients with thyroid carcinoma having undergone high-dose I-131 therapy. Clin Nucl Med 1989;14:793–800.
23. Fatourechi V, Hay ID, Mullan BP, et al. Are posttherapy radioiodine scans informative and do they influence subsequent therapy of patients with differentiated thyroid cancer? Thyroid 2000;10:573–7.
24. Pineda JD, Lee T, Ain K, et al. Iodine-131 therapy for thyroid cancer patients with elevated thyroglobulin and negative diagnostic scan. J Clin Endocrinol Metab 1995;80:1488–92.
25. Souza Rosario PW, Barroso AL, Rezende LL, et al. Post I-131 therapy scanning in patients with thyroid carcinoma metastases: an unnecessary cost or a relevant contribution? Clin Nucl Med 2004;29:795–8.
26. Van Nostrand D. Remnant ablation, adjuvant treatment and treatment of locoregional metastases with 131I. In: Wartofsky L, Van Nostrand D, editors. Thyroid cancer: a comprehensive guide to clinical management. New York: Springer New York; 2016. p. 395–409.
27. Kim BW, Yousman W, Wong WX, et al. Less is more: comparing the 2015 and 2009 American Thyroid Association guidelines for thyroid nodules and cancer. Thyroid 2016;26:759–64.
28. Van Nostrand D. Festina lente and the "crab and the butterfly". J Transl Int Med 2016;4:58–60.
29. Castagna MG, Cevenini G, Theodoropoulou A, et al. Post-surgical thyroid ablation with low or high radioiodine activities results in similar outcomes in intermediate risk differentiated thyroid cancer patients. Eur J Endocrinol 2013;169:23–9.
30. Klubo-Gwiezdzinska J, Van Nostrand D, Atkins F, et al. Efficacy of dosimetric versus empiric prescribed activity of 131I for therapy of differentiated thyroid cancer. J Clin Endocrinol Metab 2011;96:3217–25.
31. Van Nostrand D, Atkins F, Moreau S, et al. Utility of the radioiodine whole-body retention at 48 hours for modifying empiric activity of 131-iodine for the treatment of metastatic well-differentiated thyroid carcinoma. Thyroid 2009;19:1093–8.
32. Hanscheid H, Lassmann M, Luster M, et al. Blood dosimetry from a single measurement of the whole body radioiodine retention in patients with differentiated thyroid carcinoma. Endocr Relat Cancer 2009;16:1283–9.
33. Jentzen W, Bockisch A, Ruhlmann M. Assessment of simplified blood dose protocols for the estimation of the maximum tolerable activity in thyroid cancer patients undergoing radioiodine therapy using 124I. J Nucl Med 2015;56:832–8.
34. Schlumberger M, Catargi B, Borget I, et al. Strategies of radioiodine ablation in patients with low-risk thyroid cancer. N Engl J Med 2012;366:1663–73.
35. Mallick U, Harmer C, Yap B, et al. Ablation with low-dose radioiodine and thyrotropin alfa in thyroid cancer. N Engl J Med 2012;36:1674–85.
36. Ho AL, Grewal RK, Leboeuf R, et al. Selumetinib-enhanced radioiodine uptake in advanced thyroid cancer. N Engl J Med 2013;368:623–32.
37. Wells K, Moreau S, Shin Y-R, et al. Positive (+) post-treatment (tx) scans after the radioiodine (RAI) tx of patients who have well-differentiated thyroid cancer (WDTC), positive serum thyroglobulin levels (TG+), and negative diagnostic (dx) RAI whole body scans (WBS-): predictive values and frequency. J Nucl Med 2008;49(supplement 1):238P.

# Imaging of Neuroendocrine Tumors

## Indications, Interpretations, Limits, and Pitfalls

Run Yu, MD, PhD[a],*, Ashley Wachsman, MD[b]

## KEYWORDS

- Neuroendocrine tumor • Anatomic imaging • Functional imaging • CT • MRI
- Octreotide scan • Gallium-68 somatostatin analog PET

## KEY POINTS

- Imaging plays critical and indispensable roles in the diagnosis, prognosis, and management of neuroendocrine tumors (NETs).
- Each imaging modality has its strengths and limits, and may give false-negative or false-positive results.
- NETs share common imaging features, but each type of NET exhibits unique imaging features.
- Computed tomography and MRI are used routinely to assess tumor burden; functional imaging with octreotide scan or Gallium-68 somatostatin analog PET is used selectively to confirm diagnosis and guide therapy.
- Open, frank, and inquisitive discussions among radiologists and clinicians are required to give a consistent, well-explained interpretation of the latest imaging findings to patients.

## GENERAL PRINCIPLES ON IMAGING OF NEUROENDOCRINE TUMORS
### Neuroendocrine Tumors

Neuroendocrine tumors (NETs) are a group of unique tumors and are defined in various ways.[1–3] Based on cellular origin, NETs are tumors derived from neuroendocrine cells, which share common features such as secreting peptide hormones, harboring dense core vesicles, and lack of neural structures. Based on histology, NETs are tumors composed of cells with stippled ("salt-and-pepper") chromatin and arranged in trabecular growth pattern; NETs are also positive for specific markers such as chromogranin A. Based on clinical behavior, NETs are usually indolent, but

Disclosure Statement: The authors have nothing to disclose.
[a] Division of Endocrinology, Diabetes & Metabolism, UCLA David Geffen School of Medicine, 200 Medical Plaza Driveway #530, Los Angeles, CA 90095, USA; [b] Department of Imaging, Cedars-Sinai Medical Center, 8700 Beverly Boulevard #M335, Los Angeles, CA 90048, USA
* Corresponding author.
E-mail address: runyu@mednet.ucla.edu

have malignant potential and may secrete hormones that cause certain syndromes (eg, carcinoid syndrome). NETs can arise in virtually every organ but are most commonly found in the gastrointestinal (GI) tract, pancreas, and lungs. The clinical behavior, treatment, and prognosis of NETs largely depend on the organ of origin, hormonal secretion, tumor grade, and tumor stage, on most of which imaging provides invaluable information.

### Roles of Imaging in Neuroendocrine Tumor Diagnosis, Prognosis, and Management

The roles of imaging in the diagnosis, prognosis, and management of NETs are critical and indispensable (**Box 1**). Imaging is important for NET diagnosis. In patients with hormonal hypersecretion syndromes such as carcinoid syndrome, positive biochemical test results per se are not sufficient to establish NET diagnosis because false-positive test results are common owing to interferences from other diseases, medications, and laboratory and cleric errors.[4–6] Imaging is required to locate the potential tumor and assess overall tumor burden. If extensive imaging studies cannot find the suspected tumor, the NET diagnosis is seriously challenged and alternative diagnoses need to be entertained. When a tumor is identified incidentally by imaging for other purposes, the imaging characteristics of the tumor often give helpful clues to the potential NET diagnosis.[7,8] Sometimes the imaging features are so unique that they can make an NET diagnosis. For example, focal hepatic steatosis around an enhancing mass is pathognomonic for malignant insulinoma liver metastasis.[9]

Once an NET is diagnosed, imaging further characterizes the NET to guide prognosis and management. Because the organ of origin often is informative of prognosis and treatment, identifying the organ of NET origin by imaging is routine in clinical practice.[8,10] Because NET staging is anatomically based, imaging is the most important and easiest means of establishing stage.[11] Although imaging itself cannot tell if an NET is functional or not, large tumor burden identified by imaging in a patient without specific symptoms strongly suggests that the tumor is nonfunctional; a small tumor burden in a similar patient cannot exclude a functional NET. Even for tumor grade, which is defined by proliferative markers in tumor specimen,[12] imaging still helps to confirm or dispute the tumor grade by documenting tumor growth speed. Functional imaging can also suggest tumor grade (see section on F-18 fluorodeoxyglucose [FDG] PET).

NET treatment is composed of surgical resection, liver-directed therapy, systemic therapy, and complication prevention and control.[1,3] Specific treatment and order of treatment need to be individualized, largely based on imaging findings in most patients. Patients with NETs limited to the primary organ or 1 liver lobe are often treated with surgical resection, those with a large liver tumor burden are treated

---

**Box 1**
**Roles of imaging in NET diagnosis, prognosis, and management**

- Finding an NET by imaging is required for NET diagnosis in most patients.
- Imaging is the predominant means of NET staging and contributes to prognosticating.
- NET imaging characteristics help guide therapeutic options.
- Imaging is the most reliable way to monitor treatment response and disease progression.

*Abbreviation:* NET, neuroendocrine tumor.

with liver-directed therapy, those with any tumor burden after surgical resection and liver-directed therapy are treated with systemic therapy, and those with bone metastasis can be treated with external beam radiation. Functional imaging can determine the appropriateness of some systemic therapies such as peptide receptor radionuclide therapy.[13] Furthermore, the roles of functional imaging agent as cancer theranostics hold promise to precision medicine for NET patients.[14]

Imaging is the most reliable way to monitor treatment response and disease progression in both clinical practice and clinical research. NET symptoms are often nonspecific and NET biochemical markers are subject to interferences.[4–6] In clinical practice, periodic imaging studies compare the number, size, and imaging characteristics of individual tumor lesions, thus documenting disease progression and treatment response.[15] In clinical research, the RECIST (Response Evaluation Criteria In Solid Tumors) criteria, assessed by imaging, are the most frequently used method to study response to an experimental therapy.[16]

Finally, imaging is also the most reliable method for NET surveillance in patients who are carriers of mutations that predispose them to familial NETs such as multiple endocrine neoplasia syndrome type 1.[17] NET symptoms and routine biochemical tests are often inaccurate, especially when NETs are small, and thus have generally low sensitivity and specificity of identifying early stage NETs. Because NETs have specific imaging characteristics (discussed elsewhere in this article), imaging usually identifies NETs years before symptoms occur and biochemical test results become definitively positive.

### Incidental Findings and False-Positive Findings

Incidental imaging findings should always be expected and their clinical significance determined in the context of the patient's general health condition. For example, small thyroid or adrenal nodules without suspicious imaging features in a patient with metastatic NET probably should not be specifically worked up.[18,19] Some apparently incidental findings may suggest undiagnosed familiar NET syndromes. For example, an adrenal mass in a patient with multiple skin nodules may suggest neurofibromatosis type 1 with pheochromocytoma.[20]

False-positive imaging findings can lead to patient anxiety, unnecessary further testing and imaging, and even invasive interventions.[21,22] In patients with confirmed or suspected NETs, the pretest probability of finding NETs or metastatic lesions is high so that any positive findings are treated seriously. When there is disagreement between clinical condition and imaging findings or between findings from 2 imaging modalities, false-positive findings should also be suspected. Most false-positive findings are from functional imaging. Familiarity with common false-positive findings greatly facilitates identification of these benign or normal entities.

### Collaborations Between Clinicians and Radiologists

Because imaging plays critical and indispensable roles in NETs diagnosis, prognosis, and management, radiologists are important members of the multidisciplinary NET team.[23] Open, frank, and inquisitive discussions among radiologists and clinicians are required to resolve the frequent discrepancies between radiologic findings and clinical conditions or biochemical maker levels, between readings from 2 different radiologists, between results from 2 different imaging modalities, and between results from 2 serial imaging studies. NET patients often view imaging findings as infallible; thus, it is important for the NET team to give a consistent, well-explained interpretation of the latest imaging findings to patients, addressing any potential discrepancies as described.

## NEUROENDOCRINE TUMOR IMAGING MODALITIES

Imaging modalities can be anatomic, which are based on the physical characteristics, or functional or nuclear, which are based on the biochemical characteristics of the tissue to be imaged (**Box 2**). The use of contrast in anatomic imaging also helps to elucidate the biochemical characteristics of the imaged tissue to some extent. Rather than using signals from X-ray energy attenuation or nuclear magnetic resonance to form images as in anatomic imaging, functional imaging uses biological molecules linked to radioisotopes that emit $\gamma$ rays or positron. For NET imaging in contemporary clinical practice, computed tomography (CT) scans and MRI are the anatomic imaging modalities and In-111 octreotide scan, Ga-68 somatostatin analogue PET, and FDG PET the functional imaging modalities most commonly used.

### Anatomic Imaging

CT is the best imaging modality for the lungs, and is sufficient for most solid organ imaging needs if intravenous contrast is also given and multiphase images are recorded (**Fig. 1**). For the GI tract, oral contrast or contrast through enema increases the probability of identifying mucosa lesions such as NETs. For the small bowel imaging, CT enterography, which is CT with large-volume, neutral or low-density oral contrast (to distend the small bowel) and intravenous contrast to achieve better visualization of the small bowel wall and mucosa[24,25] (see **Fig. 1**). NETs as small as 0.5 cm can be detected by CT enterography.

MRI offers multiple imaging protocols and contrasts. For evaluating NET liver metastasis, T2-weighted images without or with fat suppression, diffusion-weighted imaging, and multiphase imaging are often used[26,27] (**Fig. 2**). T2-weighted images with fast spin echo sequence and diffusion-weighted imaging are both fast to acquire images and do not need contrast. T2-weighted images differentiates metastatic NETs from normal liver by the content of tissue fluid (tumor usually having more), and diffusion-weighted imaging by the freedom of water molecule random movement (tumors having less). Multiphase imaging requires intravenous contrast. The regular extracellular gadolinium contrasts (eg, gadoterate) allow early arterial phase, late arterial phase (early portal phase), and portal phase imaging to draw difference between tumors and liver (tumor appearing brighter than liver), whereas the hepatobiliary contrasts (eg, gadoxetic acid) are increasingly used to achieve a delayed, hepatobiliary phase to further differentiate metastatic NET lesions from normal liver parenchyma (tumor appearing darker than liver).[27,28] For imaging of the small bowel, MRI enterography can also be used.[29,30] Numerous other MRI protocols are available but less commonly used.

---

**Box 2**
**Essential NET imaging modalities**

*Anatomic imaging*

- CT (including CT enterography)
- MRI (including MRI enterography)

*Functional imaging*

- In-111 octreotide scan
- Ga-68 somatostatin analog PET

*Abbreviations:* CT, computed tomography; NET, neuroendocrine tumor.

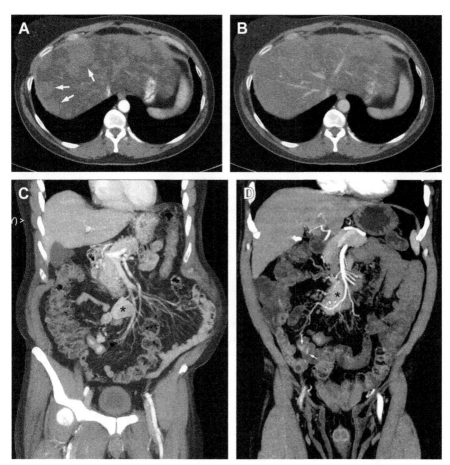

**Fig. 1.** Computed tomography (CT) imaging features of neuroendocrine tumors (NETs). (*A*) Metastatic pancreatic NET in the liver at early arterial phase, axial view (*thick arrows*). (*B*) The same view at late arterial phase. Note the multiple enhancing liver lesions. (*C*) CT urogram of a mesenteric lymph node (*asterisk*) in a patient with multifocal small bowel carcinoids, coronal view. Note the desmoplastic reaction and tethering of bowel loop with bowel wall thickening around the lymph node. (*D*) CT enterography of the same patient, coronal view. Note the dilated stomach and small bowel and small enhancing small bowel mural lesions (*thin arrows*).

### Comparison of computed tomography and MRI

CT has been used for many years, is widely available, and is less expensive than MRI (**Box 3**). CT images are intuitive to most nonradiologist physicians, which facilitates the communication before radiologists and clinicians. CT, however, subjects patients to radiation exposure and is less sensitive than MRI in NET imaging in solid organs[31,32] (see **Figs. 1** and **2**). MRI images are more challenging to be understood by nonradiologists and the MRI protocols can be complex and time consuming to perform. The MRI procedure is also hard to tolerate by patients with claustrophobia. Given these considerations, it is generally agreed that CT is better for chest NET imaging, MRI is better for imaging NET liver metastasis, and CT and MRI enterography are equally effective for imaging small bowel NETs.[30] When MRI is not available or unaffordable,

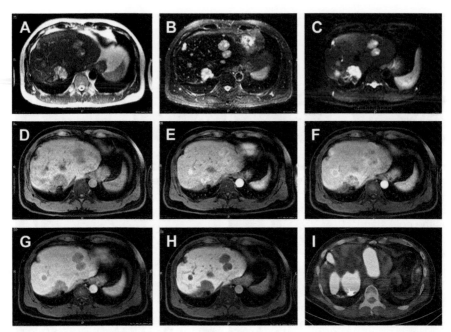

**Fig. 2.** MRI imaging features of liver metastatic lesions from a small bowel neuroendocrine tumor. Images of about the same axial section are shown. (*A*) T2-weighted image. (*B*) T2-weighted image with turbo inversion recovery magnitude sequence (a method of fat suppression). (*C*) Diffusion weighted imaging. (*D–H*) Multiphase T1-weighted imaging with intravenous contrast gadoxetic acid. (*D*) Precontrast image. (*E*) Early arterial phase. (*F*) Late arterial phase (early portal phase). (*G*) Portal phase. (*H*) Hepatobiliary phase. (*I*) Octreotide scan single-photon emission computed tomography image showing the strong expression of somatostatin receptors in these lesions.

CT is satisfactory for imaging NET liver metastasis in most patients. When clinical and biochemical data are inconsistent with CT findings in solid organs, MRI should be sought to get definitive imaging conclusions.

One particular issue on NET imaging is long-term safety, because patients with NETs usually survive many years after diagnosis and require many imaging studies. Radiation exposure owing to CT and possible secondary malignancy are legitimate concerns.[31] The use of contrast agent for both CT and MRI can cause renal compromise and nephrogenic systemic fibrosis, respectively.[33,34] Recently, gadolinium-based contrast agents have been shown to be deposited in the brains of patients

---

**Box 3**
**CT or MRI for NET imaging?**

- CT images are easier to read for nonradiologists.
- CT is better for imaging of lung NETs.
- MRI is better for imaging of NET liver metastasis.
- CT and MRI enterography are both satisfactory for small bowel NETs.

*Abbreviations:* CT, computed tomography; NET, neuroendocrine tumor.

with repetitive MRI studies,[35] although it is not clear if the brain deposits have clinical consequences. Thus, the benefits and risks of frequent imaging follow-ups need to be balanced in individual patients.

## Functional Imaging

Indium-111 (In-111) octreotide scan is a nuclear scintigraphy using In-111–labeled octreotide through a DTPA-D-Phe group (also called pentetreotide).[36] Octreotide is a synthetic analogue of somatostatin and has preferential affinity with the subtypes 2 and 5 of the somatostatin receptor (sst2 and sst5).[37] In-111–labeled octreotide binds to any tissue expressing sst2 and sst5. Because most NETs strongly express sst2, an In-111 octreotide scan localizes NETs.[38] After intravenous injection of In-111–labeled octreotide, planar images are taken at 4 and 24 hours. Single-photon emission computed tomography may be performed at 24 hours to increase the accuracy of NET localization. Octreotide scan has been in clinical use for about 30 years and was the gold standard for NET functional imaging until recently. Although the sensitivity and specificity of octreotide scan in localizing large NETs can be close to 100% (highest for small bowel NET and gastrinoma), the success of octreotide scan is limited by the intrinsic low resolution of $\gamma$ ray scintigraphy, which has a spatial resolution of about 1 cm.[39,40] Octreotide scan thus usually cannot reliably detect NETs less than 1 cm. Another limit is that the signal intensity on octreotide scan can only be determined qualitatively.

To overcome the limits of octreotide scan, PET scans using a positron-emitting radioisotope-labeled somatostatin analogue has been developed.[41] PET has a spatial resolution of 3 to 6 mm depending on the tissue where the positron is emitted.[42] The PET signal intensity can be objectively determined and expressed as a standardized uptake value. Gallium-68 is the positron emitter of choice owing to the ease of generation and labeling of the somatostatin analogue; the spatial resolution of Ga-68–based PET, however, is slightly lower than that of F-18–based PET.[42] Another advantage of PET is that the procedure is completed within 2 hours of intravenous injection of tracer. Presently, PET is usually combined with CT to provide better signal localization. Ga-68–labeled somatostatin analogue PET/CT (Ga-68 SA PET) has proven to be a superb functional imaging modality[41,43] (**Fig. 3**). Currently 2 Ga-68 labeled tracers, DOTA-TATE (tetraazacyclododecane tetraacetic acid–octreotate) and DOTATOC (DOTA$^0$-D-Phe$^1$-Tyr$^3$-octreotide), are used clinically with approximately equal accuracy, even though the former has an approximately 10-fold higher affinity with sst2 than the latter.[44] Numerous studies have shown that Ga-68 SA PET has higher sensitivity in NET detection than octreotide scan[45–48] or in paraganglioma detection than other functional imaging modalities.[49] Ga-68 DOTATATE was approved as a PET imaging agent by the US Food and Drug Administration in June 2016. Other Ga-68–labeled somatostatin analogues (including antagonists) are being developed for clinical use.[50] Currently, wide use of Ga-68 SA PET may be limited by its cost and availability. In the future, Ga-68 SA PET will likely replace octreotide scan as the first-line NET functional imaging modality.[51]

Although Ga-68 SA PET certainly is superior to octreotide scan in localizing NETs, the extra clinical benefits of Ga-68 SA PET need to be carefully evaluated in an individual patient (**Box 4**). The use of Ga-68 SA PET indeed changes management in some patients, but whether it confers clinical benefits is not clear.[52] In our clinical experience, octreotide scan is sufficient in a large number of NET patients. Ga-68 SA PET, by virtue of its higher sensitivity, has clear clinical benefits in patients with metastatic NETs of unknown origin by finding the primary tumor, in patients being considered for liver transplant by searching for extrahepatic metastatic lesion, in

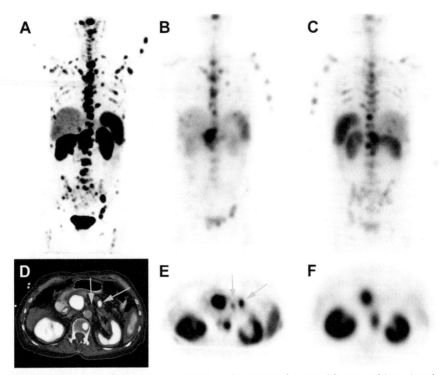

**Fig. 3.** Comparison of Ga-68 somatostatin analog PET and octreotide scan. This patient has widely metastasized small bowel neuroendocrine tumor. (*A*) Ga-68 tetraazacyclododecane tetraacetic acid–octreotate (DOTATATE) PET, coronal maximum intensity projection view. (*B*) Octreotide scan, coronal anterior planar view. (*C*) Octreotide scan, coronal posterior planar view. (*D*) Ga-68 DOTATATE PET/computed tomography fusion, axial view. (*E*) Ga-68 DOTATATE PET, axial view. (*F*) Octreotide scan single-photon emission computed tomography (SPECT), axial view. Arrows, pancreatic tail and celiac node lesions detected by Ga-68 DOTATATE PET (*D, E*) but not seen on octreotide scan SPECT (*F*). (*Courtesy of* Dr Martin Allen-Auerbach, Department of Molecular and Medical Pharmacology, UCLA David Geffen School of Medicine, Los Angeles, CA.)

patients with only small suspicious liver or lymph node lesions by determining their NET nature, and in patients with biochemical evidence of NET but without anatomic imaging findings by finding the occult NET or reassessing the NET diagnosis. Because octreotide scan and Ga-68 SA PET are both based on sst2 and sst5 expression,

---

**Box 4**
**Which patients benefit most from Ga-68 somatostatin analog PET?**

- Patients with metastatic NET of unknown origin, if finding the primary NET is important to guide treatment.

- Patients being considered for liver transplant to rule out extrahepatic metastatic lesions.

- Patients with only small suspicious liver or lymph node lesions to determine their NET nature.

- Patients with biochemical evidence of NET but without anatomic imaging findings to search for the occult NET or to reevaluate the NET diagnosis.

*Abbreviation:* NET, neuroendocrine tumor.

non-NET tumors, nontumor lesions, and normal tissue expressing high levels of these receptors can be detected by both, but especially by Ga-68 SA PET owing to the high sensitivity.[43,53] Common tumors that may seem to be positive on Ga-68 SA PET and less likely on octreotide scan include various thyroid cancers, breast cancer, melanoma, and hemangioma[54,55]; nontumor lesions include granuloma and postoperative changes[56]; and physiologic uptakes include ectopic spleen, and pancreatic polypeptide cell pseudohyperplasia in the uncinate process of pancreas.[57,58] Owing to the high image quality of Ga-68 SA PET, the false-positive signals can be deceivingly impressive and lead to overdiagnosis by an unsuspecting reader. Interpretation of Ga-68 SA PET will likely improve over time with increased clinical experience.

FDG PET is a general PET for characterizing and locating a potential malignancy. The intensity of the FDG PET signal depends on the avidity of a tissue for taking up glucose and is expressed as the standardized uptake value. Most NETs do not exhibit high standardized uptake values so that FDG PET is not routinely used for NET imaging.[59,60] In a few specific situations, FDG PET gives valuable information of an NET.[61–63] First, FDG PET is used to assess overall tumor burden of high-grade NETs, which usually are very avid in taking up glucose thus exhibit very high standardized uptake values (**Fig. 4**). Second, when an NET metastatic lesion suddenly grows fast, suggesting dedifferentiation, FDG PET can be used to confirm that and further determine the dedifferentiation potential of other metastatic lesions. Third, if FDG PET is performed for another indication, the signal intensity of a NET can be used to suggest tumor grade: low signal suggests a low or intermediate grade and high signal suggests a high grade.

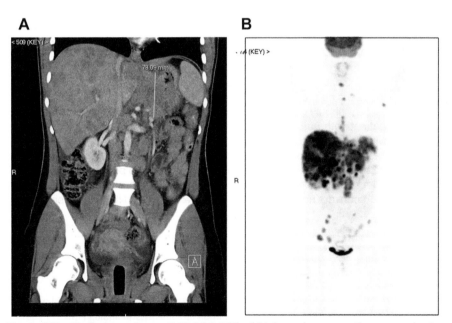

**A**

**B**

**Fig. 4.** PET with fludeoxyglucose F 18 (FDG PET) of high-grade pancreatic neuroendocrine tumor (NET) with wide metastasis. (*A*) Computed tomography scan of the abdomen and pelvis with enhancement, coronal view. The green line marks the craniocaudal dimension of the primary pancreatic NET. (*B*) FDG PET, coronal maximum intensity projection view. Highest tumor standardized uptake value was 10.

## Other functional imaging modalities

Numerous functional imaging modalities are in experimental or selected use for NET imaging. F-18–labeled dihydroxyphenylalanine (DOPA) PET is based on tissue uptake and decarboxylation of DOPA through L amino acid transporters and amino acid decarboxylase, and can be used for NET imaging.[64,65] The practical indication of F-18 DOPA PET, however, is not well-defined, because octreotide scan or Ga-68 SA PET is usually sufficient for NET imaging in most patients. F-18 DOPA PET may be used in patients with NETs suspected not to express somatostatin receptor or in patients with metastatic NETs of unknown origin.[10] C-11–labeled 5-hydroxytryptophan PET is similar to F-18 DOPA PET in that they use the same mechanism to image NET, are both more sensitive than octreotide scan, and their practical clinical indications are not well-defined.[66,67] Glucagon-like peptide-1 receptor scintigraphy has been increasingly used for insulinoma localization. For more details, please see Mark Masciocchi's article, "Pancreatic Imaging," in this issue. I-123 or I-131–labeled metaiodobenzylguanidine scan and F-18–labeled dopamine PET are used to localize pheochromocytoma/paraganglioma. Please see N. Reed Dunnick and colleagues' article, "Adrenal Imaging," in this issue, for more details.

## COMMON NEUROENDOCRINE TUMOR IMAGING CHARACTERISTICS AND STRATEGIES

NETs share common imaging characteristics (**Box 5**). NETs are usually solid tumors, but may show central cystic components if the size is large. Primary pancreatic NETs may occasionally have a relatively large or predominant cystic components even when the size is small (please see Mark Masciocchi's article, "Pancreatic Imaging," in this issue). Because NETs have rich vasculature, they often exhibit early arterial phase enhancement on CT scans and MRI (see **Figs. 1** and **2**). Larger NETs or NETs with a cystic or degenerative center tend to exhibit peripheral (or rim) enhancement.[68–70] As described earlier, NETs are usually positive on octreotide scan and Ga-68 SA PET but negative on FDG PET.

NET imaging strategies should meet the goals of imaging for NET diagnosis and follow-up (**Box 6**). Goals of imaging at the initial diagnosis are establishing the NET diagnosis and assessing the overall NET tumor burden and stage. Anatomic imaging by CT scan or MRI should target the body regions based on clinical suspicion. For example, a patient with carcinoid syndrome should undergo abdominal and pelvic CT scan or MRI with optional enterography to search for primary small bowel NET and liver metastasis, whereas a patient with ectopic Cushing syndrome should proceed with a CT scan of the chest. Functional imaging should be performed and octreotide scan is the practical choice. Ga-68 SA PET can be considered if anatomic imaging and octreotide scan do not give definitive answers to the NET diagnosis, tumor

---

**Box 5**
**Common NET imaging characteristics**

- NETs are usually solid tumors.

- NETs often exhibit early arterial phase general or rim enhancement on CT scans and MRI.

- NETs are usually positive on octreotide scan and Ga-68 somatostatin analog PET.

- NETs are usually negative on FDG-PET.

*Abbreviations:* CT, computed tomography; FDG-PET, PET with fludeoxyglucose F 18; NET, neuroendocrine tumor.

---

**Box 6**
**NET imaging strategies**

*Initial diagnosis*

- Goals of imaging: establishing the NET diagnosis and assessing the overall NET tumor burden and stage.

- Anatomic imaging of body regions based on clinical suspicion and functional imaging with octreotide scan or Ga-68 somatostatin analog PET.

*Follow-up*

- Goals of imaging: monitoring NET tumor recurrence, metastasis, and progression, and assessing treatment appropriateness and treatment response.

- Anatomic imaging of body regions based on clinical suspicion and selected use of functional imaging with octreotide scan or Ga-68 somatostatin analog PET.

- Frequency of imaging studies need to be individualized.

*Abbreviation:* NET, neuroendocrine tumor.

---

burden, or stage. During NET follow-up, the goals of imaging are to monitor NET tumor recurrence, metastasis, and progression, and to assess treatment appropriateness and treatment response (**Fig. 5**). Because the NET diagnosis is already established, new tumors are usually owing to recurrence or metastasis and anatomic imaging of

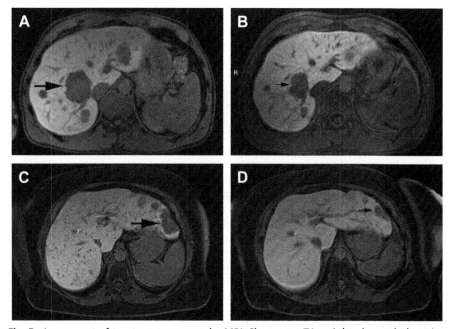

**Fig. 5.** Assessment of treatment response by MRI. Shown are T1-weighted portal phase images after intravenous contrast gadoxetic acid, axial view. (*A, B*) Metastatic pancreatic neuroendocrine tumor (NET) before (*A*) and after (*B*) 2 cycles of peptide receptor radionuclide therapy (PRRT). (*C, D*) Metastatic small bowel NET before (*C*) and after (*D*) 4 cycles of PRRT. Note the shrinkage of large metastatic lesions (*B, D*) and the disappearance of small lesions (*D*). Arrows, index lesions.

body regions based on clinical suspicion is usually sufficient. Functional imaging is usually only needed in a few situations: octreotide scan or Ga-68 SA PET to assess sst2 and sst5 expression if peptide receptor radionuclide therapy is considered, and to evaluate NET response to therapy, and FDG PET to assess the extent of aggressive transformation if tumor exhibits explosive growth.[60,71,72]

The frequency or interval of imaging studies during follow-up needs to be individualized, considering clinical benefits, long-term risk of imaging or contrast exposure, and costs. As a rule, the more aggressive a NET is, the more frequent it needs imaging follow-up. NETs with mostly benign behaviors, such as those less than 1 cm in the appendix or rectum and the usual insulinoma, do not require imaging follow-up after complete resection, whereas those of low grade and metastasis may need imaging follow-up every 6 to 12 months.[15,73,74] Because most NETs are indolent but have malignant potential, long-term follow-up is required for most patients. The risks of imaging and contrast exposure and the cost of imaging may limit the number of a certain kind of imaging study that can be given to a patient. We believe that the same number of a certain imaging study give more clinical benefits if done less frequently but over longer period of time than if done more frequently but over a shorter period of time.

## IMAGING OF SPECIFIC NEUROENDOCRINE TUMORS
### Gastrointestinal Tract Neuroendocrine Tumors

Endoscopy and endoscopic ultrasound imaging directly examine mucosal and mural lesions and can biopsy lesions in upper (esophagus, stomach, and duodenum) and lower (colon and rectum) GI tract; capsule endoscopy and double balloon enteroscopy fulfill the same purpose in the jejunum and ileum; they are usually the initial approaches to working up GI tract NETs. Imaging is needed to evaluate local invasion or lymph node or remote metastasis. Barium studies are seldom used nowadays.

Esophageal NETs are very rare, usually high grade, and seen as a lower esophageal invasive mass with lymph node metastasis on anatomic imaging and high standardized uptake value on FDG PET.[75]

Types 1 and 2 of gastric NETs are caused by hypergastrinemia, usually benign, and seen as small (<2 cm) and multiple mucosal/submucosal tumors without lymph node involvement on anatomic imaging, and do not require functional imaging. Type 3 gastric NETs are not related to hypergastrinemia, usually aggressive, seen as solitary, large lesions (>2 cm) often with lymph node involvement on anatomic imaging, and positive on both octreotide scan and FDG PET.[76]

Duodenal NETs are rare and usually small, and may secrete gastrin. They are more commonly found in the proximal duodenum. On anatomic imaging, duodenal NETs appear as intraluminal polypoid or mural masses; rarely, local invasion and lymph node metastasis may be seen. Functional imaging is needed when remote metastasis is a concern.[77]

Small bowel NETs (midgut, excluding duodenum but including ascending colon) are some of the most clinically important NETs. They are often called carcinoids and can cause carcinoid syndrome after metastasizing to liver. They commonly arise from the terminal ileum (**Fig. 6**). Multifocal primary tumors are also possible, but they are usually small (see **Fig. 1**). On anatomic imaging, especially on CT or MRI enterography, the primary tumor is usually intraluminal but with mural involvement.[24,29,78] The mesentery around the primary tumor may contain a large lymph node with metastasis (often larger than the primary tumor) and exhibits desmoplastic changes with extensive

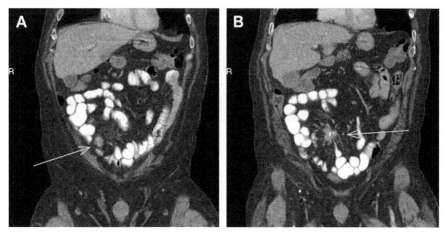

**Fig. 6.** Computed tomography (CT) images of small bowel neuroendocrine tumor (NET). The CT was done with intravenous contrast and barium enema. Shown are coronal images of the abdomen and pelvis. (*A*) Primary ileal NET (*arrow*). (*B*) Mesenteric lymph node (*arrow*) with calcification and desmoplastic reaction.

fibrosis and contraction (see **Figs. 1** and **6**). Partial small bowel obstruction may be incidentally found. At times, the mesentery vasculature is distorted, resulting in bowel ischemia. Functional imaging with octreotide scan is always done to search for lymph node or remote metastasis (mainly to the liver).

Most appendiceal NETs are small and incidental findings on surgical specimens from appendectomy or colectomy. Preoperative diagnosis is unlikely. Retrospective review of the preoperative CT images of appendix can identify a small (<1 cm) round mass at the tip of appendix.[79] Functional imaging is only needed if metastasis is suspected.

Transverse and descending colon NETs, viewed on anatomic imaging, tend to be large solitary intraluminal mass or circumferential thickening with lymph node or liver metastasis, indistinguishable from the usual adenocarcinoma.[80] Functional imaging with FDG PET is used to assess whole-body tumor burden.

Rectal NETs are usually found incidentally through screening colonoscopy. Most of them are small (<1 cm) and hard to be found on imaging, even on CT colonography.[81] Large rectal NETs may invade surrounding organs and metastasize to lymph node or the liver.

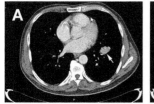
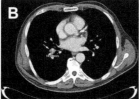
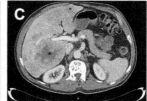

**Fig. 7.** Computed tomography (CT) images of lung carcinoid. The CT was done with intravenous contrast. Shown are axial images of the chest or abdomen. (*A*) Primary lung carcinoid (*thick arrow*). (*B*) Hilar lymph node (*thin arrow*). (*C*) Multiple metastatic lesions in liver (*asterisks*). Note the largest liver lesion has peripheral enhancement.

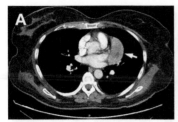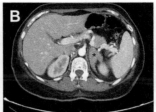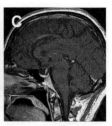

**Fig. 8.** Computed tomography (CT) images of thymic neuroendocrine tumor (NET) causing ectopic Cushing syndrome. The CT was done with intravenous contrast. (*A*) Thymic NET (*arrow*), axial view. (*B*) Hyperplastic left adrenal gland (*asterisk*) (with prior right adrenalectomy), axial view. (*C*) Contrast-enhanced MRI of the normal pituitary gland, sagittal view.

### *Other Neuroendocrine Tumors*

Pulmonary NETs are usually nonfunctional but can cause ectopic Cushing syndrome, and divided into typical (low-grade) and atypical (intermediate-grade) carcinoid, and high-grade neuroendocrine lung carcinoma. Typical and atypical lung carcinoids are generally indistinguishable on CT and functional imaging.[82,83] They usually present as solitary lung nodule either centrally or in the lung periphery with smooth borders and occasionally with hilar or mediastinal lymphadenopathy (**Fig. 7**). High-grade neuroendocrine carcinomas (including large cell and small cell lung cancers) cannot be differentiated from non–small-cell lung cancers on CT scans and FDG PET. Diffuse idiopathic pulmonary neuroendocrine cell hyperplasia appears as multiple small pulmonary nodules (< ~ 1 cm) on CT scans, which may coexist with a gross lung carcinoid.[84] Functional imaging even with Ga-68 SA PET rarely detects the nodules of diffuse idiopathic pulmonary neuroendocrine cell hyperplasia.

Thymic NETs tend to be aggressive and, like pulmonary NETs, are usually nonfunctional but can cause ectopic Cushing syndrome. The imaging features on anatomic imaging such as enhancement and local invasion are not specific (**Fig. 8**); octreotide scan has variable sensitivity in detecting thymic NETs but FDG PET has higher sensitivity.[85,86]

NETs of unknown origin are defined as NETs with liver metastasis but initial anatomic imaging with routine CT scans or MRI does not identify a primary tumor. Finding the primary NET can guide therapy. Additional anatomic imaging such as CT or MRI enterography and endoscopy may help to identify the primary tumor; functional imaging with octreotide scan often is insufficient, but Ga-68 SA PET and F-18 DOPA PET are more sensitive.[10]

For imaging pancreatic NETs and paragangliomas, see Mark Masciocchi's article, "Pancreatic Imaging," and N. Reed Dunnick's and colleagues article, "Adrenal Imaging," respectively, in this issue. Less common NETs such as those from the ovary, uterus, prostate, presacral space, kidney, skin, and skull base are usually under the purview of specialists other than endocrinologists and thus not discussed here.

### SUMMARY AND FUTURE DIRECTIONS

At present, the judicious use of routine anatomic and functional imaging has already satisfied most clinical needs of patients with NETs. Clinicians and radiologists who take care of patients with NETs should be familiar with the indications and interpretations of common imaging modalities and be mindful of limits and pitfalls (**Box 7**). The future of imaging probably belongs to novel functional imaging modalities. For NET

---

**Box 7**
**Limits and common pitfalls of NET imaging**

*Limits*

- Imaging suggests but cannot make the NET diagnosis.
- Imaging suggests but cannot determine NET grade.
- Each modality has its intrinsic limit on physical resolution.
- Some protocols provide limited tissue contrast.

*Common pitfalls*

- Misuse of imaging modality or protocol.
- False-positive findings.
- Variations in imaging results from the same study done at different times and from different studies.
- Randomness in defining the dimensions of mass.
- Subjectivity in judging whether there is a small mass.
- Inconsistent use of descriptive terms (eg, strong enhancement, intense uptake, innumerable lesions).

*Abbreviation:* NET, neuroendocrine tumor.

---

imaging, we believe that novel functional imaging modalities will be developed, based on certain cell surface receptors or metabolic processes of NETs, to detect small NETs of a particular kind, to predict prognosis of NETs, and to guide therapeutic choice and design novel therapies.

## ACKNOWLEDGMENTS

The authors thank Drs Anthony Heaney, Randy Hecht, and Martin Allen-Auerbach, UCLA David Geffen School of Medicine, and Drs Nicholas Nissen, Andrew Hendifar, and Marc Friedman, Cedars-Sinai Medical Center, for discussion and for help on retrieving images.

## REFERENCES

1. Yu R. Chapter 150 - Neuroendocrine tumor syndromes. In: Jameson JL, DeGroot LJ, editors. Endocrinology: adult and pediatric. seventh edition. Philadelphia: Elsevier Saunders; 2016. p. 2606–14.e4.
2. Kloppel G. Classification and pathology of gastroenteropancreatic neuroendocrine neoplasms. Endocr Relat Cancer 2011;18:S1–16.
3. Ro C, Chai W, Yu VE, et al. Pancreatic neuroendocrine tumors: biology, diagnosis, and treatment. Chin J Cancer 2013;32:312–24.
4. Lawrence B, Gustafsson BI, Kidd M, et al. The clinical relevance of chromogranin A as a biomarker for gastroenteropancreatic neuroendocrine tumors. Endocrinol Metab Clin North Am 2011;40:111–34.
5. Yu R, Wolin E. Ghost carcinoid in a patient with 120-fold elevated 5-hydroxyindoacetic acid. Endocr Pract 2012;18:803–4.
6. Yu R, Wei M. False positive test results for pheochromocytoma from 2000 to 2008. Exp Clin Endocrinol Diabetes 2010;118:577–85.

7. Gallotti A, Johnston RP, Bonaffini PA, et al. Incidental neuroendocrine tumors of the pancreas: MDCT findings and features of malignancy. AJR Am J Roentgenol 2013;200:355–62.

8. Polish A, Vergo MT, Agulnik M. Management of neuroendocrine tumors of unknown origin. J Natl Compr Canc Netw 2011;9:1397–402.

9. Yu R, Wachsman A, Nissen NN. Visual vignette: focal hepatic steatosis around malignant insulinoma. Endocr Pract 2016;22:117.

10. Santhanam P, Chandramahanti S, Kroiss A, et al. Nuclear imaging of neuroendocrine tumors with unknown primary: why, when and how? Eur J Nucl Med Mol Imaging 2015;42:1144–55.

11. Rindi G. The ENETS guidelines: the new TNM classification system. Tumori 2010; 96:806–9.

12. Klöppel G, Perren A, Heitz PU. The gastroenteropancreatic neuroendocrine cell system and its tumors: the WHO classification. Ann N Y Acad Sci 2004;1014: 13–27.

13. Brabander T, Teunissen JJ, Van Eijck CH, et al. Peptide receptor radionuclide therapy of neuroendocrine tumours. Best Pract Res Clin Endocrinol Metab 2016;30:103–14.

14. Taieb D, Hicks RJ, Pacak K. Nuclear medicine in cancer theranostics: beyond the target. J Nucl Med 2016;57(11):1659–60.

15. Kunz PL, Reidy-Lagunes D, Anthony LB, et al. Consensus guidelines for the management and treatment of neuroendocrine tumors. Pancreas 2013;42:557–77.

16. Therasse P, Eisenhauer EA, Verweij J. RECIST revisited: a review of validation studies on tumour assessment. Eur J Cancer 2006;42:1031–9.

17. Thakker RV, Newey PJ, Walls GV, et al. Clinical practice guidelines for multiple endocrine neoplasia type 1 (MEN1). J Clin Endocrinol Metab 2012;97: 2990–3011.

18. Hoang JK, Langer JE, Middleton WD, et al. Managing incidental thyroid nodules detected on imaging: white paper of the ACR incidental thyroid findings committee. J Am Coll Radiol 2015;12:143–50.

19. Yu R, Nissen NN, Dhall D, et al. Pheochromocytoma in patients suspected of harboring adrenal metastasis: management and clinical predictors. Endocr Pract 2008;14:967–72.

20. Yu VE, Yu R. Visual vignette: neurofibromatosis type 1 (NF1) with pheochromocytoma. Endocr Pract 2014;20:97.

21. Gibril F, Reynolds JC, Chen CC, et al. Specificity of somatostatin receptor scintigraphy: a prospective study and effects of false-positive localizations on management in patients with gastrinomas. J Nucl Med 1999;40:539–53.

22. Lev I, Kelekar G, Waxman A, et al. Clinical use and utility of metaiodobenzylguanidine scintigraphy in pheochromocytoma diagnosis. Endocr Pract 2010;16: 398–407.

23. Metz DC, Choi J, Strosberg J, et al. A rationale for multidisciplinary care in treating neuroendocrine tumours. Curr Opin Endocrinol Diabetes Obes 2012;19: 306–13.

24. Hakim FA, Alexander JA, Huprich JE, et al. CT-enterography may identify small bowel tumors not detected by capsule endoscopy: eight years experience at Mayo Clinic Rochester. Dig Dis Sci 2011;56:2914–9.

25. Ilangovan R, Burling D, George A, et al. CT enterography: review of technique and practical tips. Br J Radiol 2012;85:876–86.

26. d'Assignies G, Fina P, Bruno O, et al. High sensitivity of diffusion-weighted MR imaging for the detection of liver metastases from neuroendocrine tumors:

comparison with T2-weighted and dynamic gadolinium-enhanced MR imaging. Radiology 2013;268:390–9.

27. Armbruster M, Sourbron S, Haug A, et al. Evaluation of neuroendocrine liver metastases: a comparison of dynamic contrast-enhanced magnetic resonance imaging and positron emission tomography/computed tomography. Invest Radiol 2014;49:7–14.

28. Armbruster M, Zech CJ, Sourbron S, et al. Diagnostic accuracy of dynamic gadoxetic-acid-enhanced MRI and PET/CT compared in patients with liver metastases from neuroendocrine neoplasms. J Magn Reson Imaging 2014;40: 457–66.

29. Dohan A, El Fattach H, Barat M, et al. Neuroendocrine tumors of the small bowel: evaluation with MR-enterography. Clin Imaging 2016;40:541–7.

30. Masselli G, Gualdi G. CT and MR enterography in evaluating small bowel diseases: when to use which modality? Abdom Imaging 2013;38:249–59.

31. Fletcher JG, Kofler JM, Coburn JA, et al. Perspective on radiation risk in CT imaging. Abdom Imaging 2013;38:22–31.

32. Dromain C, de Baere T, Lumbroso J, et al. Detection of liver metastases from endocrine tumors: a prospective comparison of somatostatin receptor scintigraphy, computed tomography, and magnetic resonance imaging. J Clin Oncol 2005;23:70–8.

33. Moos SI, van Vemde DN, Stoker J, et al. Contrast induced nephropathy in patients undergoing intravenous (IV) contrast enhanced computed tomography (CECT) and the relationship with risk factors: a meta-analysis. Eur J Radiol 2013;82:e387–99.

34. Thomsen HS. Nephrogenic systemic fibrosis: a serious adverse reaction to gadolinium - 1997-2006-2016. Part 1. Acta Radiol 2016;57:515–20.

35. Murata N, Gonzalez-Cuyar LF, Murata K, et al. Macrocyclic and other non-group 1 gadolinium contrast agents deposit low levels of gadolinium in brain and bone tissue: preliminary results from 9 patients with normal renal function. Invest Radiol 2016;51:447–53.

36. Balon HR, Brown TL, Goldsmith SJ, et al. The SNM practice guideline for somatostatin receptor scintigraphy 2.0. J Nucl Med Technol 2011;39:317–24.

37. Reubi JC, Schonbrunn A. Illuminating somatostatin analog action at neuroendocrine tumor receptors. Trends Pharmacol Sci 2013;34:676–88.

38. de Herder WW, Hofland LJ, van der Lely AJ, et al. Somatostatin receptors in gastroentero-pancreatic neuroendocrine tumours. Endocr Relat Cancer 2003; 10:451–8.

39. Gibril F, Jensen RT. Diagnostic uses of radiolabelled somatostatin receptor analogues in gastroenteropancreatic endocrine tumours. Dig Liver Dis 2004;36: S106–20.

40. Lubberink M, Tolmachev V, Widström C, et al. 110mIn-DTPA-D-Phe1-octreotide for imaging of neuroendocrine tumors with PET. J Nucl Med 2002;43:1391–7.

41. Ambrosini V, Nanni C, Fanti S. The use of gallium-68 labeled somatostatin receptors in PET/CT imaging. PET Clin 2014;9:323–9.

42. Sánchez-Crespo A, Andreo P, Larsson SA. Positron flight in human tissues and its influence on PET image spatial resolution. Eur J Nucl Med Mol Imaging 2004;31: 44–51.

43. Hofman MS, Lau WF, Hicks RJ. Somatostatin receptor imaging with 68Ga DOTA-TATE PET/CT: clinical utility, normal patterns, pearls, and pitfalls in interpretation. Radiographics 2015;35:500–16.

44. Poeppel TD, Binse I, Petersenn S, et al. 68Ga-DOTATOC versus 68Ga-DOTATATE PET/CT in functional imaging of neuroendocrine tumors. J Nucl Med 2011;52: 1864–70.

45. Gabriel M, Decristoforo C, Kendler D, et al. 68Ga-DOTA-Tyr3-octreotide PET in neuroendocrine tumors: comparison with somatostatin receptor scintigraphy and CT. J Nucl Med 2007;48:508–18.

46. Buchmann I, Henze M, Engelbrecht S, et al. Comparison of 68Ga-DOTATOC PET and 111In-DTPAOC (Octreoscan) SPECT in patients with neuroendocrine tumours. Eur J Nucl Med Mol Imaging 2007;34:1617–26.

47. Geijer H, Breimer LH. Somatostatin receptor PET/CT in neuroendocrine tumours: update on systematic review and meta-analysis. Eur J Nucl Med Mol Imaging 2013;40:1770–80.

48. Sadowski SM, Neychev V, Millo C, et al. Prospective study of 68Ga-DOTATATE positron emission tomography/computed tomography for detecting gastro-entero-pancreatic neuroendocrine tumors and unknown primary sites. J Clin Oncol 2016;34:588–96.

49. Janssen I, Blanchet EM, Adams K, et al. Superiority of [68Ga]-DOTATATE PET/CT to other functional imaging modalities in the localization of SDHB-associated metastatic pheochromocytoma and paraganglioma. Clin Cancer Res 2015;21: 3888–95.

50. Smith DL, Breeman WA, Sims-Mourtada J. The untapped potential of Gallium 68-PET: the next wave of [68]Ga-agents. Appl Radiat Isot 2013;76:14–23.

51. Öberg K. Gallium-68 somatostatin receptor PET/CT: is it time to replace (111)Indium DTPA octreotide for patients with neuroendocrine tumors? Endocrine 2012; 42:3–4.

52. Herrmann K, Czernin J, Wolin EM, et al. Impact of 68Ga-DOTATATE PET/CT on the management of neuroendocrine tumors: the referring physician's perspective. J Nucl Med 2015;56:70–5.

53. Kuyumcu S, Özkan ZG, Sanli Y, et al. Physiological and tumoral uptake of (68)Ga-DOTATATE: standardized uptake values and challenges in interpretation. Ann Nucl Med 2013;27:538–45.

54. Sollini M, Erba PA, Fraternali A, et al. PET and PET/CT with 68gallium-labeled somatostatin analogues in non GEP-NETs tumors. ScientificWorldJournal 2014; 2014:194123.

55. Skoura E, Alshammari A, Syed R, et al. Adolescent with 68Ga DOTATATE-avid vertebral hemangioma mimicking metastasis in PET imaging. Clin Nucl Med 2015;40:e378–9.

56. Taneja S, Jena A, Kaul S, et al. Somatostatin receptor-positive granulomatous inflammation mimicking as meningioma on simultaneous PET/MRI. Clin Nucl Med 2015;40:e71–2.

57. Collarino A, del Ciello A, Perotti G, et al. Intrapancreatic accessory spleen detected by 68Ga DOTANOC PET/CT and 99mTc-colloid SPECT/CT scintigraphy. Clin Nucl Med 2015;40:415–8.

58. Castellucci P, Pou Ucha J, Fuccio, et al. Incidence of increased 68Ga-DOTANOC uptake in the pancreatic head in a large series of extrapancreatic NET patients studied with sequential PET/CT. J Nucl Med 2011;52:886–90.

59. Adams S, Baum R, Rink T, et al. Limited value of fluorine-18 fluorodeoxyglucose positron emission tomography for the imaging of neuroendocrine tumours. Eur J Nucl Med 1998;25:79–83.

60. Panagiotidis E, Bomanji J. Role of 18F-fluorodeoxyglucose PET in the study of neuroendocrine tumors. PET Clin 2014;9:43–55.

61. Zalom ML, Waxman AD, Yu R, et al. Metabolic and receptor imaging in patients with neuroendocrine tumors: comparison of fludeoxyglucose-positron emission tomography and computed tomography with indium in 111 pentetreotide. Endocr Pract 2009;15:521–7.

62. Squires MH 3rd, Volkan Adsay N, Schuster DM, et al. Octreoscan versus FDG PET for neuroendocrine tumor staging: a biological approach. Ann Surg Oncol 2015;22:2295–301.

63. Nilica B, Waitz D, Stevanovic V, et al. Direct comparison of (68)Ga-DOTA-TOC and (18)F-FDG PET/CT in the follow-up of patients with neuroendocrine tumour treated with the first full peptide receptor radionuclide therapy cycle. Eur J Nucl Med Mol Imaging 2016;43:1585–892.

64. Becherer A, Szabó M, Karanikas G, et al. Imaging of advanced neuroendocrine tumors with (18)F-FDOPA PET. J Nucl Med 2004;45:1161–7.

65. Santhanam P, Taïeb D. Role of (18) F-FDOPA PET/CT imaging in endocrinology. Clin Endocrinol (Oxf) 2014;81:789–98.

66. Orlefors H, Sundin A, Garske U, et al. Whole-body (11)C-5-hydroxytryptophan positron emission tomography as a universal imaging technique for neuroendocrine tumors: comparison with somatostatin receptor scintigraphy and computed tomography. J Clin Endocrinol Metab 2005;90:3392–400.

67. Ambrosini V, Morigi JJ, Nanni C, et al. Current status of PET imaging of neuroendocrine tumours ([18F]FDOPA, [68Ga]tracers, [11C]/[18F]-HTP). Q J Nucl Med Mol Imaging 2015;59:58–69.

68. Chang S, Choi D, Lee SJ, et al. Neuroendocrine neoplasms of the gastrointestinal tract: classification, pathologic basis, and imaging features. Radiographics 2007; 27:1667–79.

69. Lewis RB, Lattin GE Jr, Paal E. Pancreatic endocrine tumors: radiologic-clinicopathologic correlation. Radiographics 2010;30:1445–64.

70. Sahani DV, Kalva SP. Imaging the liver. Oncologist 2004;9:385–97.

71. Lapa C, Werner RA, Schmid JS, et al. Prognostic value of positron emission tomography-assessed tumor heterogeneity in patients with thyroid cancer undergoing treatment with radiopeptide therapy. Nucl Med Biol 2015;42:349–54.

72. Wulfert S, Kratochwil C, Choyke PL, et al. Multimodal imaging for early functional response assessment of (90)Y-/(177)Lu-DOTATOC peptide receptor targeted radiotherapy with DW-MRI and (68)Ga-DOTATOC-PET/CT. Mol Imaging Biol 2014;16:586–94.

73. Alexandraki KI, Kaltsas GA, Grozinsky-Glasberg S, et al. Appendiceal neuroendocrine neoplasms: diagnosis and management. Endocr Relat Cancer 2016; 23:R27–41.

74. Mehrabi A, Fischer L, Hafezi M, et al. A systematic review of localization, surgical treatment options, and outcome of insulinoma. Pancreas 2014;43:675–86.

75. Lewis RB, Mehrotra AK, Rodriguez P, et al. From the radiologic pathology archives: esophageal neoplasms: radiologic-pathologic correlation. Radiographics 2013;33:1083–108.

76. Hargunani R, Maclachlan J, Kaniyur S, et al. Cross-sectional imaging of gastric neoplasia. Clin Radiol 2009;64:420–9.

77. Levy AD, Taylor LD, Abbott RM, et al. Duodenal carcinoids: imaging features with clinical-pathologic comparison. Radiology 2005;237:967–72.

78. Woodbridge LR, Murtagh BM, Yu DF, et al. Midgut neuroendocrine tumors: imaging assessment for surgical resection. Radiographics 2014;34:413–26.

79. Coursey CA, Nelson RC, Moreno RD, et al. Carcinoid tumors of the appendix: are these tumors identifiable prospectively on preoperative CT? Am Surg 2010;76: 273–5.
80. Ganeshan D, Bhosale P, Yang T, et al. Imaging features of carcinoid tumors of the gastrointestinal tract. AJR Am J Roentgenol 2013;201:773–86.
81. Tsurumaru D, Kawanami S, Nishimuta Y, et al. Contrast-enhanced CT colonography features of rectal carcinoid tumors. Adv Comput Tomogr 2014;3:24–30.
82. Chong S, Lee KS, Chung MJ, et al. Neuroendocrine tumors of the lung: clinical, pathologic, and imaging findings. Radiographics 2006;26:41–57.
83. Prasad V, Steffen IG, Pavel M, et al. Somatostatin receptor PET/CT in restaging of typical and atypical lung carcinoids. EJNMMI Res 2015;5:53.
84. Foran PJ, Hayes SA, Blair DJ, et al. Imaging appearances of diffuse idiopathic pulmonary neuroendocrine cell hyperplasia. Clin Imaging 2015;39:243–6.
85. Nasseri F, Eftekhari F. Clinical and radiologic review of the normal and abnormal thymus: pearls and pitfalls. Radiographics 2010;30:413–28.
86. Guidoccio F, Grosso M, Maccauro M, et al. Current role of 111In-DTPA-octreotide scintigraphy in diagnosis of thymic masses. Tumori 2011;97:191–5.

# Moving?

## Make sure your subscription moves with you!

To notify us of your new address, find your **Clinics Account Number** (located on your mailing label above your name), and contact customer service at:

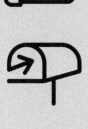

Email: **journalscustomerservice-usa@elsevier.com**

**800-654-2452** (subscribers in the U.S. & Canada)
**314-447-8871** (subscribers outside of the U.S. & Canada)

Fax number: 314-447-8029

**Elsevier Health Sciences Division**
**Subscription Customer Service**
**3251 Riverport Lane**
**Maryland Heights, MO 63043**

*To ensure uninterrupted delivery of your subscription, please notify us at least 4 weeks in advance of move.

Printed and bound by CPI Group (UK) Ltd, Croydon, CR0 4YY

08/05/2025

01864701-0002